THE MUCOSAL IMMUNE SYSTEM

CURRENT TOPICS IN VETERINARY MEDICINE AND ANIMAL
SCIENCE

VOLUME 12

THE MUCOSAL IMMUNE SYSTEM

Series ISBN-13:978-94-009-8333-5

THE MUCOSAL IMMUNE SYSTEM

Proceedings of a Seminar in the EEC Programme of Coordination of Agricultural Research on Protection of the Young Animal against Perinatal Diseases, held at the University of Bristol, School of Veterinary Science, Langford, Nr. Bristol, United Kingdom on September 9-11, 1980

Sponsored by the Commission of the European Communities, Directorate-General for Agriculture, Coordination of Agricultural Research

Edited by

F.J. Bourne

Department of Animal Husbandry,
Langford House,
Langford,
Bristol, United Kingdom

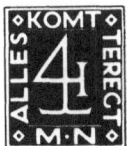

1981
MARTINUS NIJHOFF PUBLISHERS
THE HAGUE / BOSTON / LONDON

for

THE COMMISSION OF THE EUROPEAN COMMUNITIES

Distributors

for the United States and Canada
Kluwer Boston, Inc.
190 Old Derby Street
Hingham, MA 02043
USA

for all other countries
Kluwer Academic Publishers Group
Distribution Center
P.O. Box 322
3300 AH Dordrecht
The Netherlands

ISBN-13: 978-94-009-8333-5   e-ISBN-13: 978-94-009-8331-1
DOI: 10.1007/978-94-009-8331-1

Publication arranged by
Commission of the European Communities,
Directorate-General Information Market and Innovation, Luxembourg

EUR 7341

Manuscript Preparation by
Janssen Services, 33a High Street, Chislehurst, Kent BR7 5AE, UK

LEGAL NOTICE

CONTENTS

SESSION III: IMMUNE RESPONSE TO MICRO-ORGANISMS AND
            PROTECTION

VIII

POSTER PRESENTATIONS

PREFACE

This publication contains the proceedings of a Seminar on 'The Mucosal Immune System' held by the Commission of the European Communities (CEC) at the University of Bristol, School of Veterinary Science, Langford, Bristol on September 9th - 11th, 1980. The seminar formed part of the CEC programme of co-ordinated agricultural research on Protection of the Young Animal against Perinatal Disease and was organised by Professor F.J. Bourne and his colleagues Dr. T.J. Newby and Dr. C.R. Stokes. The Proceedings were edited by the organisers assisted by Janssen Services, 33a High Street, Chislehurst, Kent and provide an authoritative and up-to-date account of this rapidly moving research area.

Serious economic loss from diseases of mucosal surfaces - particularly the enteric and respiratory tracts - occurs in young farm animals throughout the EEC. Protection against these diseases is based on an understanding of their epidemiology including host defence mechanisms. Mucosal vaccines have in the main given disappointing field results with, however, some notable exceptions. This seminar rationalises methods used to stimulate mucosal immune defence and indicates likely areas for future research and development.

The CEC wishes to thank the organisers and the participants who contributed to the success of the seminar.

OPENING SESSION

Chairman : F.J. Bourne

OPENING REMARKS

F.J. Bourne

On behalf of the University of Bristol and the European Economic Community my colleagues and I welcome you to the Langford Veterinary School.

As you will appreciate from the list of speakers and delegates we are fortunate in having attracted immunologists from most of the leading laboratories working in the field of mucosal immunity and I look forward to a successful meeting.

This symposium is part of a European Economic Community research programme on 'Protection of the young farm animal against infectious disease' and I would like to express my gratitude to the EEC staff involved in this project, and in particular to Dr. Jim Connell, for the help and support that we have received.

MUCOSAL IMMUNITY

J. Bienenstock, A.D. Befus and M. McDermott

McMaster University Health Sciences Centre,
Hamilton, Ontario, Canada, L8N 3Z5.

INTRODUCTION

In the last two decades considerable attention has been focussed on immune mechanisms of mucosal tissues. Perhaps this is not surprising since mucosal surfaces are intimately associated with potentially pathogenic organisms and continuous antigenic bombardment with products of the environment and dietary antigens. Because of the size of the subject, we will only discuss selected components of the mucosal immune system and will focus on the intestine since more is known about this organ in respect to mucosal immunity. For a more extensive treatment, readers are referred elsewhere (Tomasi and Bienenstock, 1968; Tomasi and Grey, 1972; Heremans, 1974; Ciba Symposium 46, 1977; Asquith, 1979; Bienenstock and Befus, 1980).

Although secretory IgA (sIgA) predominates in most mucosal secretions, IgA is only one component of the local mucosal immune response. It may mark that response but any consideration of mucosal immunity is incomplete without a consideration of cellular and other humoral mechanisms. Mucosal tissues are under different antigenic loads and the GI tract is under continuous stimulation and may be thought to be in a state of mild chronic inflammation. The concept of 'pathotopic potentiation' (Fazekas and Donnelly, 1950) must always be remembered. Parenteral immunisation with subsequent specific local challenge led to circulating immunity localised at that mucosal site. The physiological integrity of any tissue must be considered when assessing the significance of mucosal immunity. Inflammation will change the normal balance by involvement of systemic humoral and cellular elements.

Elsewhere we have categorised mucosal tissues into three classes (Bienenstock et al., 1980); the first in which evidence of a local predominance of plasma cells and secretory component (SC) is well established; the second (class two) in which evidence of local SC in the absence of IgA plasma cells has been determined; and the third, in which tissues are bathed by secretions containing sIgA but in which neither local SC nor local IgA plasma cell localisation has been found. The current distribution of tissues according to this classification can be found in Table 1. Although the actual classification may be considered to be artificial, it may serve a useful purpose to focus discussion and some predictions may be made from its consideration.

TABLE 1

COMPONENTS OF MUCOSAL SYSTEM BATHED BY FLUIDS CONTAINING SECRETORY IgA

Class 1   Evidence for local predominance of IgA plasma cells and secretory component

Glands	Tissues
Salivary	Gastrointestinal tract
Mammary	Upper respiratory tract
Lacrimal	Nose
Prostate	Middle ear
	Gall bladder
	Cervix
	Biliary duct

Class 2   Evidence for local secretory component but no evidence for local IgA plasma cells

Skin (sweat glands)	Amnion
Kidney	Fallopian tube
Urinary bladder	Uterine mucosa
Hepatic parenchymal cell	Thymus

TABLE 1 (CONTINUED)

COMPONENTS OF MUCOSAL SYSTEM BATHED BY FLUIDS CONTAINING SECRETORY IgA

Class 3   No evidence for either local secretory component or

           local IgA plasma cells

               Ureter

               Oesophagus

               Vagina

               Buccal squamous epithelium

Tomasi & Bienenstock, 1968;   Heremans, 1974

IgA

Selective transport

        The studies of several groups (Hall, Vaerman and Underdown)
have shown that the hepatic parenchymal cell appears to have
the selective capacity to transport dimeric IgA to the bile, at
least in the rat (Lemaitre-Coelho et al., 1978;   Orlans et al.,
1978;   and Socken et al., 1979). Thus, dimeric IgA antibody
synthesised at one mucosal site may be selectively secreted via
the bile into the intestinal secretions. Ligation of the
common bile duct in rats leads to an exponential rise of dimeric
IgA in serum and the transport is dependent upon the expression
of secretory component on the hepatic parenchymal cell (Socken
et al., 1979). At this time SC has not been identified for
certain on the human hepatic parenchymal cell, although
selective IgA transport appears to occur in the biliary
epithelium.   Monomeric and secretory IgA are not transported
selectively across the liver and this may explain the
observations on lack of transport of radiolabelled 7S or 11S
IgA into secretions in some of the original IgA metabolic
studies.   It is not known whether this selective transport
system may also exist for IgM, since IgM appears to have a high
affinity for secretory component in man (Socken and Underdown,
1978). We now do know that the same system appears to occur in
the salivary gland (Coelho et al., 1974;   Montgomery et al.,
1977) as well as the breast (Halsey et al., 1980). It may be
expected that this transport system will apply to those tissues

of class 1, Table 1. It may also account for the presence of secretory IgA in class 2 tissue, Table 1, in the absence of local IgA plasma cell infiltrates. In the kidney, no free secretory component is found in the urine (Bienenstock and Poortmans, 1970), whereas in physiological proteinuria secretory and serum IgA, but no free secretory component, is found in the urine, suggesting that this system may be saturated via the circulation.

It is important to note that the presence of sIgA into secretions may indeed indicate local synthesis and local secretion by local mucosal plasma cells but, alternatively, local secretion with distant synthesis may have occurred. The exact extent to which this system exists in glandular tissues remains to be defined.

Antibody activity

Local mucosal IgA antibody correlates better with resistance to infection than the presence of antibody in serum. The mode of its function is unknown but sIgA does not activate complement by the classical pathway and considerable questions exist as to its ability to activate the alternate pathway (Colten and Bienenstock, 1974) except when chemically denatured. sIgA does not support opsonisation although there appear to be IgA receptors on polymorphonuclear leukocytes (Van Epps et al., 1978). It is resistant to proteolysis, prevents adherence and colonisation of bacteria on epithelia, may block complement fixation by complement fixing antibodies, act as a blocking antibody in hypersensitivity reactions, and may exclude macromolecular uptake by both GI and respiratory tracts ('immune exclusion'). The role of sIgA in the regulation of dietary antigen ingress across the intestinal mucosal epithelium has been extensively analysed (Walker and Issel- bacher, 1977). The way in which this antibody may exert its effect and control access to the local and systemic immune systems and the significance of this to the subsequent develop- ment of allergy to environmental antigens will not be explored in the present study but the readers are recommended to pursue this significant area for themselves (Matthew et al., 1977).

The pathogenicity of certain organisms found in the upper respiratory and GI tracts may be correlated with the capacity to secrete a protease capable of selectively cleaving IgAl (Mulks and Plaut, 1978). Since IgA2 is present in secretions in about equivalent amounts to the IgAl subclass, the significance of this observation is not known. The functional role of the proteolytic fragments in the possible regulation of the synthesis of secretory component or IgA has not been explored but may be expected to be a fruitful area of invest-

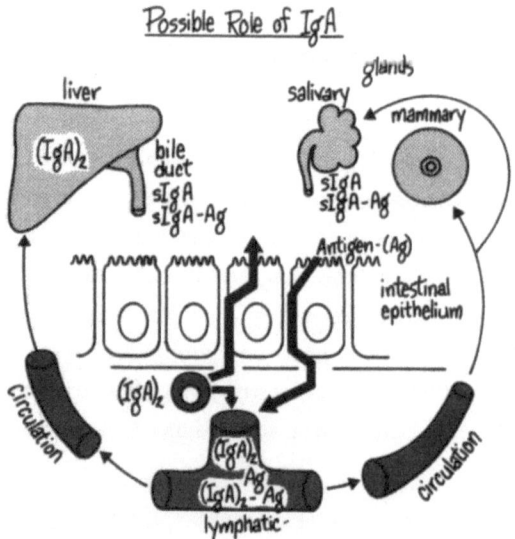

Fig. 1. The possible primary role of dimeric IgA is to act as defence
against ingress of dietary macromolecules. Complexing of
locally synthesised or transported IgA may occur locally but
selective secretion may occur in distal sites and cause rapid
clearance. This system may also provide the antigenic drive
for mucosal tissues not normally exposed to antigen.

derived lymphocytes from other mucosal sites, might in addition
provide transport of IgA dimers complexed to antigen and in
this way provide an additional antigenic drive for proliferation
and retention of such cells locally in salivary glands. Thus,
some of them might be seeded from one mucosal site to another
(see Traffic of Lymphocytes) and antigen also might find its
way suitably packaged to those sites and concentrated in distal
mucosal sites by this mechanism. The lactating breast possesses
this selective transport system for IgA (Halsey et al., 1980),
as do the salivary glands (Montgomery et al., 1977) and antigen
intravenously administered may be selectively secreted into the
milk of lactating mothers (Halsey and Benjamin, 1976). The
intestinal absorption of immune complexes by neonatal rats from
mothers' milk is a mechanism whereby increased antigen uptake
may occur (Abrahamson et al., 1979) and this may also be
involved in the regulation of the subsequent immune response.
Although there has been a suggestion that IgA immune complexes
after oral immunisation may be tolerogenic (André et al., 1975),
no confirmation of this has occurred. Indeed, IgA immune
complexes are rapidly cleared from the circulation and enhance
subsequent IgG and IgM responses (Stokes et al., 1980).

MUCOSA ASSOCIATED LYMPHOID TISSUES (MALT)

Two types of lymphoid aggregates are found in mammalian
lung and gut. The first consists of multiple aggregates and
is known as Peyer's patches in the intestine and in some
mammals exists also in the mucosa of the respiratory tract.
The second consists of isolated lymphoid follicles, scattered
throughout the intestine, often prominent in the colon, which
have been termed solitary lymphoid nodules (Keren et al., 1978).
These are found more commonly in the respiratory tract. Both
tissues have a specialised epithelium containing M cells which
have the capacity selectively to concentrate luminally administered antigen (Owen, 1977; Tenner-Racz et al., 1979).
According to Ham (1969) isolated lymphoid follicles are
characteristic of wet mucosal epithelial membranes and are
also found in the urinary bladder. For further discussion of

this area, see Bienenstock et al., 1973a; Bienenstock et al., 1973b; Bienenstock et al., 1976).

TRAFFIC OF LYMPHOCYTES

B blasts - IgA

Lymphoblasts from mesenteric node (MLN) or thoracic duct (TD) have a selective localisation potential for the small intestine (Gowans and Knight, 1964; Hall and Smith 1970). The majority of these cells after adoptive transfer are found in the small intestine, although a half to a third as many localise in the colon. The Peyer's patches contain a population of precursor cells bearing IgA which subsequently are found in various mucosal sites (Craig and Cebra, 1971; Rudzik et al., 1975). These cells migrate via the MLN to the TD (Roux et al., 1979). These cells with IgA on their cell surface may already be primed (Gearhard and Cebra, 1979) suggesting that priming for IgA may occur elsewhere than Peyer's patches.

Common mucosal system

GALT derived cells will repopulate the bronchial mucosa. Cells from BALT will repopulate spleen, bowel and lung with IgA containing cells. Because of this, and functional and morphologic similarities between BALT and GALT, we coined the term common mucosal immune system (Bienenstock, 1974). Goldblum et al., 1975, showed that IgA containing cells with specific activity against a non-pathogenic *E. coli* with which they had been fed appeared in the milk of lactating females. This may have been an over-representation in terms of numbers (Mestecky et al., 1980) but MLN B blasts localise in mammary glands where they selectively make IgA (Roux et al., 1977). Further support for this concept came from evidence showing selective localisation of MLN blasts in both bronchial and cervical mucosa with predominant IgA synthesis (McDermott and Bienenstock, 1979). The organ derivation of the cells appeared important since the majority of BLN blasts went back to the lung. Similarly, MLN blasts showed selectivity for the gut.

We predict that other mucosal tissues of class 1, Table 1, will eventually be shown to be part of this system. Weisz-Carrington et al.(1979) showed that after ferritin feeding, IgA antibody containing cells were found in gut, lung, mammary and parotid glands.

Factors affecting localisation of IgA blasts

Two models may be addressed to account for these experimental findings. The first suggests that lymphocyte surface characteristics may account for localisation according to complementary receptors expressed on the vascular endothelium of mucosal tissues. The second is that relatively random migration of blasts occurs from the vascular compartment and subsequent selective retention by factors in the tissues occurs. Although antigen amplifies the localisation of primed mucosal IgA precursors, these blasts do selectively localise in germ-free animals and in foetal intestine transplanted under the kidney capsule. It seems reasonable to accept that B blasts destined to make dimeric IgA, wherever primed, will traffic from mucosal tissues of one site to another with a tendency to return to their site of origin. The actual candidate factors for this localisation are numerous but it is fair to say that no single factor has so far been shown to account for these observations.

IgG and IgM

The tendency to emphasise the importance of IgA in dealing with mucosal immunity has obscured the possibility that other precursor isotypes might also selectively lodge in mucosal tissues (see Jacobson et al., 1961, and Perey et al., 1968). We showed (McDermott et al., 1979) when compared to peripheral nodes that MLN are a major source of intestinal IgG and IgM precursor cells. Since these cells may be presumed to be in the same evolutionary line of development as the IgA class, the pressures affecting the selective mucosal localisation of IgM or IgG may be similar. In ruminants IgG_1 is the predominant immunoglobulin in milk and a selective glandular transport

system exists for this subclass. A subpopulation of IgG
containing cells is found in human intestine which also contains
the J chain (Nagura et al., 1979). The selective mucosal
localisation of IgG, the J chain content and subclass specificity
could possibly be related.

IgE

This class of immunoglobulin is the major reaginic
antibody present in secretions of mucosal target organs such
as nose, eyes, bronchial and intestinal mucosa. These cells
are synthesised in GALT, MLN and BLN (Ngan and Kind, 1978;
Gerbrandy and Bienenstock, 1976), as well as the lamina propria
of the mucosa of the upper respiratory and intestinal tracts
(Tada and Ishizaka, 1970).

IgE is not found associated with secretory component and
not all mucosal secretions contain this antibody. For example,
IgE is not found in mammary secretions (Underdown et al., 1976).
The factors controlling the distribution of IgE containing
cells, their migration, localisation and differentiation are
totally unexplored at present.

T BLASTS

T immunoblasts from normal MLN and TD localise
selectively in the intestinal lamina propria and the villous
epithelium of normal gut and foetal gut isografts under the
kidney capsule (Guy-Grand et al., 1974; Sprent, 1976). Only
when intestines were infected with *Trichinella* did PLN T blasts
localise in the intestine to any extent (Rose et al., 1976).

The population of lymphocytes above the epithelium basement membrane in the intestine amounts to about 10% of total
epithelial cell numbers. These cells increase in number of
patients with coeliac disease, are reduced in remission and
increase on challenge with gluten (Ferguson, 1977). They are
thought to be exclusively T cells, often are recently divided
(Marsh, 1975), have a different half life than the epithelial

cells which migrate over their top (Darlington and Rogers, 1966), possess a number of metachromatic granules (Collan, 1972; Rudzik and Bienenstock, 1974) and contain low concentrations of histamine and serotonin (Guy-Grand et al., 1978). The relation-ship of these cells to mucosal mast cells, globule leukocytes and lymphocytes, and to the epithelial lymphocytes in other mucosal tissues (Seelig et al., 1979) is unknown. The factors controlling migration and localisation of T blasts into mucosal tissues is unfortunately not known. The presence of free cells in the lumen of the intestine has been known for some time (Harris et al., 1972; Owen et al., 1979) and lymphocytes are commonly found in the secretions of the breast and respiratory tract (Seeling et al., 1979). We have suggested that these cells in the lung may be derived from the BALT follicles and recent observations on the rabbit appendix suggests that the GALT may be a prime source of some of these gut luminal cells (Heatley and Bienenstock, 1980).

Antigen uptake

The mucosal epithelium does not serve as a barrier to macromolecules and particulate material; even asbestos fibres can be eliminated from the urine by the use of filtered drinking water (Cooke and Olsen, 1979). Substances such as carageenan which can cause mucosal ulceration can be found in macrophages in the intestinal lamina propria after feeding (Abraham et al., 1974) and after feeding of latex particles diameter 2 μ to mice they were found in Peyer's patches, villi and mesenteric nodes. Despite the selective antigen uptake by M cells in MALT, there appears to be a defect in antigen processing in this tissue (Kagnoff and Campbell, 1974); Challacombe et al., 1980) and since GALT appears to contain cells already primed, the functional purpose of these cells may be to cause proliferation only of primed cells.

It is interesting that macrophages from the intestine do migrate and may be found in the thoracic duct (Macpherson and Steer, 1979) under abnormal circumstances such as mesenteric adenectomy. The possibility that such cells may have a migration pattern themselves which could influence the subsequent quality of the immune response is an intriguing one which should be explored.

IMMUNISATION

Because Dr. Pierce elsewhere in these proceedings will be dealing with approaches to immunisation, we will not cover this area in our contribution from the standpoint of antibody synthesis.

Cellular immunity

Oral immunisation can lead to systemic delayed hypersensitivity (Perrotto et al., 1974) and the generation of cytotoxic T cells (Kagnoff, 1978). Lamina propria cells in rabbit and man may both stimulate and respond in mixed lymphocyte reactions (Singal, et al., 1976; Goodacre et al., 1979). Clancy and Pucci (1978) suggested that lymphocytes from the intestinal lamina propria were unable to react in antibody dependent cytotoxic model and this has been confirmed (Fiocchi et al., 1979). In the guinea pig, we have shown (Arnaud-Battandier et al., 1978) that T cell (mitogen induced cellular cytotoxicity: MICC), natural killer (NK) and ADCC activities were all present in lymphocyte populations contaminated with epithelial 'granular' lymphocytes, but this was not so for lymphocytes obtained from deeper in the lamina propria. Here, whereas ADCC and NK activity were absent at any effector cell target cell ratio, the MICC response was reduced. Thus, cells derived from different portions of the intestinal lamina propria may have different functional cellular activities.

The possibility that T cell mediated hypersensitivity may contribute to partial villous atrophy in nematode infections and/or coeliac and tropical sprue is an interesting one (Ferguson and Macdonald, 1977) and Miller and Nawa (1979) showed it was possible to transfer a goblet cell response in nematode

infected rats by the use of thoracic duct cells presumed to be
T cells on the basis of deficiency in membrane immunoglobulin.
Thus the possibility exists that circulating lymphocytes might
indirectly affect the nature and numbers of a variety of cell
types in the intestine not normally associated with immune
activity, such as goblet cells, etc.

REGULATION OF IMMUNITY

Immunity as a negative event

Both Swarbrick et al. (1979) and Pierce and Koster (1980)
have shown that oral immunisation produces humoral positive
responses as well as concurrent suppression or negative
influence. The mechanism whereby regulation and potential
suppression of the immune response occurs after mucosal
presentation of antigen is highly complex. Many of the
experiments performed have not looked at the effect of cells
or substances on the local immune response in the intestine
but suppressor phenomena have been identified in the spleen or
orally immunised animals specific for IgG, IgM and cell
mediated responses. Some of these have been antigen specific,
some have shown cells capable of suppression with a sequential
appearance in Peyer's patches, mesenteric node and spleen. The
variability of the factors involved, which include T suppressor
cells as well as B cells and adherent macrophage-like cells,
serve only to delineate the complexity of these systems. Some
of these activities may be mediated by prostaglandins released
by macrophages under the influence of a non-adherent presumed
T cell, and may be reversed by the administration of indomethacin
(Mattingly et al., 1979). (See Asherson et al., 1977; Hanson
et al., 1979; Thomas and Parrott, 1974; Mattingly and Waksman,
1978). It is interesting that this type of mucosal tolerance
may not be peculiar to the intestine since Parker and Turk (1978)
showed that the instillation of soluble metal salts into the
respiratory tract rendered mice tolerant to subsequent challenge
with this specific chemical.

REGULATION OF THE IMMUNE RESPONSE BY THE EXTERNAL ENVIRONMENT

Diet

Protein and calorie malnutrition may markedly depress both mucosal and systemic immune responses (Chandra, 1980). Specific amino acid deficiencies may influence the function of suppressor cells (Bounous and Kongshavn, 1978) and specific trace metal deficiency, such as zinc, may cause the generation of helper T cells to be depressed (Fraker et al., 1978). We have recently shown, (McDermott et al., 1980) that blast cells from the mesenteric nodes of vitamin A deficient animals, as well as pair fed protein calorie malnourished animals, are at one-third of the capacity of normals to localise in the intestinal mucosa. This may be one of the reasons for the known susceptibility to mucosal infection of protein mal-nourished and vitamin A deficient humans.

Products of digestion such as simple sugars (e.g. L-fucose and L-rhamnose) or complex carbohydrates containing these substances may totally inhibit various lymphocyte activities both *in vivo* and *in vitro*. These include cutaneous and peritoneal manifestations of cell mediated immunity (Amsden et al., 1978; Baba et al., 1979) and the inhibition of migration inhibition factor and neutrophil chemotactic factor amongst others. Therefore, the diet and dietary products may have marked immunoregulatory influence.

Flora

Germfree animals have little capacity to generate suppression of the secondary immune response *in vitro*. It may be that this deficit is contained in the lack of the microbial induced signal from a non-adherent cell to an adherent cell population and that the suppressive influence may be a prostaglandin. Mattingly et al., (1979) showed that this activity could be eradicated by indomethacin, an inhibitor of prostaglandin synthetase. Germfree mice are more able to response to lipopolysaccharide than conventional animals and mono-contaminated mice are intermediate between the two groups (Kiyono et al., 1980). Conventionalisation restores the relative depression (McGhee et al., 1980). Endotoxin also has been shown to depress the development of cell mediated cytotoxicity but this may be through an effect on a regulatory B cell.

In germfree animals, the number of IgE bearing cells found in GALT is much higher than in conventionals. Many factors have been described in the colostrum and milk which may effect immune responses. Delayed hypersensitivity reactions may be transferred from mother to child by factors either soluble or cellular found in colostrum. Pittard and Bill (1979) have shown a factor in human milk which may promote IgA synthesis and secretion and similar factors have been described in pigs (Hoerlein, 1957). Jarrett and Hall (1979) showed that there may be a factor in milk which is capable of suppressing the offspring's capacity to mount an IgE immune response.

From the above, it is clear that mucosal and systemic immune responses will be influenced both directly and indirectly by both dietary and environmental products in our intestine, and possibly respiratory tract, and also the flora contained within these two mucosal sites. The extent to which they may affect normal health and allow maintenance of the integrity of the mucosa is incompletely understood and this exciting area promises to be a fruitful arena for students of mucosal immunity.

ACKNOWLEDGEMENTS

We wish to thank Mrs. J. Merness for her expert help with the manuscript, and the Medical Research Council of Canada for grant support of the research described herein.

REFERENCES

Abraham, R., Fabian, R.J., Goldberg, L. and Coulston, F., 1974. Role of lysosomes in carrageenian-induced cecal ulceration. Gastroenterology 67, 1169.

Abrahamson, D.R., Powers, A. and Rodewald, R., 1979. Intestinal absorption of immune complexes by neonatal rats: a route of antigen transfer from mother to young. Science 206, 657.

Amsden, A., Ewan, V., Yoshida, T. and Cohen, S., 1978. Studies on cellular receptors for lymphokines. I. Interaction of chemotactic factors with monosaccharides. J. Immunol. 120, 542.

André, C., Heremans, J.F., Vaerman, J.P. and Cambiaso, C.L., 1975. A mechanism for the induction of immunological tolerance by antigen feeding: antigen-antibody complexes. J. Exp. Med. 142, 1509.

Arnaud-Battandier, F., Bundy, B.M., O'Neill, M., Bienenstock, J. and Nelson, D.L., 1978. Cytotoxic activities of gut mucosal lymphoid cells in guinea pigs. J. Immunol. 121, 1059.

Asherson, G.L., Zembela, M., Perera, M., Mayhew, B. and Thomas, W.R., 1977. Production of immunity and unresponsiveness in the mouse by feeding contact sensitizing agents and the role of suppressor cells in the Peyer's patches, mesenteric lymph nodes and other lymphoid tissues. Cell Immunol. 33, 145.

Asquith, P., 1979. Immunology of the Gastrointestinal Tract. Churchill Livingston, London. 348 pp

Baba T., Yoshida, T., Yoshida, T. and Cohen, S., 1979. Suppression of cell-mediated immune reactions by monosaccharides. J. Immunol., 122, 838.

Bienenstock, J., 1974. The physiology of the local immune response and the gastrointestinal tract. In: Progress in Immunology II. vol. 4. (eds. L. Brent & J. Holborow). North-Holland Publishing. p 197.

Bienenstock, J. and Befus, A.D., 1980. Mucosal immunology. Immunology (in press)

Bienenstock, J., Clancy, R.L. and Perey, D.Y.E., 1976. Bronchus associated lymphoid tissue (BALT): its relationship to mucosal immunity. In: Immunologic and Infectious Reactions in the Lung (eds. C.H. Kirkpatrick and H.Y. Reynolds). Marcel Dekker Inc., New York. p 29.

Bienenstock, J., Johnston, N. and Perey, D.Y.E., 1973a. Bronchial lymphoid tissue. I. Morphologic characteristics. Lab. Invest. 28, 686.

Bienenstock, J., Johnston, N. and Perey, D.Y.E., 1973b. Bronchial lymphoid tissue. II. Functional characteristics. Lab. Invest. 28, 693.

Bienenstock, J. and Poortmans, J., 1970. γA in exercise proteinuria. Proc. Soc. Exp. Biol. Med. 134, 138.

Bounous, G. and Kongshavn, P.A.L., 1978. The effect of dietary amino acids on immune reactivity. Immunology 35, 257.

Challacombe, S., Krco, C.J., David, C.S. and Tomasi, T.B., 1980. Defective antigen presentation by adherent Ia positive Peyer's patch cells. (submitted for publication)

Chandra, R.K., 1980. Mucosal immunity in nutritional deficiency. In: Mucosal Immune System in Health and Disease. Proceedings of the 81st Ross Conference on Pediatric Research. (In press)

Ciba Foundation Symposium 46, 1977. Immunology of the Gut (eds. R. Porter and J. Knight). Elsevier, Excerpta Medica, Amsterdam.

Clancy, R.L., and Pucci, A., 1978. Absence of K cells in human gut mucosa. Gut 19, 273.

Coelho, I.M., Pereira, M.T. and Virella, G., 1974. Analytical study of salivary immunoglobulins in multiple myeloma. Clin. Exp. Immunol. 17, 417.

Collan, Y., 1972. Characteristics of non epithelial cells in the epithelium of normal rat ileum. Scand. J. Gastroenterol. 7 (Suppl. 18, 5.)

Colten, H.R. and Bienenstock, J., 1974. Lack of C3 activation through classical or alternate pathways by human secretory IgA anti blood group A antibody. In: The Immunologlobulin A System (eds. J. Mestecky and A.R. Lawton). Plenum Publishing, New York. p 305.

Cook, P.M. and Olson, G.F., 1979. Ingested mineral fibers: elimination in human urine. Science 204, 194.

Craig, S.W. and Cebra, J.J., 1971. Peyer's patches: an enriched source of precursors for IgA-producing immunocytes in the rabbit. J. Exp. Med. 134, 188.

Darlington, D. and Rogers, A.W., 1966. Epithelial lymphocytes in the small intestine of the mouse. J. Anat. 100, 813.

Fazekas de St. Groth and Donnelly, M., 1950. Studies in experimental immunology of influenza: enhancement of immunity by pathotopic vaccination. Austr. J. Exp. Biol. 28, 77.

22

Ferguson, A., 1977. Intraepithelial lymphocytes of the small intestine.
     Gut 18, 921.

Ferguson, A. and Macdonald, T.T., 1977. Effects of local delayed
     hypersensitivity on the small intestine. In: Immunology of the
     Gut. Elsevier North-Holland. p 305.

Fiocchi, C., Battisto, J.R. and Farmer, R.G., 1979. Gut mucosal
     lymphocytes in inflammatory bowel disease: isolation and
     preliminary functional characteristics. Dig. Dis. Sci. 24, 705.

Fraker, P.J., Depasquale-Jardieu, P., Zwickl, C.M. and Luecke, R.W., 1978.
     Regeneration of T-cell helper function in zinc-deficient adult mice.
     Proc. Natl. Acad. Sci. 75, 5660.

Gearhard, P.J. and Cebra, J.J., 1979. Differentiated B lymphocytes:
     potential to express particular antibody variable and constant
     regions depends on site of lymphoid tissue and antigen load.
     J. Exp. Med. 149, 216.

Gerbrandy, J.L.F. and Bienenstock, J., 1976. Kinetics and localization
     of IgE tetanus antibody response in mice immunized by the
     intratracheal, intraperitoneal and subcutaneous routes. Immunology
     31, 913.

Goldblum, R.M., Ahlstedt, S., Carlsson, B., Hanson, L.A., Jodal, V.,
     Lidin-Janson, G. and Sohl-Åkerlund, A., 1975. Antibody-forming
     cells in human colostrum after oral immunization. Nature 257, 797.

Goodacre, R., Davidson, R., Singal, D. and Bienenstock, J., 1979.
     Morphologic and functional characteristics of human intestinal
     lymphoid cells isolated by a mechanical technique. Gastroenterology
     76, 300.

Gowans, J.L. and Knight, E.J., 1964. The route of re-circulation of
     lymphocytes in the rat. Proc. Roy. Soc. Ser. B. Biol. Sci.,
     159, 257.

Guy-Grand, D., Griscelli, C. and Vassali, P., 1978. The mouse gut T
     lymphocyte, a novel type of T cell. Nature, origin and traffic in
     mice in normal and graft-versus-host conditions. J. Exp. Med.
     148, 1661.

Guy-Grand, D., Griscelli, C. and Vassalli, P., 1974. The gut-associated
     lymphoid system: nature and properties of the large dividing cells.
     Eur. J. Immunol. 4, 435.

Hall, J.G. and Smith, M.E., 1970. Homing of lymph-borne immunoblasts to
     the gut. Nature 226, 262.

Halsey, J.F., Johnson, B.H. and Cebra, J.J., 1980. Transport of
immunoglobulins from serum into colostrum. J. Exp. Med. 151, 767.

Halsey, J.R. and Benjamin, D.C., 1976. Induction of immunologic tolerance
in bursing neonates by absorption of tolerogen from colostrum.
J. Immunol. 116, 1204.

Ham, A.W., 1969. In: Histology by A.W. Ham. Lippincott Co.,
Philadelphia. p 313.

Hanson, D.G., Vaz, N.M., Rawlings, L.A. and Lynch, J.M., 1979. Inhibition
of specific immune responses by feeding protein antigens. II.
Effects of prior passive and active immunization. J. Immunol.
122, 2261.

Harris, J.G., Dupont, H.L. and Hornick, R.B., 1972. Fecal leukocytes in
diarrheal illness. Ann. Intern. Med. 76, 697.

Heatley, R.V. and Bienenstock, J., 1980. Lymphocytes in the lumen of the
rabbit appendix. (Submitted for publication)

Heremans, J.G., 1974. Immunoglobulin A. In: The Antigens vol. II.
(ed. M. Sela). Academic Press, New York. p 365

Hoerlein, A.B., 1957. The influence of colostrum on antibody response
in baby pigs. J. Immunol. 78, 112.

Jacobson, L.O., Marks, E.K., Simmons, E.L. and Gaston, E.O., 1961. Immune
response in irradiated mice with Peyer's patch shielding. Proc.
Soc. Exp. Biol. Med. 108, 487.

Jarrett, E.E.E. and Hall, E., 1979. Selective suppression of IgE antibody
responsiveness by maternal influence. Nature 280, 145.

Kagnoff, M.F., 1978. Effects of antigen-feeding on intestinal and
systemic immune responses. I. Priming of precursor cytotoxic T
cells by antigen feeding. J. Immunol. 120, 395.

Kagnoff, M.F. and Campbell, S., 1974. Functional characteristics of
Peyer's patch lymphoid cells. I. Induction of humoral antibody
and cell mediated allograft reactions. J. Exp. Med. 139, 398.

Keren, D.F., Holt, P.S., Collins, H.H., Gemski, P. and Formal, S.B., 1978.
The role of Peyer's patches in the local immune response of rabbit
ileum to live bacteria. J. Immunol. 120, 1892.

Kiyono, H., McGhee, J.R., and Michalek, S.M., 1980. Lipopolysaccharide
regulation of the immune response: comparison of responses to LPS
in germfree *Escherichia Coli* - monoassociated and conventional mice.
J. Immunol. 124, 36.

Lawton, A.R., Asofsky, R. and Mage, R.G., 1970. Synthesis of secretory IgA in the rabbit. 3. Interaction of colostral IgA fragments with T chain. J. Immunol. 104, 397.

Lemaitre-Coelho, I., Jackson, G.D.F. and Vaerman, J.P., 1978. High levels of secretory IgA and free secretory component in the serum of rats with bile duct obstruction. J. Exp. Med. 147, 934.

Macpherson, G.G. and Steer, H.W., 1979. Properties of mononuclear phagocytes derived from the small intestinal wall of rats. In: Function and Structure of the Immune System (eds. W. Muller-Bucholtz and H.K. Muller-Hermelink). Plenum Press, New York. p 433.

Marsh, M.N., 1975. Studies of intestinal lymphoid tissue. I. Electron microscopic evidence of 'blast transformation' in epithelial lymphocytes of mouse small intestinal mucosa. Gut 16, 665.

Matthew, D.J., Taylor, B., Norman, A.P., Turner, M.W. and Soothill, J.F., 1977. Prevention of Eczema. Lancet 1, 321.

Mattingly, J.A., Eardley, D.D., Kemp, J.D. and Gershon, R.K., 1979. Induction of suppressor cells in rat spleen: influence of microbial stimulation. J. Immunol. 122, 787.

Mattingly, J.A. and Waksman, B.H., 1978. Immunologic suppression after oral administration of antigen. I. Specific suppressor cells formed in rat Peyer's patches after oral administration of sheep erythrocytes and their systemic migration. J. Immunol. 121, 1878.

McDermott, M.R. and Bienenstock, J., 1979. Evidence for a common mucosal immunologic system. I. Migration of B immunoblasts into intestinal, respiratory and genital tissues. J. Immunol. 122, 1892.

McDermott, M.R., Bienenstock, J., Mark, D.A. and Suskind, R., 1980. Depressed intestinal localization of mucosal lymphoblasts during vitamin A and protein calorie deficiency. (In preparation)

McGhee, J.R., Kiyono, H., Michalek, S.M., Babb, J.L., Rosenstreich, D.L. and Mergenhagen, S.E., 1980. Lipopolysaccharide (LPS) regulation of the immune response: T lymphocytes from normal mice suppress mitogenic and immunogenic responses to LPS. J. Immunol. 124, 1603.

Mestecky, J., Crago, S.S., Laven, G.T. and McGhee, J.R., 1980. Immunoglobulin-containing cells and non-cellular elements of human colostrum. In: Mucosal Immune System in Health and Disease. Proceedings of the 81st Ross Conference on Pediatric Research (In press)

Miller, H.R.P. and Nawa, Y., 1979. *Nippostrongylus brasiliensis:*
intestinal goblet-cell response in adoptively immunized rats.
Exp. Parasit. 47, 81.

Montgomery, P.C., Khaleel, S.A., Goudswaard, J. and Virella, G., 1977.
Selective transport of an oligomeric IgA into canine saliva.
Immunol. Commun. 6, 633.

Mulks, M.H. and Plaut, A.G., 1978. IgA protease production as a
characteristic distinguishing pathogenic from harmless
neisseriaceae. N. Engl. J. Med. 299, 973.

Nagura H., Brandtzaeg, P., Nakane, P.K. and Brown, W.R., 1979.
Ultrastructural localization of J chain in human intestinal
mucosa. J. Immunol. 123, 1004.

Ngan, J. and Kind, L.S., 1978. Suppressor T cells for IgE and IgG in
Peyer's patches of mice made tolerant by the oral administration
of ovalbumin. J. Immunol. 120, 861.

Orlans, E., Peppard, J., Reynolds, J. and Hall, J., 1978. Rapid active
transport of immunoglobulin A from blood to bile. J. Exp. Med.
147, 588.

Owen, R.L., 1977. Sequential uptake of horseradish peroxidase by lymphoid
follicle epithelium of Peyer's patches in the normal unobstructed
mouse intestine: an ultrastructural study. Gastroenterology
72, 440.

Owen, R.L., Nenamic, P.C. and Stevens, D.P., 1979. Ultrastructural
observations on giardiasis in a murine model. I. Intestinal
distribution attachment and relationship to the immune system of
Giardia muris. Gastroenterology 76, 757.

Parker, D. and Turk, J.L., 1978. Delay in the development of the allergic
response to metals following intratracheal instillation. Int. Arch.
Allergy Appl. Immunol., 57, 289.

Perey, D.Y.E., Cooper, M.D. and Good. R.A., 1968. The mammalian homologue
of the avian bursa. I. Neonatal extirpation of Peyer's patch-type
lymphoepithelial tissues in rabbits. Method and inhibition of
development of humoral immunity. Surgery 64, 614.

Perrotto, J.L., Hang, L.M., Isselbacher, K.J. and Warren, K.S., 1974.
Systemic cecular hypersensitivity induced by an intestinally
absorbed antigen. J. Exp. Med., 140, 296.

Pierce, N.J. and Koster, F.T., 1980. Priming and suppression of the intestinal immune response to cholera toxoid-toxin by parenteral toxoid in rats. J. Immunol., 124, 307.

Pittard, W.B. and Bill, K., 1979. Immunoregulation by breast milk cells. Cell Immunol., 42, 437.

Rose, M.L., Parrott, D.M.V. and Bruce, R.G., 1976. Migration of lymphoblasts to the small intestine. II. Divergent migration of mesenteric and peripheral immunoblasts to sites of inflammation in the mouse. Cell Immunol. 27, 36.

Roux, M.E., McWilliams, M., Lamm, M.E. and Phillips-Quagliata, J.M., 1979. Site of maturation of IgA plasma cell precursors. Fed. Proc., 38, 1081.

Roux, M.E., McWilliams, M., Phillips-Quagliata, J.M., Weisz-Carrington, P. and Lamm, M.E., 1977. Origin of IgA-secreting plasma cells in the mammary gland. J. Exp. Med. 146, 1311.

Rudzik, O. and Bienenstock, J., 1974. Isolation and characteristics of gut mucosal lymphocytes. Lab. Invest., 30, 260.

Rudzik, O., Clancy, R.L., Perey, D.Y.E., Day, R.P. and Bienenstock, J., 1975. Repopulation with IgA-containing cells of bronchial and intestinal lamina propria after the transfer of homologous Peyer's patch and bronchial lymphocytes. J. Immunol., 114, 1599.

Seelig, L.L., Holt, R.G. and Beer, A.E., 1979. Cell kinetics and transepithelial migration of leukocytes in rat mammary epithelium during pregnancy and lactation. In: Immunology of Breast Milk (eds. P.L. Ogra and D. Dayton). Raven Press, New York. p 159.

Singal, D.P., O'Neill, M., Clancy, R. and Bienenstock, J., 1976. Functional T cells in rabbits gut mucosal lymphocytes. Gut 17, 325.

Socken, D.J., Jeejeebhoy, K.N., Bazin, H. and Underdown, B.J., 1979. Identification of secretory component as an IgA receptor on rat hepatocytes. J. Exp. Med. 50, 1538.

Socken, D.J. and Underdown, B.J., 1978. Comparison of human, bovine and rabbit secretory component-immunoglobulin interactions. Immunochemistry 15, 499.

Sprent, J., 1976. Fate of H2-activated T lymphocytes in syngeneic hosts. I. Fate in lymphoid tissue and intestines traced with ^{3}H-thymidine, ^{125}I-Deoxyuridine and [51]Chromium. Cell Immunol., 21, 278.

Stokes, C.R., Swarbrick, E.T. and Soothill, J.F., 1980. Immune elimination
    and enhanced antibody responses: functions of circulating IgA
    Immunology 40, 455.

Swarbrick, E.T., Stokes, C.R. and Soothill, J.F., 1979. Absorption of
    antigens after oral immunization and the simultaneous induction of
    specific systemic tolerance. Gut 20, 121.

Tada, T. and Ishizaka, K., 1970. Distribution of gamma E-forming cells in
    lymphoid tissues of the human and monkey. J. Immunol., 104, 377.

Tenner-Racz, K., Racz, P., Myrvik, Q.N., Ockers, J.R. and Geister, R., 1979.
    Uptake and transport of horseradish peroxidase by lymphoepithelium
    of the bronchial associated lymphoid tissue in normal and bacillus
    Calmette-Guérin-immunized and challenged rabbits. Lab. Invest.
    41, 106.

Thomas, H.C. and Parrott, D.M.V., 1974. The induction of tolerance to a
    soluble protein antigen by oral administration. Immunology 27, 631.

Tomasi, T.B. and Bienenstock, J., 1968. Secretory immunoglobulins.
    In: Advances in Immunology vol. 9. Academic Press, New York. p 1.

Tomasi, T.B. and Grey, H.M., 1972. Structure and function of
    immunoglobulin A. Progr. Allergy 16, 81.

Underdown, B.J., Knight, A. and Papsin, F.R., 1976. Relative paucity of
    IgE in human milk. J. Immunol., 116, 1435.

Van Epps, D.E., Reed, K. and Williams, R.C., 1978. Suppression of human
    PMN bactericidal activity by human IgA paraproteins. Cell Immunol.,
    36, 363.

Walker, W.A. and Isselbacher, K.J., 1977. Intestinal antibodies.
    N. Engl. J. Med., 297, 767.

Weisz-Carrington, P., Roux, M.E., McWilliams, M., Phillips-Quagliata, J.M.
    and Lamm, M.E., 1979. Organ and isotype distribution of plasma
    cells producing specific antibody after oral immunization:
    evidence for a generalized secretory immune system. J. Immunol.,
    123, 1705.

SESSION I

IgA SECRETION AND TRANSPORT

Chairman : F.J. Bourne

COMPARATIVE ASPECTS OF SECRETORY IMMUNITY: THE TRANSPORT OF HETEROLOGOUS IgA FROM BLOOD TO BILE IN EXPERIMENTAL ANIMALS

J.G. Hall, L.A. Gyure, A.W.R. Payne and E. Andrew

Block X, Institute of Cancer Research, Downs Road, Clifton Avenue, Sutton, Surrey, UK.

ABSTRACT

Polymeric IgA was isolated from human and rat IgA myeloma sera and labelled with ^{125}I. When injected intravenously into rats and rabbits these materials were, like native IgA antibodies, rapidly transported from blood to bile so that up to half the injected dose was recovered in the bile within 5 h.

When the same materials were injected into either sheep or guinea-pigs, they remained in the vascular compartments and were not transported into the bile to any significant extent.

Thus there seems to be a functional homology between the Immunoglobulin A-secretory component system of some animals but this is far from universal, and the reasons for this odd distribution are not immediately apparent.

INTRODUCTION

Since 1977, it has become apparent that in the rat, and probably in man and many other animals, much of the IgA that enters the gut does so by way of the bile. Rat bile is a rich source of IgA (Lemaitre-Coelho et al, 1977) because when this immunoglobulin is in a polymeric or dimeric form it is actively transported from blood to bile (Jackson et al, 1978) by the hepatocytes (Birbeck et al, 1979) which display SC on their surfaces (Orlans et al, 1979) and transport the SC-(IgA)$_{2+}$ complex in endocytic vesicles (Mullock et al, 1979). In other words, the hepatocytes transport IgA in the same way as do enterocytes (Brown, 1978) with which they share a common developmental origin. However, there are large numbers of hepatocytes and because of the fenestrations in the portal sinusoids they are essentially in direct contact with humoral factors in the blood and are thus able to clear IgA antibodies from the blood very rapidly. There is no doubt that naturally occurring, polyclonal IgA antibodies produced by antigenic stimulation of the GALT, leave the blood by this route (Hall et al, 1979; Reynolds et al, 1980) and, most importantly, this can happen even when the IgA is in the form of an immune complex (Peppard et al, in press). Thus the hepato-biliary transport of IgA may be doubly important; first as an additional means of combating freshly ingested pathogenic micro-organisms, and second as means of quickly eliminating from the circulation as immune complexes those dietary antigens that have succeeded in penetrating the mucosae in an intact and potentially allergenic form. It is likely that such important functions would have appeared early enough in evolution for the mechanism to be fairly widely distributed, and it is the purpose of this paper to begin to explore this question. Since it is relatively easy to study the extent and kinetics of the IgA transport by collecting bile, and since there is evidence that IgA and SC from different species will interact *in vitro* (Mach, 1970; Socken and Underdown, 1978) we have used this method to study the transport of heterologous IgA in 4 mammalian species.

MATERIALS AND METHODS

General plan

All experiments involved injecting intravenously immunoglobins labelled either with ^{125}I or with defined anti-body activity, and the extent of the trans-hepatic transport of the injected material was monitored by collecting hepatic bile quantitatively. Recipient animals were prepared with an indwelling i.v. cannula so that an accurately measured and timed dose of the test immunoglobulin could be given and later samples of blood obtained. The recipients were provided also with a cannula in the common bile duct; the cannulae were placed as high as possible to avoid contaminating the bile with pancreatic secretions and, in those species which possess them, the gall bladders were either tied off or excised.

The surgical techniques and the methods of isolating and labelling monoclonal (myeloma) or polyclonal immunoglobulins have all been described elsewhere (Orlans et al, 1978; Hall et al, 1979; Reynolds et al, 1980; Hall et al, 1980; Hall et al, 1977).

RESULTS

Experiments with rats

The standard against which all results were judged was the extent and kinetics with which rats transport homologous, polymeric myeloma IgA, labelled with ^{125}I, from blood to bile. When rats received a single i.v. dose of about 1 mg of such material it became detectable in the bile within 30 minutes and reached high levels in this fluid in $\frac{1}{2}$ - $1\frac{1}{2}$ h, thereafter levels of activity declined quickly so that by 5 h, between 20 and 40% of the injected dose was recovered in the bile in an antigenically intact form. This sequence of events is illustrated in the upper graph in Figure 1. It is important to note that the peak of biliary excretion, the specific radioactivity of the bile (counts per unit time per ml), was always higher than that of the blood. It is also important to note that neither monomeric IqA nor IqG or IgM ever appeared significantly in the bile after the i.v. injection.

When polymeric human myeloma IgA was injected i.v. into a rat, it appeared in the recipient's bile in just the same way as did the homologous material, and this is shown in the lower graph in Figure 1. Again, neither monomeric human IgA nor human IgG were transported into the bile. It seemed that, in terms of hepatic transport, the rat cannot distinguish between its own IgA and human IgA.

Experiments with rabbits

When either polymeric rat IgA or polymeric human IgA were injected i.v. into rabbits they disappeared rapidly from the blood and appeared in the bile just as they had in the experiments on rats. This is shown in Figure 2. Again, monomeric heterologous IgAs or heterologous IgGs were not transported from blood to bile.

Experiments with sheep and guinea-pigs

Neither of these species transported any class of heterologous polymeric or monomeric immunoglobulin from blood to bile; all experiments gave uniformly negative results.

An examination of guinea-pig bile by electrophoresis in a polyacrylamide gel in the presence of sodium dodecylsulphate, showed that a protein corresponding to the α chains of other mammals was unequivocally present. It seems likely, therefore, that guinea-pig transport their own IgA from blood to bile but, nevertheless, are unable to transport heterologous material.

The situation in sheep is more complicated. In this species IgG_1 accounts always for at least half of the Ig in secretions (Lascelles and Macdowell, 1974) and from our own experience this is certainly true of bile. The means by which

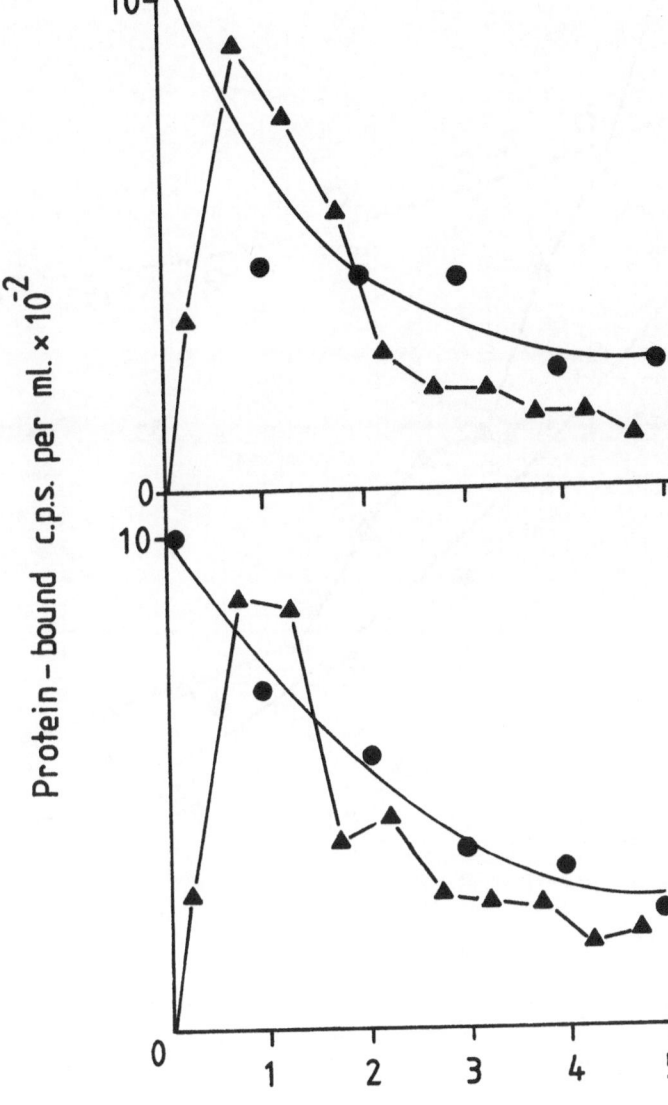

Fig. 1. The protein-bound radioactivity (counts/second/ml) of whole blood (●——●) and bile (▲——▲) of rats after ^{125}I polymeric IgA had been injected intravenously at time zero. The upper graph shows the results from an experiment where homologous (rat) IgA had been injected; the lower graph shows the results of injecting heterologous (human) IgA. In both experiments just over 30% of the injected radioactivity was recovered in the bile. (By courtesy of 'Immunology').

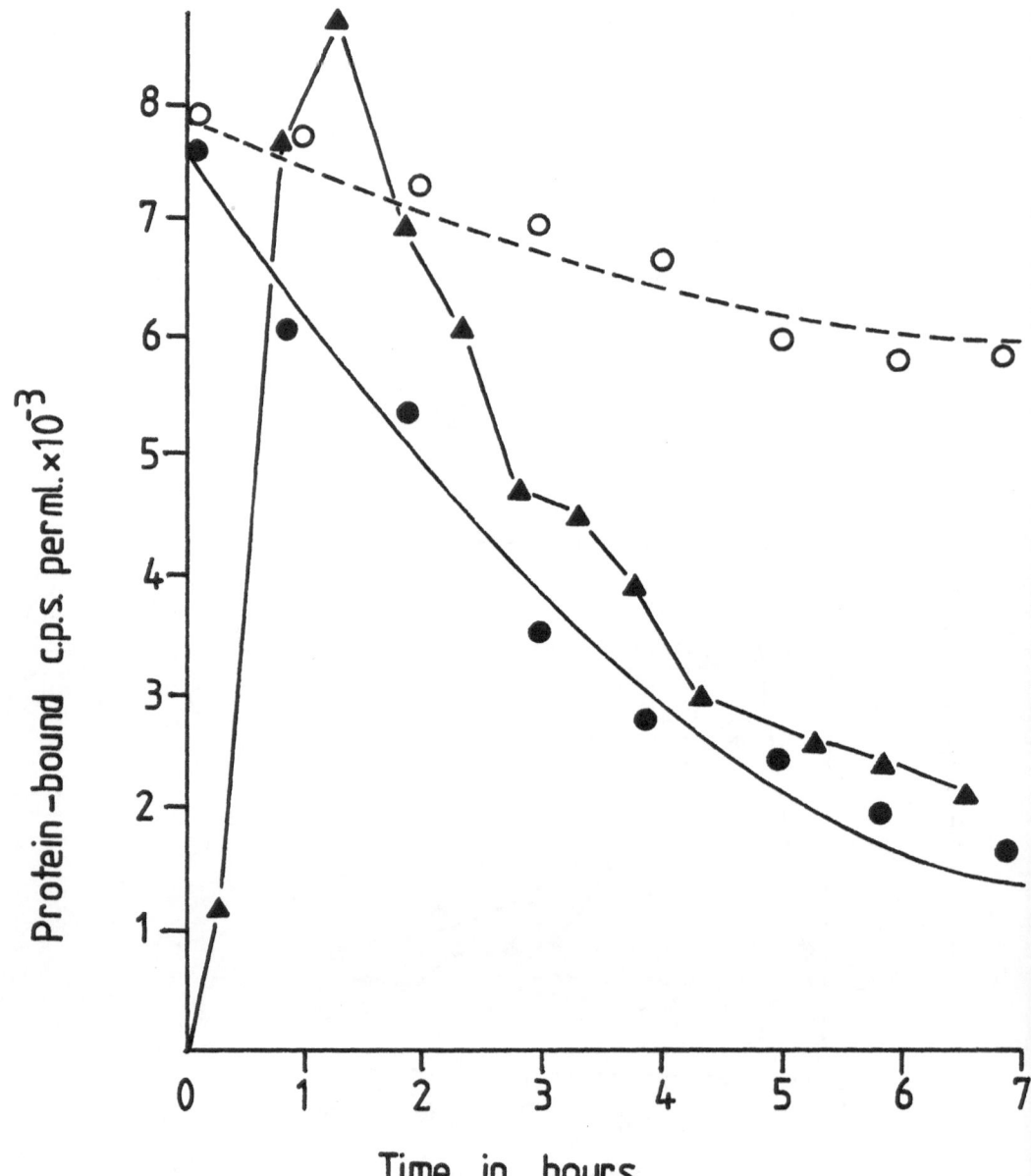

Fig. 2. The protein-bound radioactivity (counts/second/ml) of the blood plasma
(●——●) and bile (▲——▲) of a rabbit after ^{125}I polymeric rat IgA
had been injected intravenously at time zero. During the 7 hours of
the experiment, 35% of the injected dose of IgA was recovered in the
bile. An identical set of results was obtained when ^{125}I polymeric
human IgA was injected. The broken line (O----O) shows the
radioactivity in the blood of a rabbit after ^{125}I rat IgG$_2$ had been
injected; none of this material appeared in the recipients's bile.
(By courtesy of 'Immunology').

either IgA or IgG$_1$ get into sheep bile remains to be discovered.
However, by providing the recipient sheep with a cannula in the
efferent lymph duct from either the popliteal or prefemoral
node it was possible to show that the heterologous IgA polymers
that were injected, equilibrated normally between blood and
lymph. Thus, their failure to enter the bile cannot be
attributed to an inability to circulate and diffuse normally.

The transport of sheep immuloglobulins in the rat

Because it was clear that sheep could not transport rat
IgA from blood to bile (and perhaps could not even transport
their own), it was thought important to discover whether or
not rats could transport sheep IgA. Unfortunately, myelomata
do not occur commonly in sheep, and the isolation of sheep IgA
from normal body fluids is laborious. Our first experiments
were therefore carried out using impure immunoglobulin
preparations with defined antibody activity.

A donor sheep was immunised with killed *Brucella abortus*
organisms (Hall et al, 1977) by injecting a bacterial
suspension into multiple sites in the wall of the ileum as well
as subcutaneously into the lower leg. Cannulation of the
intestinal lymphatic provided lymph rich in antibodies produced
by the GALT (which were a mixture of IgGs and IgA), while
cannulation of the efferent popliteal duct provided lymph
containing conventional IgG antibodies. A crude globulin fraction
was prepared from each type of lymph plasma by salt fractionation
and, after dialysis, a sample of each was injected i.v. into
rats and the partitioning of the antibody activity between blood
and bile was monitored. The results of such an experiment are
shown in Figure 3. It can be seen that only after intestinal
lymph antibodies had been injected did antibody activity appear
in the bile, although in both types of experiment a comparable
titre had been established in the blood. This type of
experiment provided *prima facie* evidence that an Ig in sheep
intestinal lymph was actively transported from blood to bile
by the hepatocytes of the rat, and the detection by immunodif-

38

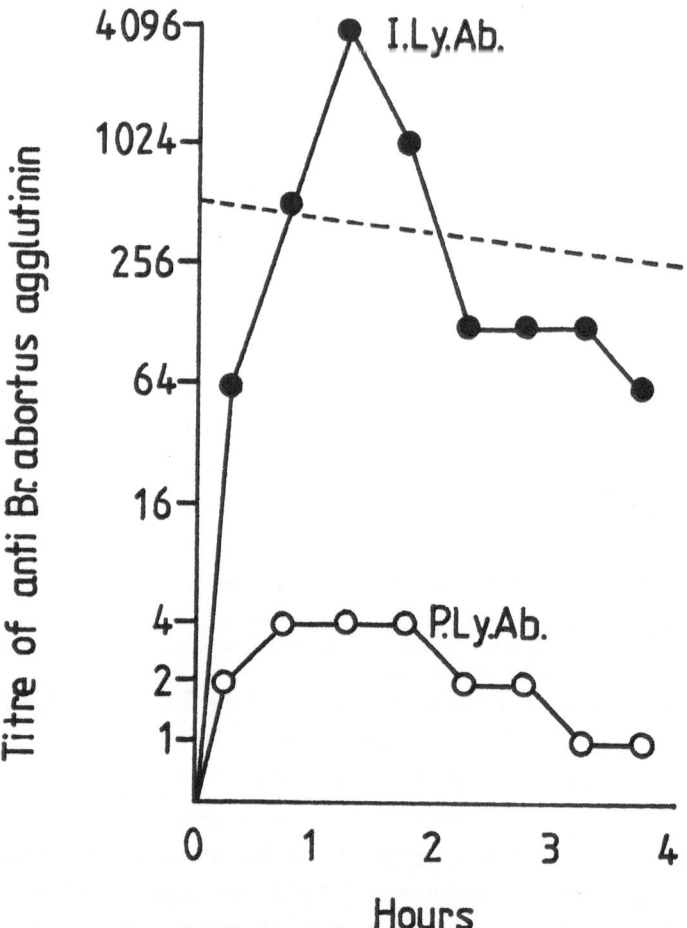

Fig. 3. The appearance of passively acquired antibodies in the bile of rats
that had received an i.v. injection of lymph globulins from a sheep
that had been immunised with *Br. abortus*.

Substantial titres of antibody appeared in the recipient's bile
only after intestinal lymph antibody had been injected (●——●).
After the injection of popliteal lymph antibody only trivial amounts
of antibody entered the bile (○——○), although in both experiments
comparable, high titres of antibody were present in the blood
throughout. (----).

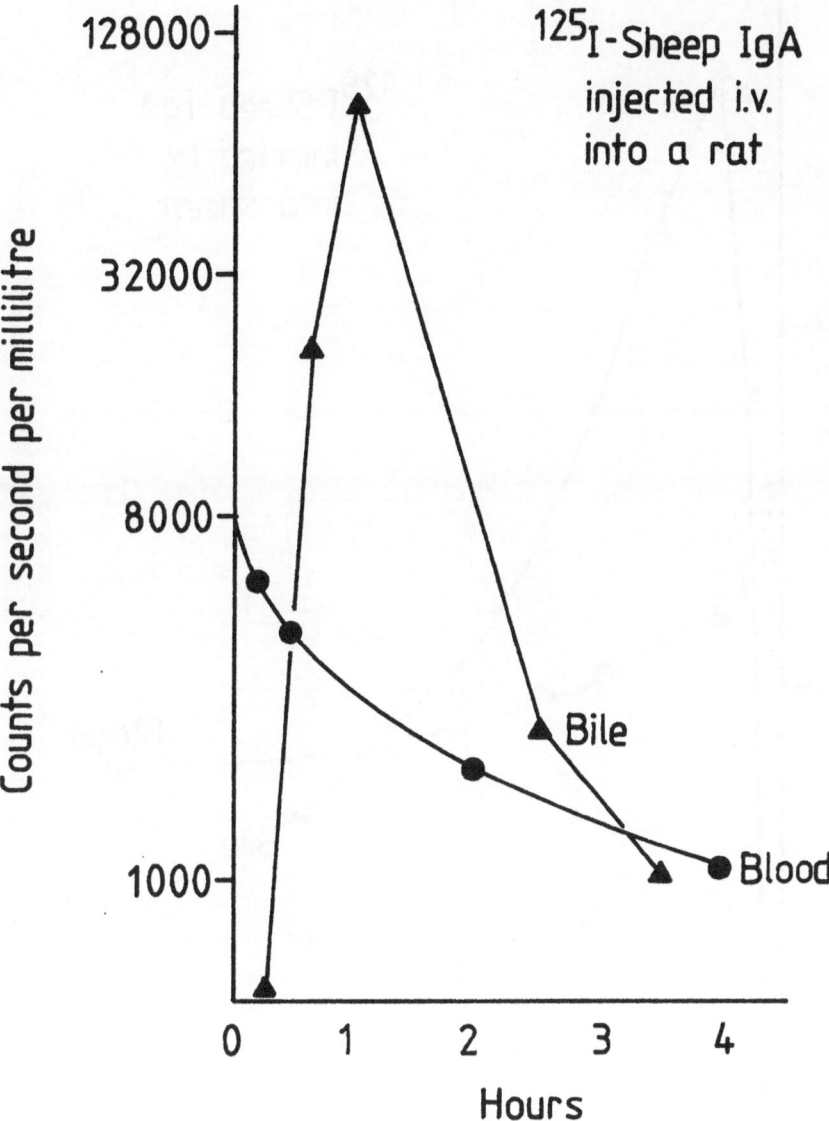

Fig. 4. The partitioning of intravenously injected ^{125}I-sheep IgA between the blood (●——●) and bile (▲——▲) of a rat during the 4 hours after the injection; within this time, 21% of the injected dose was recovered in the bile, and the maximum specific radioactivity of the bile was more than 10 times greater than that of the blood.

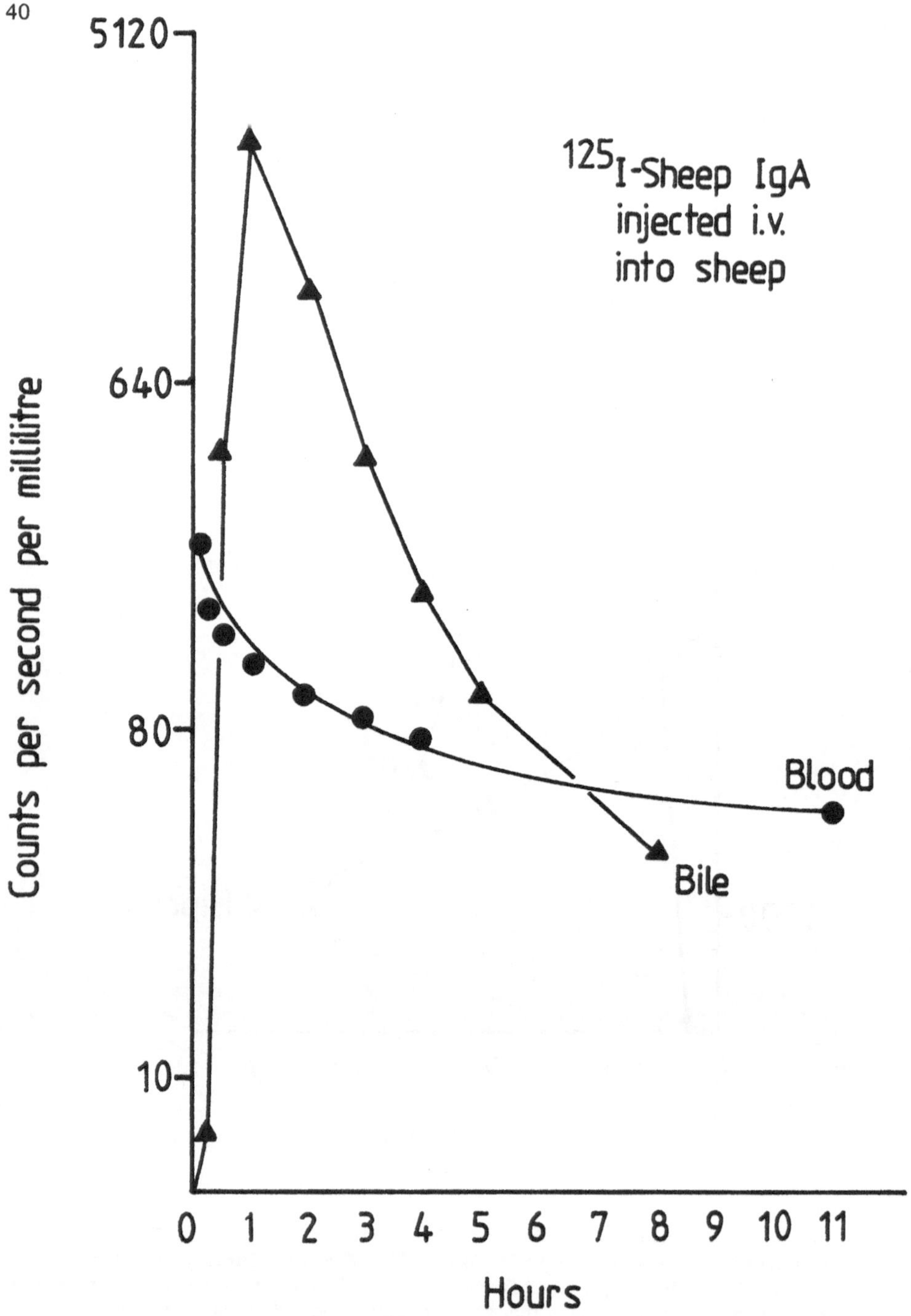

^{125}I-Sheep IgA
injected i.v.
into sheep

Blood

Bile

Counts per second per millilitre

Hours

Fig. 5. The partitioning of intravenously injected ^{125}I-sheep IgA between
the blood (●——●) and the bile (▲——▲) of a sheep during the 11
hours after the injection. Although the maximum specific
radioactivity of the bile was much greater than that of the blood,
only 5% of the injected dose was recovered in the bile in the
entire course of the experiment.

fusion of sheep α determinants in the recipients' bile indicated
that this Ig was of the IgA class. Thus encouraged, we isolated
and purified a small amount of IgA from the intestinal lymph of
sheep by affinity chromatography and, after labelling it with
^{125}I, injected it i.v. into a rat. The results of this
experiment are shown in Figure 4; they cannot be distinguished
from the results obtained after injecting the homologous material,
and 20% of the injected dose of sheep IgA was recovered from the
bile of the recipient rat within 5 h of the injection.

The transport of homologous IgA in sheep

A portion of the same preparation of ^{125}I-sheep IgA that
had been injected into a rat was injected i.v. into a sheep;
the results are shown in Figure 5, and they are rather difficult
to interpret. The kinetics of the transport of the IgA from
blood to bile were identical to those seen in the rat, and at the
peak of the transport process the specific radioactivity of the
bile was greater than that of the blood by an order of magnitude.
However, although it was obvious that a moiety of the ^{125}I-sheep
IgA had been actively transported, only 5% of the injected
material was recovered in the bile, the remainder remained
circulating in the blood.

DISCUSSION

The failure of sheep and guinea-pigs to transport polymers
of heterologous IgA from blood to bile, contrasts with the
ability of rats and rabbits to do so. This confirms a previous
report (Vaerman and Lemaitre-Coelho, 1979) that rat liver can
transport human myeloma IgA and, in addition, shows that the
kinetics of the process are similar in both species.

Because the transport process is mediated by the SC on
hepatocytes, acting as a receptor for IgA, one is bound to
assume that rat SC does not distinguish between its own IgA and
that of humans or sheep. On the other hand, it seems that SC
of sheep (and of guinea-pigs) has much more critical requirements

and only recognises a minority even of its own IgA. This could be an experimental artefact; given that sheep SC genuinely requires a very precise configuration in the IgA for which it is the receptor, it may be that the damage inflicted on many of the IgA molecules during their isolation and labelling is enough to prevent their engagement with sheep (but not with rat) SC. Alternatively, IgA transport in the sheep may be limited to a special sub-class which sheep SC can discern but rat SC cannot. Further speculation on the limited *in vivo* data will remain unprofitable until the results of further experiments are available. Even so, it should not be concluded that the relevant phenomena are restricted to mammals, for it has been discovered recently that the domestic fowl can transport human IgA from blood to bile as rapidly and abundantly as it does its own (Orlans and Rose, personal communication).

ACKNOWLEDGEMENTS

We thank Christine Winstanley for carrying out the electrophoresis of guinea-pig bile in polyacrylamide gel, Eva Orlans and Jane Peppard for helpful advice and discussion, and the editor of 'Immunology' for permission to reproduce Figures 1 and 2.

The experimental work was supported by programme and project grants from the Medical Research Council and Cancer Research Campaign.

REFERENCES

Birbeck, M.S.C., Cartwright, P., Hall, J.G., Orlans, E. and Peppard, J., 1979.
The transport by hepatocytes of Immunoglobulin A from blood to bile
visualised by autoradiography and electron microscopy. Immunology,
37, 477.

Brown, W.R., 1978. Relationships between immunoglobulins and intestinal
epithelium. Gastroenterology, 75, 129.

Hall, J.G., Gyure, L.A. and Payne, A.W.R., 1980. Comparative aspects of
the transport of Immunoglobulin A from blood to bile. Immunology,
in press.

Hall, J.G., Hopkins, J. and Orlans, E., 1977. Studies on the lymphocytes of
sheep. III. The destination of lymph-borne immunoblasts according
to theri tissue of origin. Europ. J. Immunol. 7, 30.

Hall, J.G., Orlans, E., Reynolds, J., Dean, C., Peppard, J., Gyure, L.
and Hobbs, S, 1979. Specific antibodies of the IgA class in the
bile of rats. Int. Archs. Allergy. appl. Immunol. 59, 75.

Jackson, G.D.F., Lemaitre-Coelho, I., Vaerman, J-P., Bazin, H, and Beckers, A.,
1978. Rapid disappearance from the serum of intravenously injected
rat myeloma IgA and its secretion into the bile. Europ. J. Immunol.
8, 123.

Lascelles, A.K. and MacDowell, G.H., 1976. Localised humoral immunity with
particular reference to ruminants. Transplant. Revs. 19, 170.

Lemaitre-Coelho, I., Jackson, G.D.F. and Vaerman, J.P., 1977. Rat bile
as a convenient source of secretory IgA and free secretory
component. Europ. J. Immunol. 8, 588.

Mach, J-P., 1970. *In vitro* combination of human and bovine free secretory
component with IgA of various species. Nature, Lond. 228, 1278.

Mullock, B.M., Hinton, R.H., Dobrota, M., Peppard, J. and Orlans, E. 1979.
Endocytic vesicles in liver carry polymeric IgA from serum to bile.
Biochem. Biophys. Acta. 587, 381.

Orlans, E., Peppard, J., Fry, J.F., Hinton, R.H. and Mullock, B.M., 1979.
Secretory component as the receptor for polymeric IgA on rat
hepatocytes. J. exp. Med. 150, 1577.

Orlans, E., Peppard, J., Reynolds, J. and Hall, J.G., 1978. Rapid active
transport of Immunoglobulin A from blood to bile. J. exp. Med. 147, 588.

Peppard, J., Orlans, E., Payne, A.W.R. and Andrew, E., 1980. The elimination
of circulating complexes containing polymeric IgA by excretion in the
bile. Immunology, in press.

Reynolds, J., Gyure, L., Andrew, E. and Hall, J.G., 1980. Studies of the transport of polyclonal IgA antibody from blood to bile in rats. Immunology, 39, 463.

Socken, D.J. and Underdown, B.J., 1978. Comparison of human, bovine and rabbit secretory component-immunoglobulin interactions. Immunochemistry, 15, 499.

Vaerman, J-P. and Lemaitre-Coelho, I., 1979. Transfer of circulating human IgA across the rat liver into the bile, pp 383-398. In: Protein transmission through living membranes. W.A. Hemmings (Ed.) Elsevier/ North Holland Biomedical press.

DISCUSSION

H. Miller *(UK)*

Dr. Hall, have you ever looked at the amount of bile secreted after your challenge with immune complexes? Is there any alteration in the rate of flow of bile?

J. Hall *(UK)*

No, not that we can measure. It is fairly variable in the rat but it is difficult to compare flow rates from one animal to another. In an individual we have seen nothing of that so far. Of course, our experiments are really only just starting in that field.

W. Leibold *(FRG)*

Does IgA pass through the gut epithelium at the same rate as it does through the bile into the gut lumen? What proportion of IgA passes through the bile?

J. Hall

I don't think I can answer this question very accurately. I believe there is some work by Brown's group from Colorado which would suggest that intestinal epithelial cells will transport IgA just as quickly as hepatic cells, probably in about half an hour or so. Now, the question as to how much IgA gets into the gut via the bile is something that Dr. Vaerman and I were talking about just before I started to speak; we both agreed that this is a very difficult question to answer. I think it is about 50 - 50 in the rat but that is just a guess. I believe there are claims that none of it gets in via the epithelium, that it all comes via the bile. I really don't know. We have certainly found IgA in isolated loops of gut, and I think other people have done the same in the rat. So some certainly gets through but I can't tell you the proportions.

F.J. Bourne *(UK)*

This does raise the question of the biological significance
of the liver secreted IgA. You could argue that it would be more
exposed to proteolysis and thereby be biologically less significant than that reaching the gut through the enterocyte.

J. Hall

Well, presumably, if it distributes itself along the gut
wall and into the mucous monolayer, it may be well protected.
There are obvious advantages in having it come in in concert
with the gastric emptying, when you have a sudden influx of
antigens and pathogens; having a sudden influx of IgA would
make some sense. Also, the antigen elimination may be the
most important biological function but we aren't in a position
to say that for sure.

R. Levinsky *(UK)*

This system can only work for dimeric IgA. In man, for
instance, the maximum amount of dimeric IgA is in the order of
5%. How do you invoke the clearance of IgA immune complexes
in that situation?

J. Hall

Here I am speculating but I suspect that the level of
dimeric IgA is so low in man simply because it is cleared. Most
animals do not produce much monomer; in this man is somewhat
different. So far we have been unable to show in the rat that
complexes involving IgA monomer are transported. If a lot of
the antibody activity was in the monomer I would expect that
not to be transported. I suspect that the dimeric antibodies
are cleared very rapidly which is why, when you look at the
blood at any one instant of time, the amount of IgA dimer or
polymer is extremely low. This applies to rats, guinea pigs
and even sheep to a certain extent. But that doesn't mean
that in the course of a day an awful lot of IgA dimer has not
passed through the blood compartments. We have to think in terms
of turnover, rather than a concentration at a given time.

P. Brandtzaeg *(Norway)*

I have a question for Dr. Hall and Dr. Vaerman on the point about transport of monomers to bile. I believe Dr. Vaerman has some experiments showing that some selectivity is also present for monomeric transport in the bile of the rat. But Dr. Hall says there is none.

J. Hall

Well, we haven't found it. Of course, we are using myeloma monomer and that may not be quite typical. We haven't yet produced polyclonal monomer in concentrations necessary to do the experiment.

J.P. Vaerman *(Belgium)*

We found some transfer of monomeric IgA using human myelomas but when we carefully purified rat myeloma monomer the amount of transfer was very, very low.

J. Hall

That has been our experience; we have found some human myelomas which do seem to have abnormal chain lengths and conceivably some of these may behave differently. But the human monomers we have have not been transported.

J. Soothill *(UK)*

May I suggest that you have put forward a number of ideas and two perfectly straightforward experiments could explore them. One is to prepare the monomer from MOPc 315 complexed with antigen-like material and inject it and see if it transported. The second one would be to make differential clearance studies of monomer and dimer IgA. Are you telling me that no one has done the latter? If you are right in your hypothesis, the half time of dimer IgA ought to be extremely short and this could be done by a simple metabolic study.

J. Hall

It is certainly so in the rat; the half life of dimeric
IgA is extremely short. That was published a long time ago.
But thank you for those very kind suggestions.

F.J. Bourne

Thank you Dr. Hall.

BINDING, UPTAKE AND PROCESSING OF POLYMERIC IgA BY CULTURED RAT HEPATOCYTES

J.N. Limet*, Y.-J. Schneider, A. Trouet and J.P. Vaerman

Université Catholique de Louvain
(Laboratoires de Chimie Physiologique et de Médecine
Expérimentale) and International Institute of Cellular
and Molecular Pathology, ICP, 75, Avenue Hippocrate,
B 1200, Brussels, Belgium.

ABSTRACT

The binding, uptake and processing of polymeric IgA (pIgA) by cultured rat hepatocytes have been studied in conditions where the cells reassociate into hepatic-like trabeculae and reform bile caniculi.

The cells synthesise secretory component (SC), partly secreted in the culture medium, and partly exposed at the cell surface. At 4°, hepatocytes bind specifically pIgA and competition experiments indicate that SC is the receptor responsible for the major part of this binding.

Lactoferrin but not asialofetuin inhibits both the low temperature binding and the uptake at 37°. This suggests that in our in vitro conditions ^{3}H-labelled pIgA is taken up for a part through binding sites which recognise also lactoferrin possibly through the presence of exposed fucose residues.

At 37°, pIgA is taken up by the cells and rapidly interiorised. A minor part of the cell bound pIgA reappears after a lag phase into the culture medium as low molecular weight labelled material; another major part reappears more rapidly as secretory IgA, most probably after its secretion at the biliary pole of the hepatocyte.

* J.N.L. is Aspirant of the Belgian FNRS.

INTRODUCTION

In rats, hepatic bile is rich in secretory IgA (sIgA) and free secretory component (SC) (Lemaître-Coelho et al., 1977), while the serum level of IgA is about 10-fold lower. In addition, thoracic duct lymph which drains the small gut lymph contains also much higher IgA levels than serum (Vaerman and Heremans, 1970; Vaerman et al., 1973). These data led to the discovery of an active transport of rat or human polymeric IgA (pIgA) from blood to bile (Vaerman and Lemaître-Coelho, 1979; Jackson et al., 1978; Orlans et al., 1978). This transport is mediated by rat hepatocytes (Birbeck et al., 1979; Renston et al., 1980; Fisher et al., 1979), the SC located at the sinus-oidal membrane serving as a receptor for pIgA (Socken et al., 1979; Orlans et al., 1979) in a model similar to that proposed for the translocation of human pIgA through differentiated neoplastic colon cells (Nagura et al., 1979).

We have used cultured hepatocytes as a well defined *in vitro* model in an attempt to improve our knowledge of the cellular mechanism by which pIgA is taken up, processed and finally released into the bile as sIgA. We have first invest-igated the presence of SC at the cell surface of the hepat-ocytes and its role in the binding of pIgA at 4°. We have further determined the kinetics of interiorisation, uptake, digestion and release of pIgA at 37°.

MATERIALS AND METHODS

Purification and labelling of proteins

Rat pIgA was isolated from the serum or the ascitic fluid of rats bearing IgA secreting myeloma (IR 22 tumour) or from the serum of a patient with an IgA secreting myeloma as already described (Acosta-Altamirano et al., 1980; Vaerman and Lemaître-Coelho, 1979), by gel filtration on Ultrogel AcA 22 (LKB Instruments, Villeneuve-la-Garenne, France), followed by preparative Pevikon block electrophoresis and immuno-adsorption

on anti-rat albumin IgG immobilised (Cambiaso et al., 1975) on
Sepharose CL-4B (Pharmacia, Uppsala, Sweden). Labelling of
pIgA was carried out by reductive methylation (Means and
Feeney, 1968) with Na^3H borohydride (The Radiochemical Centre,
Amersham, England); ^3H-labelled monomeric IgA was then
separated by ultracentrifugation in isokinetic sucrose grad-
ients. Antisera against IgA were raised in rabbits by repeated
multisite injections of IgA; to achieve monospecificity for α-
chains antisera were immuno-adsorbed on rat IgG and rat IgM
immobilised on Sepharose CL-4B. The specific antibodies were
isolated by immuno-adsorption and labelled by reductive
methylation with ^{14}C-formaldehyde (The Radiochemical Centre,
Amersham, England). sIgA and SC were purified from rat bile
as previously described (Acosta-Altamirano et al., 1980).
Antisera against SC were raised in rabbits by repeated
multisite injections of SC partially purified from rat bile.
To obtain monospecificity, the antisera were immuno-adsorbed
with normal rat serum immobilised on Sepharose CL-4B. The
monospecificity of the antibodies was checked by immunoelectrophoresis and Ouchterlony analysis using rat bile and
rat serum as antigens.

The IgG fractions were isolated from different sera
either by ammonium sulphate precipitation and DEAE-cellulose
chromatography or by affinity chromatography on Sepharose CL-
4B-protein A (Pharmacia, Uppsala, Sweden) and elution with
0.58% acetic acid in 0.15 M NaCl. The IgG fractions were then
labelled by reductive methylation using either ^{14}C-formaldehyde
or Na^3H borohydride. $F(ab')_2$ fragments were prepared according
to Limet et al. (1979). Human lactoferrin was isolated from
human milk (Querinjean et al., 1971) and freed from SC by
immuno-adsorption on anti-SC IgG immobilised on Sepharose CL-
4B. Asialofetuin was kindly provided by M. Masquelier (this
Institute).

Immunological assays

The concentration of free SC in the culture medium was
determined by a particle counting immunoassay technique

(Cambiaso et al., 1977) using ^{14}C-labelled F(ab')$_2$ coated
latex particles (Limet et al., 1979) and purified SC as standard.

In order to determine the concentration of ^{3}H-labelled
sIgA released in the medium, 0.1 μl of culture medium diluted
2 to 4 times was incubated for 3 to 4 h at 25°, under constant
stirring, with 25 μl of a 0.1% suspension of latex particles
coated with ^{14}C-labelled anti-SC F (ab')$_2$ in glycine buffered
saline (GBS : 0.1 M glycine-NaOH, pH 9.2; 0.17 M NaCl) supplemented with 1% bovine serum albumin (BSA). The suspension was
then centrifuged for 20 minutes at 7 000 RPM in a Sorvall SS-
34 rotor (Dupont Instruments, Orsay, France), washed twice
with GBS-BSA, resuspended in 0.8 ml of the same buffer and
assayed for radioactivity in a Beckman LS 9 000 liquid
scintillation counter (Beckman, Palo Alto, Ca). The concentration of sIgA was calculated as a function of the specific
activity of the ^{3}H-labelled pIgA; a standard of sIgA was run
in parallel in order to monitor the efficiency of the antigen/
antibody reaction; determinations were corrected for the
losses of latex particles during the assay procedure as
estimated by the recovery of ^{14}C counts; blanks consisting of
pIgA diluted in control culture medium (not incubated in the
presence of cells) were performed and subtracted.

Isolation and culture of rat hepatocytes

Rat hepatocytes were isolated and cultivated essentially
as described by Wanson et al. (1977), excepted that collagen
(Type III from Sigma, St. Louis, Mo) coated Petri dishes were
used. The culture was initiated with respectively 1 or 3 x
10^6 cells per 9 cm^2 or 20 cm^2 dishes in Dulbecco's modified
Eagle medium supplemented with 15% foetal calf serum (FCS).
Plastic Petri dishes (Falcon, Becton Dickinson, Cockeysville,
Md) or Petriperm dishes (Heraeus, Germany), were used. After
a few hours the cells adhered to the dish and started to reassociate; after about 4 to 6 hours, hepatic-like trabeculae
and bile canaliculi progressively reappeared. After about 24
hours a complete monolayer was formed and maintained for at

least 4 to 5 days. For the present experiments only cells
cultured from 1 to 3 days were used.

Kinetic experiments

Hepatocyte monolayers were incubated in a culture medium
containing 15% FCS either as such for the incubations at 37°
or supplemented with 20 mM Hepes buffered at pH 7.2, for the
incubations at 4°. At the end of the 37° incubations, the
culture medium was removed and for some experiments analysed
for the presence of sIgA as described above and of degradation
products by precipitation with an equal volume (250 to 500 µl)
of 20% trichloracetic acid (TCA) followed by ultracentrifugation and assay of the supernate for radioactivity. The
concentration of degradation products was determined by comparison to a culture medium incubated with labelled material
for the same duration in the absence of cells.

At the end of the incubation at 4°, cells were washed
twice with 2.5 ml phosphate buffered saline (PBS : 0.14 M
NaCl, 3 mM KCl, 10 mM Na_2HPO_4-KH_2PO_4, pH 7.4), once with
complete culture medium and again twice with PBS and finally
dissolved in 2 ml of 1% Na deoxycholate adjusted to pH 11.3
with NaOH; the cell lysate was then analysed for radioactivity
and protein using BSA as standard (Lowry et al., 1951).

After the incubations at 37°, cells were washed once with
2.5 ml of complete culture medium and 4 times with 2.5 ml of
PBS. For some experiments they were then incubated at 4° for
15 minutes in the presence of 0.1% trypsin in PBS, a treatment
whereby most of the cells are detached from the dish; the dish
was then flushed with 0.4 ml of complete culture medium. The
cell suspension and the washing liquid were pooled and
centrifuged through a cushion of 0.3 ml of dibutylphtalate for
2 minutes in a Microfuge (Beckman, Palo Alto, Ca). The cell
pellets were resuspended in 1 ml of Na deoxycholate and assayed
for radioactivity and protein; the supernatants were assayed
for radioactivity. For some experiments, the cells were

reincubated at 4° for 30 minutes in the presence of 40 μg/ml
of ^{14}C-labelled (anti-IgA) IgG in a volume of 0.7 ml. Cells
were then washed once with 2.5 ml of complete culture medium
and 5 times with 2.5 ml of PBS, resuspended and analysed for
protein and radioactivity. The anti-IgA to IgA antibody to
antigen ratio was estimated by incubating cell monolayers for
30 minutes at 4° with IgA (5 μg/ml in a volume of 0.7 ml.
Cells were then washed once with 2.5 ml of complete culture-
medium and 5 times with 2.5 ml of PBS, resuspended and analysed
for protein and radioactivity. The anti-IgA to IgA antibody to
antigen ratio was estimated by incubating cell monolayers for
30 minutes at 4° with IgA (5 μg/ml in a volume of 0.7 ml) and,
by reincubating them, after washing, in the presence of (anti-
IgA) IgG in the same conditions. After subtraction of the non-
specific fixation (cells incubated without pIgA and then
exposed to [14]C (anti-IgA) IgG) this ratio was found to be 1.8
in the present conditions.

RESULTS

Synthesis and secretion of free SC

In the absence of pIgA in the culture medium, hepatocytes synthesise and secrete free SC in the culture medium
as detected by a specific immunoassay. The concentration of
SC in the medium increases proportionally to the duration of
the incubation (Figure 1).

Low temperature binding of pIgA

At 4°, cultured hepatocytes bind both rat and human pIgA
in a process nearly saturable with both the duration of the
incubation and the pIgA concentration (Figure 2). Considering
the Scatchard analysis of the binding parameters and assuming
that 1 mg of cell protein corresponds to 2.25×10^6 hepatocytes
(as determined by counting the cells after detachment by
collagenase and by assaying the protein content), these data
suggest that each cell exposes 350 000 binding sites for rat
pIgA (with an affinity constant of 0.43×10^8 M^{-1}) and 260 000

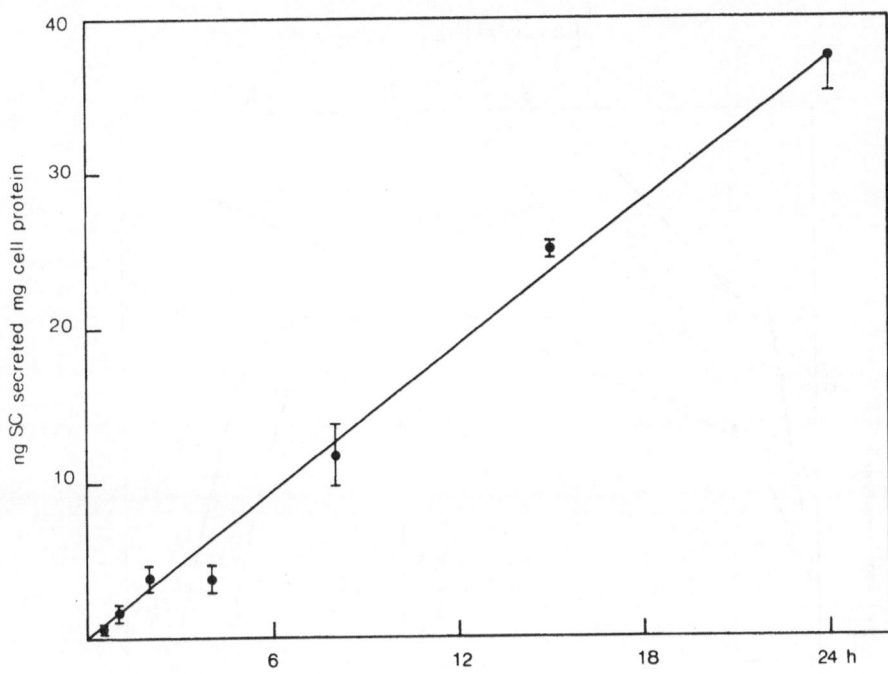

Fig. 1. Secretion of SC in the culture medium. Cells cultured 3 days in
9 cm^2 Petri dishes (<u>ca</u> 0.8 mg of protein) were washed in culture
medium and then reincubated for different durations in fresh
medium. After culture the cells were washed and analysed for
protein content whereas the media were centrifuged and assayed
for SC concentration.

sites for human pIgA (Ka = 0.19 x 10^8 M^{-1}), as well as about
125 000 sites with a Ka of 0.3 x 10^7 M^{-1} for rat pIgA and about
250 000 sites with a Ka of 0.3 x 10^6 M^{-1} for human pIgA.
Competition experiments indicate that the binding of rat ^{3}H-
labelled pIgA can be inhibited up to 90% by a 100-fold excess
of unlabelled rat pIgA (not shown). Hepatocytes bind 10 times
more pIgA than sIgA, monomeric IgA and rat IgG when exposed to
these proteins at a concentration of 10 µg per ml (not shown).

Low temperature binding of anti-SC IgG

The binding of ^{3}H-labelled anti-SC F(ab')$_2$ by cultured
hepatocytes is a process nearly saturable with the duration of
the incubation at 4°. As indicated by Figure 3, when taking
into account the binding of ^{3}H-labelled control rabbit F(ab')$_2$

56

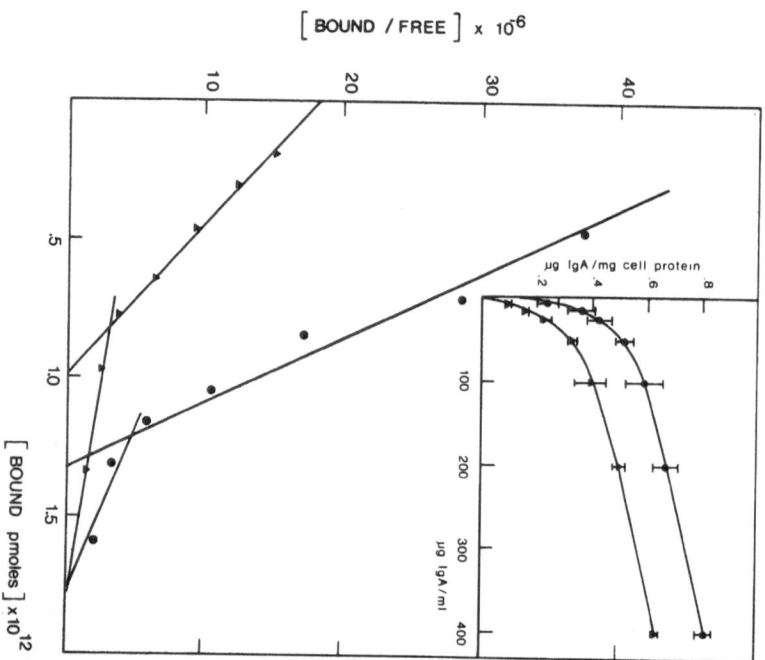

Fig. 2. Low temperature binding of ^{3}H-labelled pIgA. Cells cultured 3
days in 9 cm^2 Petri dishes (<u>ca</u> 0.8 mg of protein) were incubated
for 13 h at 4° in 0.3 ml culture medium containing ^{3}H-labelled
pIgA at concentrations ranging from 6.25 µg per ml to 400 µg per
ml. Means ± S.D. of 3 independent experiments. The Scatchard
plot was calculated according to Klotz and Hunston (1971).

● rat ^{3}H-labelled pIgA

▲ human ^{3}H-labelled pIgA

part of the binding of anti-SC F(ab')$_2$ can be considered
specific and saturable with the antibody concentration.

Competition experiments

The binding of ^{3}H-labelled pIgA to cultured hepatocytes
at 4° can be inhibited up to 80% by the presence of anti-SC
IgG (Figure 4). When the cells are preincubated in the presence of 5 mg/ml of anti-SC IgG and then exposed to ^{3}H-labelled
pIgA, the binding of pIgA is inhibited up to 80% by comparison
with an experiment performed in the presence of control IgG.

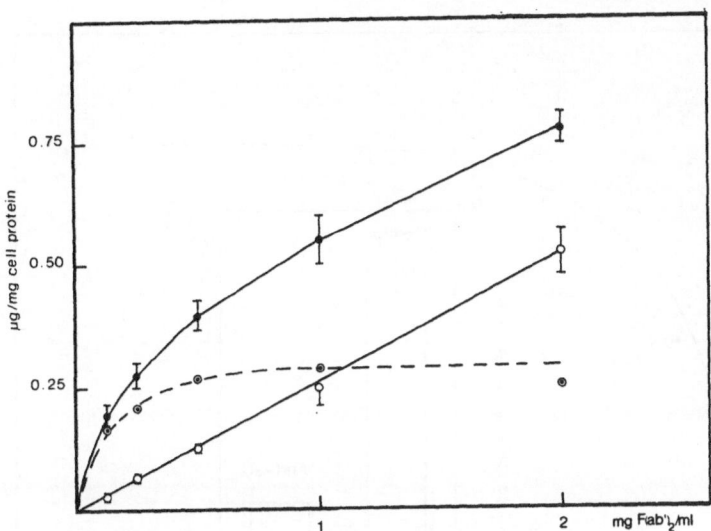

Fig. 3. Low temperature binding of ^{3}H-labelled anti-SC F(ab')$_2$.

Cells cultured 3 days in 9 cm^2 Petri dishes (ca 0.8 mg of protein) were incubated for 13 h at 4° in 0.3 ml culture medium supplemented with ^{3}H-labelled anti-SC(ab')$_2$ (●) or control F(ab')$_2$ (o) at concentrations ranging from 0.125 to 2 mg per ml. (⊙) represents the specific binding as determined after substraction of the binding of control F(ab')$_2$ from the binding of anti-SC F(ab')$_2$. Mean ± S.D. of 3 independent experiments.

On the other hand, as illustrated by Table 1, lactoferrin but not asialofetuin competes strongly with ^{3}H-labelled pIgA for the binding to cultured hepatocytes.

Uptake and processing of pIgA at 37°

In a first set of experiments, cultured hepatocytes were incubated up to 20 h at 37° in the presence of ^{3}H-labelled pIgA. As illustrated by Figure 5, the total amount of pIgA which is taken up and processed by the cells is almost proportional to the duration of the incubation: up to 3 h incubation almost all the ^{3}H-labelled material is associated to the cells, afterwards the amount of ^{3}H-labelled material processed by the cells, but recovered in the culture medium becomes predominant. The amount of cell associated label increases up to about 3 h and reaches then a plateau stable up to 20 h.

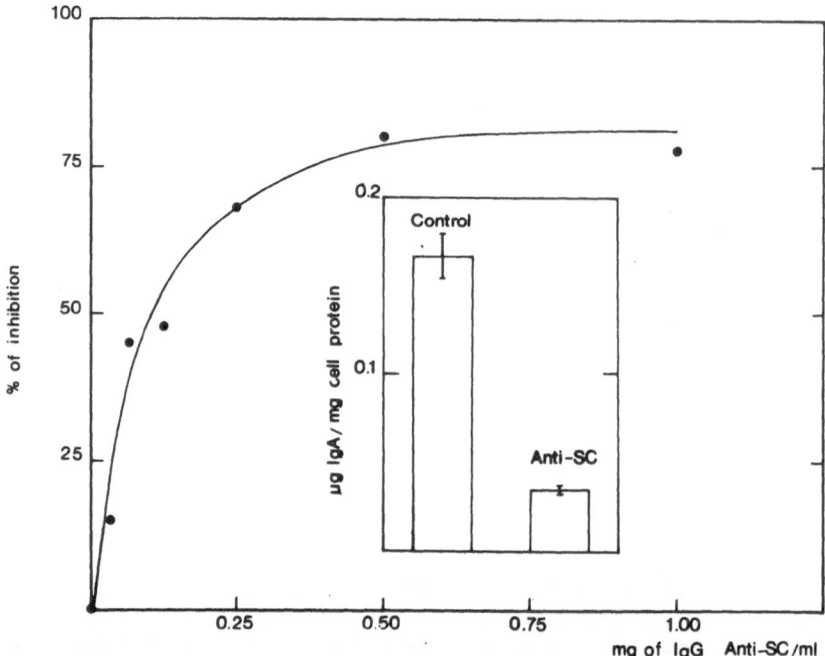

Fig. 4.   Inhibition of the binding of ^{3}H-labelled pIgA by anti-SC IgG.
Cells cultured 3 days in 9 cm^2 Petri dishes (ca 0.8 mg or protein)
were incubated simultaneously with 1 μg of ^{3}H-labelled pIgA per ml
and increasing concentrations of unlabelled anti-SC IgG ranging
from 31.25 to 1 000 μg per ml. Enclosed panel: for this experiment
cells were preincubated with control IgG or anti-SC IgG (5 mg per
ml for 3 h at 4°), washed and then exposed for 10 min at 4° to 10
μg/ml of ^{3}H-labelled pIgA.

It can be divided into two parts of about equal extent: a first
one which can be released from the cells by a short treatment
with trypsin at 4° and a second one unreleasable by this enzyme.
In the culture medium, ^{3}H-labelled material processed by the
cells appears after a lag phase of about 3 h.   A major part
consists of sIgA, the concentration of which increases with
the duration of the incubation; a minor part consists of
degradation products soluble in TCA.

    In a second set of experiments, hepatocytes were
incubated for 2 h at 37° with ^{3}H-labelled pIgA, washed and
then reincubated in a IgA free medium. The amount of ^{3}H-
labelled material which remains bound to the cells and that

TABLE 1

EFFECT OF ASIALOFETUIN AND LACTOFERRIN ON THE INTERACTION OF ^{3}H-LABELLED pIgA WITH CULTURED HEPATOCYTES

	ng of ^{3}H-labelled material (expressed as pIgA equivalents) per mg cell protein		
	Control	+ asialofetuin	+ lactoferrin
Low temperature binding (1 h at 4°)	109.5 ± 3.4	108.5 ± 7.5	27.8 ± 8.5
Cell bound ^{3}H-label (24 h at 37°)	47.7 ± 4.5	51.0 ± 6.6	30.0 ± 1.2
Digestion products in the culture medium (24 h at 37°)	24.2 ± 2.6	27.04 ± 3.6	17.8 ± 2.1

Cells cultured 2 days in 20 cm^2 Petri dishes containing ca 2.5 mg protein were incubated either for 1 h at 4° or for 24 h at 37° in a culture medium containing 5 µg per ml of ^{3}H-labelled pIgA, in the absence or the presence of 1 mg of asialofetuin or of 1 mg/ml of human lactoferrin.

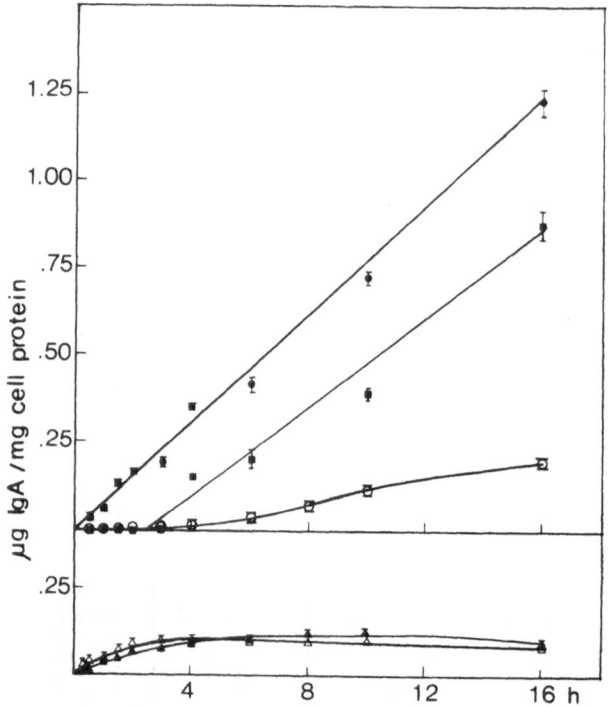

Fig. 5.   Uptake and processing of ^{3}H-labelled pIgA at 37°. Cells cultured
1 day in 20 cm^2 Petri dishes (ca 1.6 mg of protein) were incubated
for different durations at 37° in 1.5 ml of culture medium containing 2.5 µg of ^{3}H-labelled pIgA per ml.

Upper panel: ^{3}H-labelled material recovered in the culture medium.

o : TCA soluble label expressed as pIgA equivalents

■ : ^{3}H-labelled sIgA

● : total uptake and processing of pIgA by hepatocytes as deter-
      mined by summing up the accumulation results illustrated in
      the lower panel and the sIgA and TCA soluble material in the
      culture medium.

Lower panel: ^{3}H-labelled material associated with the cells
expressed as pIgA equivalents releasable (Δ) or non-releasable
(▲) by trypsin. Mean results ± S.D. of three independent
experiments.

which appears in the culture medium were determined and the
results are presented in Figure 6.   At the start of the wash-
out about 20% of the cell bound ^{3}H-labelled material is
accessible to anti-IgA antibody; this proportion decreases

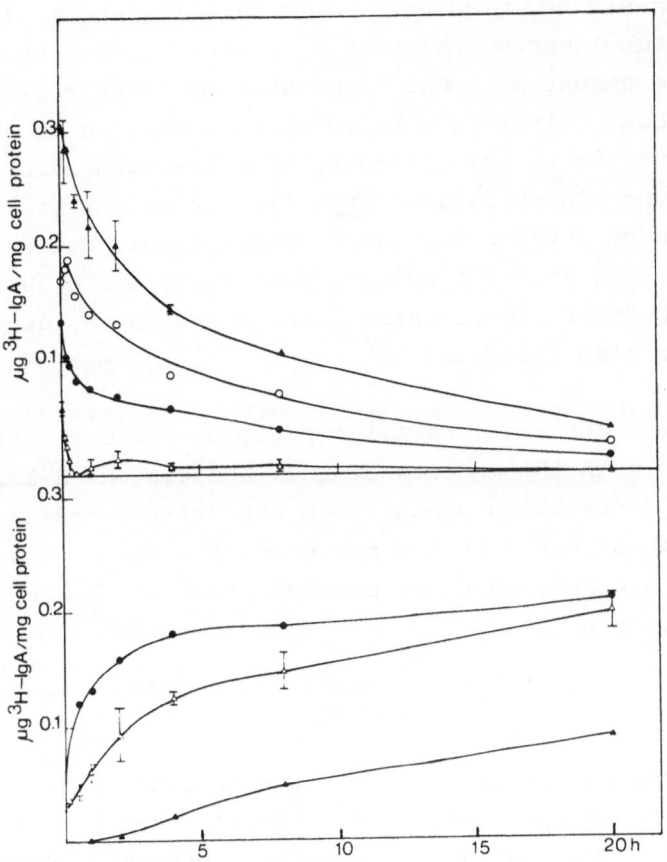

Fig. 6.   Wash-out experiment.

Cells cultured 1 day in 20 cm^2 Petri dishes (ca 2.5 mg of protein) were first incubated for 2 h at 37° in 1 ml of culture medium containing 5 µg of ^{3}H-labelled pIgA per ml.   After washings, cells were reincubated for different durations in a fresh IgA free culture medium.

Upper panel: cell associated ^{3}H-labelled material.

▲ :   total cell bound label

o :   label unreleasable by trypsin

● :   label releasable by trypsin

Δ :   label accessible to anti-IgA antibody.

Lower panel: ^{3}H-labelled material recovered in the wash-out medium, and expressed as pIgA equivalents.

▲ :   TCA soluble material

Δ :   TCA precipitable material.

● :   sum of the cell associated label releasable by trypsin and the TCA precipitable label in the culture medium.

rapidly within a few minutes. Concomitantly about 44% of the cell-bound label can be released by a short treatment with trypsin; the amount of label releasable by trypsin progress-ively decreases, first in a rapid phase completed in about 30 minutes amounting to 19% of the total cell-bound label, and then in a much slower phase. Finally the amount of label unreleasable by trypsin decreases progressively but rather slowly. In the wash-out medium, TCA precipitable ^{3}H-labelled material appears rapidly, while after a lag phase, degradation products are also released.

On the other hand, as illustrated by Table 1, after a 24 h incubation both the amounts of cell-associated ^{3}H-label and TCA soluble degradation products in the culture medium are not significantly affected by the presence of 1 mg/ml of asialo-fetuin, but are reduced to respectively 37% and 26% by 1 mg per ml of lactoferrin.

DISCUSSION

Cultured rat hepatocytes secrete free SC in the culture medium (Figure 1) and bind, at 4°, ^{3}H-pIgA in a largely specific (80 - 90%) and nearly saturable process. Human pIgA is bound to a comparable extent but with a lower affinity than rat pIgA.

Anti-SC antibody also attaches to cultured hepatocytes and furthermore it can inhibit largely but not completely the binding of pIgA. These results confirm that the specific receptor responsible for the major part of pIgA binding to hepatocytes consists in SC exposed at the cell surface (Orlans et al., 1979; Socken et al., 1979). This observation agrees with *in vivo* experiments which have shown that the hepatic transfer of sIgA is small and that purified SC inhibits the transfer of endogenous and exogenous pIgA (Fisher et al., 1979; Lemaître-Coelho et al., 1980).

Asialofetuin which is recognised by the hepatocytes through a receptor specific for glycoproteins with a terminal galactose residue (Ashwell and Morell, 1974) does not affect the binding nor the uptake of pIgA by hepatocytes. This pleads strongly against an implication of this receptor in the uptake of pIgA. In addition, treatment of rat and human pIgA with neuraminidase does not significantly alter their *in vivo* transfer into bile (Vaerman, unpublished results).

On the other hand, lactoferrin inhibits by 80% the binding of pIgA to hepatocytes at 4° and only by 26% its digestion after 24 h incubation at 37° (Table 1). These results indicate that lactoferrin competes with pIgA for the specific binding to SC while interfering much less with its digestion. Since lactoferrin is a glycoprotein with a terminal fucose residue, linked to a N-acetyl-glucosamine residue in a α 1 - 3 linkage, which is cleared rapidly from the circulation by the liver (Prieels et al., 1978), our data would suggest that SC could be the hepatocytic receptor for lactoferrin and that SC could recognise fucose moieties. A receptor with such a specificity has indeed recently been demonstrated at the surface of cultured hepatocytes (Deschuyteneer et al., 1980). It must however be emphasised that fucose is poorly (1 mole per mole of protein in a α 1 - 6 linkage) represented in human α 1-chains (Baenzinger and Kornfeld, 1974) and is not in a terminal position.

Since it has been reported (Kuhn and Kraehenbuhl, 1979) that rabbit mammary gland cells expose high affinity receptors for SC, we could also propose that lactoferrin competes with SC for a similar receptor present at the cell surface of the hepatocytes and that fucose is involved in this binding. Finally since lactoferrin is positively charged at the pH of the experiments, this protein could also bind unspecifically to a large number of sites at the plasma membrane, including SC and therefore inhibit the binding of pIgA. Experiments are in progress both *in vivo* and *in vitro* to investigate further whether the inhibition by lactoferrin of the low temperature

binding and the uptake of pIgA by hepatocytes has some
physiological relevance.

After binding to the plasma membrane, pIgA seems at 37°
to be rapidly interiorised inside the hepatocytes since during
a continuous incubation in the presence of pIgA, part of the
cell-bound ^{3}H-label becomes unreleasable by trypsin (Figure 5)
and since during a wash-out experiment, pIgA becomes inaccessible to anti-IgA antibody (Figure 6) with a t 1/2 of disappearance of about 10 minutes.

There is, however, a discrepancy between the amount of
pIgA accessible to anti-IgA antibody and the amount of pIgA
releasable by trypsin (Figure 6). These amounts should at
first sight be very similar and be related to the amount of
pIgA remaining at the surface of the cells. In order to understand these differences, one has to consider that in cultured
hepatocytes, bile canaliculi are formed which are inaccessible
to ruthenium red and to horseradish peroxidase (Wanson et al.,
1977) and swell when the cells are exposed to cholic acid
(May et al., 1979). Part of the sIgA secreted into the bile
canaliculi will thus be inaccessible to anti-IgA antibody at
4° whereas trypsin, which dissociates completely the cell
monolayer will also release the material retained inside these
canaliculi.

Two models can be proposed to explain the intracellular
processing of pIgA. In the first model previously proposed
(Kraehenbuhl and Kuhn, 1978), pIgA would be interiorised and
processed by two different routes. The first route would
involve binding sites different from SC and present at the cell
surface; the pinocytic vesicles would enclose membrane bound
pIgA but also immunoglobulin molecules taken up by fluid phase
pinocytosis and would deliver their contents to lysosomes to
be digested. Different pinocytic vesicles would be formed
enclosing pIgA bound to SC; these vesicles would escape from
fusing with lysosomes, preventing the proteolysis of sIgA and
would thereafter fuse with the plasma membrane at the biliary

pole and finally release their content into the bile
canaliculi.

As we have already discussed (Schneider et al., 1980) on
the basis of the plasma membrane recycling concept, another
model can be invoked which involves only one route but two
stations. The pIgA after its binding either to SC or to other
binding sites, would be interiorised in one unique type of
vesicles, enclosing also pIgA taken up by fluid phase pinocytosis. After fusion of these vesicles with lysosomes, pIgA
present in the fluid content of the vesicles or attached to
other sites than SC would be transferred into the lysosomes
and then be digested; pIgA linked to SC would, on the contrary,
remain bound to the membrane of the pinocytic vesicles and, so,
escape from proteolysis. The phagolysosome would then dis-
sociate and the vesicles containing membrane-bound sIgA would
be conveyed to the biliary pole of the cell and release sIgA
into the bile canaliculi.

At this stage our results do not allow to distinguish
between these two models. Biochemical and morphological
experiments are now in progress to further investigate the
intracellular processing of pIgA.

ACKNOWLEDGEMENTS

The excellent technical help of Mrs. Doumont-Tasiaux is
gratefully acknowledged. This work was supported by the
Belgian Fonds de la Recherche Scientifique Médicale (grants
n°3.4512.76, 3.4545.80 and 3.4504.70).

REFERENCES

Acosta Altamirano, G., Barranco-Acosta, C., Van Roost, E. and Vaerman, J.P., 1980. Isolation and characterisation of secretory IgA (sIgA) and free secretory component (FSC) from rat bile. Mol. Immunol. 17, in press.

Ashwell, G. and Morell, A.G., 1974. The role of surface carbohydrates in the hepatic recognition and transport of circulating glycoproteins. Adv. Enzymol. 41, 99-128.

Baenzinger, J. and Kornfeld, S., 1974. Structure of the carbohydrate units of IgAl immunoglobulin. I. Composition, glycopeptide isolation, and structure of the asparagine-linked oligosaccharide units. J. Biol. Chem. 249, 7260.

Birbeck, M.S.C., Cartwright, P., Hall, J.G., Orlans, E. and Peppard, J., 1979. The transport by hepatocytes of immunoglobulin A from blood to bile visualised by auto-radiography and electron microscopy. Immunology 37, 477.

Cambiaso, C.L., Goffinet, A., Vaerman, J.P. and Heremans, J.F., 1975. Glutaraldehyde-activated 6-aminohexyl-Sepharose as a new versatile immuno-absorbent. Immunochemistry 12, 273.

Cambiaso, C.L., Leek, A.E., De Steenwinkel, F., Billen, J. and Masson, P.L., 1977. Particle counting immunoassay (PACIA). I. A general method for the determination of antibodies, antigens and haptens. J. Immunol. Meth. 18, 33.

Deschuyteneer, M., Prieels, J.P., May, C., Perraudin, J.P. and Wanson, J.C., 1980. Presence of galactose and fucose receptors on adult rat hepatocytes in primary monolayer culture. Eur. J. Cell Biol. 22, 264.

Fisher, M.M., Nagy, B., Bazin, H. and Underdown, B.J., 1979. Biliary transport of IgA: role of secretory component. Proc. Natl Acad. Sci. USA. 76, 2008.

Jackson, G.D.F., Lemaitre-Coelho, I., Vaerman, J.P., Bazin, H. and Beckers, A., 1978. Rapid disappearance from serum of intravenously injected rat myeloma IgA and its secretion into bile. Eur. J. Immunol. 8, 123.

Klotz, I.M. and Hunston, D.L., 1971. Properties of graphical represent-ations of multiple clones of binding sites. Biochemistry 10, 3065.

Kraehenbuhl, J.P. and Kuhn, L., 1978. Transport of immunoglobulins across
        epithelia. In: 'Transport of Macro-molecules in Cellular Systems'
        (S.C. Silverstein, ed.), Dahlem Konferenzen, Abakon Verlag Ges.,
        Berlin, pp 213-228.

Kuhn, L.C. and Kraehenbuhl, J.P., 1979. Role of secretory component, a
        secreted glycoprotein, in the specific uptake of IgA dimer by
        epithelial cells. J. Biol. Chem. **254**, 11072.

Lemaitre-Coelho, I., Jackson, G.D.F. and Vaerman, J.P., 1977. Rat bile as
        a convenient source of secretory IgA and free secretory component.
        Eur. J. Immunol. **7**, 588.

Lemaitre-Coelho, I., Acosta, G., Barranco, C. and Vaerman, J.P., 1980.
        Role of secretory component (SC) in the hepatic transfer of IgA:
        in vivo experiments. In: '4th Intern. Congress of Immunology, Paris,
        July 1980' (Ed. Preud 'homme, J.L. and Hawken, V.A.L.), Abstract
        18.1.22, Amelot, Brionne.

Limet, J.N., Moussebois, C.H., Cambiaso, C.L., Vaerman, J.P. and Masson,
        P.L., 1979. Particle counting immunoassay. IV. The use of
        $F(ab')_2$ fragments and N^ε-chloroacetyl lysine N-carboxyanhydride
        for their coupling to particles. J. Immunol. Meth. **28**, 25.

Lowry, O.H., Rosebrough, N.Y., Farr, A.L. and Randall, R.J., 1951. Protein
        measurement with the folin phenol reagent. J. Biol. Chem. **193**, 265.

May, C., Bernaert, D., Mosselmans, R., Popowski, A., Penasse, W. and
        Wanson, J.C., 1979. Cell aggregates and monolayer cultures of
        adult rat hepatocytes: models for the study of the ultrastructural
        behaviour and metabolic functions of parenchymal cells. In:
        'Models for the Study of Inborn Errors of Metabolism' (F.A. Homes,
        ed), Elsevier North-Holland Biomed. Press.

Means, G.E. and Feeney, R.E., 1968. Reductive alkylation of amino groups
        in proteins. Biochemistry **7**, 2192.

Nagura, H., Nakane, P.K. and Brown, W.R., 1979. Translocation of dimeric
        IgA through neoplastic colon cells *in vitro*.J. Immunol. **123**, 2359.

Orlans, E., Peppard, J., Reynolds, J. and Hall, J.G., 1978. Rapid active
        transport of immunoglobulin A from blood to bile. J. Exptl Med.
        147, 588.

Orlans, E., Peppard, J., Fry, J.F., Hinton, R.H. and Mullock, B.M., 1979.
        Secretory component as the receptor for polymeric IgA on rat
        hepatocytes. J. Exptl Med. **150**, 1577.

68

Prieels, J.P., Pizzo, S.V., Glasgow, L.R., Paulson, J.C. and Hill, R.L.,
    1978. Hepatic receptor that specifically binds oligosaccharides
    containing fucosyl α 1-3 N-acetyl-glucosamine linkages. Proc. Natl
    Acad. Sci. USA. 75, 2215.

Querinjean, P., Masson, P.L. and Heremans, J.F., 1971. Molecular weight,
    single chain structure and aminoacid composition of human lacto-
    ferrin. Eur. J. Biochem. 20, 420.

Renston, R.H., Jones, A.L., Christiansen, W.D., Hradek, G.T. and Underdown,
    B.J., 1980. Evidence for a vesicular transport mechanism in
    hepatocytes for biliary secretion of immunoglobulin A. Science 208,
    1276.

Schneider, U.-J., Octave, J.N., Limet, J.N. and Trouet, A., 1980.
    Functional relationship between cell surface and lysosomes during
    pinocytosis. Proceedings of the Second International Congress
    on Cell Biology, Berlin, September 1980.

Socken, D.J., Jeejeebhoy, K.N., Bazin, H. and Underdown, B.J., 1979.
    Identification of secretory component as an IgA receptor on rat
    hepatocytes. J. Exptl Med. 150, 1538.

Vaerman, J.P. and Heremans, J.F., 1970. Origin and molecular size of
    immunoglobulin A in the mesenteric lymph of the dog. Immunology
    18, 27.

Vaerman, J.P., Andre, C., Bazin, H. and Heremans, J.F., 1973. Mesenteric
    lymph as a major source of serum IgA in guinea pigs and rats. Eur.
    J. Immunol. 3, 580.

Vaerman, J.P. and Lemaitre-Coelho, I., 1979. Transfer of circulating
    human IgA across the rat liver into the bile. In: 'Transmission of
    Proteins Through Living Membranes' (Hemmings, W.A., ed.), Elsevier/
    North-Holland Biomed. Press, Amsterdam, p.383.

Wanson, J.C., Drochmans, P., Mosselmans, R. and Ronveaux, M.F., 1977. Adult
    rat hepatocytes in primary monolayer culture. Ultrastructural
    characteristics of intercellular contacts and cell membrane
    differentiations. J. Cell Biol. 74, 858.

DISCUSSION

J. Bienenstock (Canada)

Underdown and his colleagues showed, in the rat, that IgM has a high affinity for secretory component, equivalent to IgA. The question is whether you or Joe Hall have done any experiments to look at IgM transport. As far as I can understand it, IgM is not transported and yet it still has an affinity for secretory component. You have shown also that the covalent bonding is not necessary for that transport to occur.

J.P. Vaerman (Belgium)

First of all, with regard to IgM, Dr. Hall will give his own results but if I remember correctly, we find some IgM in bile and it seems to be a little more than would be expected from its molecular size, but is still present in only very small amounts. Using labelled IgM, Fisher found a little transfer but, as I recall, Underdown described the affinity of IgM for the rat secretory component having an order of magnitude lower than that of IgA. So it has not the same affinity. He used this as an argument to explain that there was much less IgM in bile although you would expect that it would be transported, and there is more IgM than polymeric IgA in rat serum.

J. Bienenstock

Have you looked at human IgM in the rat system?

J.P. Vaerman

No, I haven't tried that because Underdown also reported that the affinity of rat secretory component for human IgM was also much lower.

J. Bienenstock

I realise it is an order of magnitude lower but that order of magnitude lower is several orders of magnitude higher than IgG. You are comparing this also to IgG and I think it might help us to understand if you could solve the question as to whether or not IgM is transported.

J. Hall *(UK)*

IgM *in vivo*, does not. If you label rat IgM and inject it, it is not transported to any extent. Of course, that is in the presence of the native IgA and what we need is an IgA deficient rat and then maybe we could demonstrate it. I think that is all one can say. It certainly does not happen *in vivo* and I can only assume that it is because it is blocked by the much higher affinity of the native IgA.

F.J. Bourne *(UK)*

Thank you very much Dr. Vaerman.

EPITHELIAL TRANSPORT OF HUMAN
SECRETORY IMMUNOGLOBULINS

P. Brandtzaeg

Histochemical Laboratory, Institute of Pathology,
The National Hospital, Rikshospitalet,
Oslo, Norway

ABSTRACT

According to the proposed transport model, the J ('joining') chain and epithelial SC ('secretory component') represent 'the lock and key' in the selective external translocation of dimeric IgA and pentameric IgM through serous-type secretory epithelial cells. Incorporation of J chains into these two immunoglobulin isotypes during their production in gland-associated immunocytes apparently induces a configurational fit (binding site) allowing them to combine with SC in the plasma membrane of the epithelial cell. This complexing on the basolateral surface of the cell seems to stimulate pinocytosis (adsorptive endocytosis); the completed secretory IgA and secretory IgM molecules with bound SC are then transported in cytoplasmic vesicles to the gland lumen along with an excess of free SC. The following observations that support the proposed transport model will be discussed in some detail: 1. Immunoglobulin-binding properties of SC; 2. Characteristics of the immunoglobulin products of gland-associated immunocytes; 3. Localisation of SC and immunoglobulins in normal and neoplastic secretory epithelium.

INTRODUCTION

Dimeric IgA, associated with an epithelial glycoprotein now called the 'secretory component' (SC), is the principal immunoglobulin (Ig) in human exocrine body fluids. A comprehensive literature has accumulated about the properties of secretory IgA, which is considered to function as a highly stabilised antibody molecule performing antigen exclusion at mucosal surfaces in co-operation with innate, natural immune mechanisms (for review, see Hanson and Brandtzaeg, 1980).

The small amounts of IgM and IgG that normally appear in the external secretions may likewise participate in immunological antigen exclusion, although these Ig isotypes are less stable than secretory IgA. In a pure glandular fluid, with minimum contamination by transudation of tissue fluid through surface epithelia, the IgG : IgA concentration ratio is reduced to about 0.2% of that in serum, and the IgG : IgM ratio may be reduced to less than 2% (Brandtzaeg, 1973a). This indicates that selectivity is involved in the glandular translocation of both IgA and IgM compared with IgG. Comparisons of the parotid Ig secretion in patients with selective IgA deficiency, G myeloma, or macroglobulinaemia have further attested to the selectivity inherent in the external transport of IgM compared with IgG (Brandtzaeg, 1971a). Moreover, parotid IgA and IgM show similar secretory dynamics on gustatory stimulation of the gland (Brandtzaeg, 1971c).

It was speculated in several early studies that SC may facilitate the entry of extracellular IgA into glandular epithelial cells (Tomasi et al., 1965; South et al., 1966; O'Daly et al., 1971). SC was therefore originally called "transport piece" (South et al., 1966). This suggestion was prompted by the fact that SC was a regular subunit of the secretory IgA polymer; but there was no obvious explanation for its postulated transport function.

We proposed originally that the selective external translocation of IgA and IgM takes place independently of SC, perhaps

by means of unique characteristics ('transfer sites') in the
heavy chains of these two Ig isotypes and a corresponding
epithelial receptor of unknown nature (Brandtzaeg, 1968; Brandtzaeg et al., 1970). This view was mainly influenced by our early
failure to demonstrate a regular association between SC and
secretory IgM (Brandtzaeg et al., 1968; Brandtzaeg, 1971a). Moreover, the observation that pure glandular fluids contain about ten
times more monomeric IgA than IgG indicated that the transport
mechanism was specific for the IgA isotype rather than for dimeric
IgA (Brandtzaeg et al., 1970). By analogy, an epithelial receptor
specific for IgG1 has been demonstrated in bovine mammary glands,
which preferentially transmits this Ig unchanged from serum during
the colostrum-forming period (Kemler et al., 1975). The intestinal
epithelium of some suckling animals likewise contains a specific
receptor that mediates the translocation of intact IgG from the gut
lumen into the blood circulation (Rodewald, 1976).

It should be stressed from the outset that the possible
existence of an as yet undefined glandular receptor specific
for the heavy chains of human IgA and IgM has not been
definitely excluded. Nevertheless, studies during the first
part of the last decade made it increasingly likely that
specific epithelial uptake of Ig is mediated by SC. It seemed
justified, therefore, in 1973 to propose a common glandular
transport model for dimeric IgA and pentameric IgM (Brandtzaeg
1973a,b); it was suggested that plasma-membrane associated
SC, by selective non-covalent affinity for these two J-chain-
containing Ig polymers, determines their uptake by serious-type
secretory epithelial cells. This model was further elaborated
in two subsequent publications (Brandtzaeg, 1974a,b).

A MODEL FOR GLANDULAR IMMUNOGLOBULIN TRANSPORT

As reviewed elsewhere (Brandtzaeg and Baklien, 1977), at
least six different models have been proposed for the external
transport of IgA and its mode of combination with SC. Some of
the confusion in this field has been caused by the many
conflicting reports about the cellular origin of SC. In several
studies it has been claimed that SC is produced by the goblet cell

whereas IgA is translocated through the columnar cell. However, Poger and Lamm (1974) clearly identified the latter cell type as the major intestinal source of SC, in accordance with independent studies from our laboratory (Brandtzaeg, 1973a, 1974a). Also in agreement with our studies (Brandtzaeg, 1974b), SC was found to exist in a free form in the Golgi zone but was partially complexed with IgA in the apical part of the columnar epithelial cell. Nevertheless, since Poger and Lamm found no indication of membrane-associated SC, their observations were interpreted to suggest that the assembly of secretory IgA took place inside the epithelial cell after the fusion of pinocytotic vesicles and SC-containing Golgi vesicles (Lamm, 1976).

If the epithelial uptake of IgA according to the model of Poger and Lamm (1974) should occur as 'fluid' or 'bulk' pinocytosis, it would be difficult to explain the selectivity for IgA and IgM. One possibility mentioned by Lamm (1976) was that SC protected IgA against degradation by intracellular enzymes, whereas IgG and other proteins included in the pinocytotic vesicle were degraded. Even fragments of IgG should retain some antigenicity, however, and the complete lack of cytoplasmic IgG staining in glandular epithelia (discussed in a later section) speaks against an entry of this protein into intact secretory cells. Also, secretory IgM contains SC in a more 'open' quaternary structure than secretory IgA (Brandtzaeg, 1975a), and IgM is apparently not protected against proteolytic degradation by its combination with SC (Richman and Brown, 1977) in the way described for dimeric IgA (Lindh, 1974).

IgA and IgM will according to our transport model (Brandtzaeg, 1973a,b; 1974a,b) be selected at the basolateral epithelial cell membrane owing to the SC-binding site of these J-chain-containing polymers (Figure 1). The receptor-polymer complexes formed on the cell surface are either taken up by adsorptive pinocytosis or may partially float in the plasma membrane and reach the gland lumen without entering the cytoplasm (broken arrow in Figure 1). Which route is preferred may depend on the cellular distribution of SC, which apparently varies among different glands as discussed in a subsequent section.

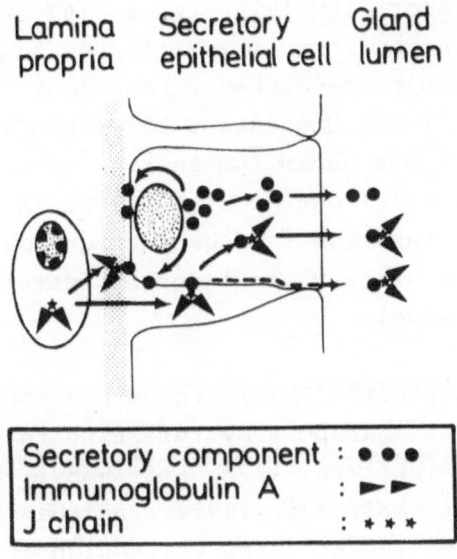

| Lamina propria | Secretory epithelial cell | Gland lumen |

Secretory component : ● ● ●
Immunoglobulin A : ► ►
J chain : ✦ ✦ ✦

Fig. 1. Schematic representation of the common glandular transport model
proposed for J-chain-containing IgA and IgM, exemplified by
external translocation of dimeric IgA from the plasma cell in the
lamina propria to the lumen. Secretory component (SC) produced
by the serous-type epithelial cell is partly incorporated into the
plasma membrane, partly secreted in a free form. SC-IgA complexes
are formed in the plasma membrane and then taken up by adsorptive
endocytosis. The possibility exists (broken arrow) that some of
the complexes floating in the plasma membrane may reach the gland
lumen without entering the cytoplasm.

SC is disulphide-linked in 75 - 80% of human 11S secretory
IgA (Brandtzaeg, 1971b, 1977a), and Lamm (1976) pointed out
that there is no other known situation where a receptor becomes
permanently attached to the transported molecule. This is
probably no valid argument against a receptor function of SC
in the glandular transport of IgA and IgM, however. Stabilisation
of SC-Ig complexes, as regularly seen for human dimeric IgA,
apparently depends on the production of a surplus of free SC
and unique possibilities for disulphide-exchange reactions
(Brandtzaeg, 1977a). In normal human saliva and colostrum the
amount of free SC may approach that of bound SC (Brandtzaeg,
1973a), whereas in pig colostrum there are only traces of free
SC and 60% of the dimeric IgA lacks SC after purification

(Bourne, 1974). SC is likewise retained in only 60 - 70% of purified human secretory IgM (Brandtzaeg, 1975a), and SC-IgM complexes formed *in vitro* show very little or no tendency to stabilisation by disulphide-exchange reactions (Brandtzaeg, 1974c, 1977a; Weicker and Underdown, 1975; Lindh and Bjork, 1976a). In this respect human IgM is also similar to rabbit IgA of the subclass g (Knight et al., 1975). A covalent interaction with SC thus seems to be a unique characteristic of human IgA instead of being an inherent feature of the proposed transport model.

Weicker and Underdown (1975) argued against a participation of SC in glandular Ig transport by referring to the lack of *in vivo* (Newcomb and Ishizaka, 1970) and *in vitro* association between SC and IgE (Brandtzaeg, 1977a); neither is this argument valid, however, since the previous assumption of selectivity in the secretion of IgE comparable to that of IgA does not hold true (Nakagima et al., 1975). A relative enrichment of IgE in some exocrine fluids compared with serum apparently depends on local synthesis combined with passive diffusion through epithelial interstices as part of 'pathothopic potentiation' of mucosal immunity (Hanson and Brandtzaeg, 1980).

In the transport model proposed on the basis of studies in our laboratory (Brandtzaeg, 1973a,b; 1974a,b) it was not possible to suggest how SC could reach the plasma membrane of the epithelial cell, although it was implied that SC was an integral membrane protein. The question of the routes of intracellular transport of secretory products from the rough endoplasmic reticulum to the plasma membrane remains vexed (Newmark, 1979). Recent extensive studies with isolated rabbit mammary cells have supported the proposed role of SC as an epithelial receptor for dimeric IgA (Kraehenbuhl and Kühn, 1978; Kühn and Kraehenbuhl, 1979b). In addition, these authors proposed that SC reaches the basolateral plasma membrane by some unexplained mechanism after initial secretion and binding to a luminal receptor specific for free SC. The alternative possibility that free SC encounters its receptor in cytoplasmic vesicles was also considered. It remains to be shown, however, that a receptor truly specific for SC is present in the plasma membrane of all types of secretory epithelial cells and in all species.

The suggestion made by the same authors (Kraehenbuhl and Kühn, 1978; Kühn and Kraehenbuhl, 1979b) that the final luminal release of dimeric IgA takes place due to displacement by free SC can definitely not hold true to the human species where dimeric IgA becomes covalently linked to SC during the glandular transport. Although a considerable amount of bound SC can be displaced from human SC-IgM complexes by addition of a large excess of free SC, this is not so for human SC-IgM complexes (Brandtzaeg, 1977a). Immunoelectron microscopy of human epithelial cells has indicated that the exteriorisation of secretory IgA occurs by opening of vesicles or extrusion of vesicles into the gland lumen (Nagura et al., 1979b). But how the SC-Ig complexes actually are released from the membranes of the vesicles to which they are bound remains unexplained.

In the following sections various observations supporting the transport model depicted in Figure 1 will be discussed in some detail.

IMMUNOGLOBULIN-BINDING PROPERTIES OF SC

The discovery of SC as a regular subunit of human secretory IgA (Tomasi et al., 1965) stimulated a series of attempts to demonstrate specific affinity between SC and IgA. Mach (1970) and Radl et al. (1971) independently reported the significance of the IgA-dimer conformation by studying the combination between human myeloma proteins and free SC isolated from colostrum. Complexing with IgM was also noted in these studies, but only polymers larger than 19S pentamers were thought to be active (Radl et al., 1971). The latter observation could not be confirmed in our laboratory (Brandtzaeg, 1974c). By contrast, it was shown that SC was able to combine with 19S IgM as readily as with dimeric IgA, and that the specific complex formation depended on non-covalent interactions rather than on the formation of disulphide bonds (Brandtzaeg, 1974c, 1977a). This observation was a prerequisite for the proposed receptor function of membrane-associated SC, and has been confirmed independently by two other research groups (Weicker and Underdown, 1975; Socken and Underdown, 1978; Lindh and Björk, 1976a,b; 1977)

When Mach published his results in 1970, the J chain had just been detected in polymeric IgA and IgM (for review, see Koshland, 1975); in an addendum to his paper he therefore postulated a role for this polypeptide in the SC-binding process. We obtained the first evidence to substantiate such a function of the J chain when we found that an IgM polymer lacking J chain failed to bind SC *in vitro* (Eskeland and Brandtzaeg, 1974). In a subsequent study the reductive release of J chain was quantified immunochemically in 24 IgA preparations (Brandtzaeg, 1976a). Five polymeric fractions that contained only 0.2 - 0.8 mg J chain per 100 mg IgA showed an SC-binding capacity of 6 - 12% compared with 69 - 82% for polymers containing more than 4.0 mg J chain per 100 mg (Table 1). The marginal SC binding properties of IgA monomer preparations could be ascribed to contaminating J-chain-containing polymers.

The report of Jerry, Kunkel and Adams (1972) has caused some confusion in this respect. They found that in the presence of a large excess of SC obtained from reduced secretory IgA, covalent complexing took place with monomeric IgA of the subclass α_2 and genetic variant Am_2 (+). It has also been reported that bovine SC, added in large excess, to some extent may become covalently complexed with certain J-chain-deficient IgA polymers *in vitro* (Tomasi and Czerwinski, 1976). These findings must be clearly distinguished from our results which are based on non-covalent interactions with small amounts of native human SC.

Although it seems justified to conclude that the J chain is mandatory for spontaneous non-covalent interaction of SC with

TABLE 1

SC-BINDING CAPACITY OF VARIOUS HUMAN SERUM IgA PREPARATIONS RELATED TO THEIR J-CHAIN CONTENT

IgA preparations	J-chain (mg/100 mg IgA)	SC-binding* (mean % ± SD)
Polyclonal polymers	7.3	75.8
Monoclonal polymers (n=7)	4.9 ± 1.5	74.4 ± 5.3
Monoclonal polymers (n=5)	0.4 ± 0.3	8.6 ± 3.1
Monoclonal monomers (n=12)	0.1 ± 0.3	7.1 ± 6.0

*Percentage of 2.5 µg ^{125}I-labelled SC bound/100 g IgA

dimeric IgA and pentameric IgM, it is not clear how this polypeptide is involved in the binding process. A direct interaction between SC and J chain is not likely since the purified dimeric polypeptide, obtained by mild reductive release without alkylation or denaturation, shows only marginal blocking of the binding of SC to the Ig polymers (Brandtzaeg, 1975b).

Weicker and Underdown (1975) initially reported that IgM pentamers and IgA dimers bind SC with similar affinity. Conversely, in our laboratory a much stronger non-covalent interaction was found between pentameric IgM and SC than between dimeric IgA and SC (Brandtzaeg, 1974c). Moreover, the apparent equilibrium constant of association (K_a) was estimated to be 2.7 - 12.5 times higher for IgM than for dimeric IgA, depending on the pair of protein preparations compared (Brandt- zaeg, 1977a). In a direct competitive SC-binding assay, which is not influenced by uncontrolled variables to the same extent as determinations of K_a, it was substantiated with the same test proteins that SC shows 5 - 30 times higher affinity for IgM than for dimeric IgA (Brandtzaeg, 1977a). Socken and Underdown (1978) subsequently confirmed these results to some extent by reporting that the binding constant of SC for IgM was 2 - 5 times higher than for dimeric IgA (Table 2). It should be noted that this difference was probably underestimated in their experiments because the measurements were performed after incubation for 1 h at room temperature (followed by 18 h at 4°C), which favours stabilisation of the SC-IgA complexes by disulphide bonding (Brandtzaeg, 1977a; Lindh and Björk, 1977). In our laboratory the separation of unassociated SC from the complexes was started as soon as possible (Brandtzaeg, 1977a).

The results of K_a determinations listed in Table 2 are in good agreement in both the human and rabbit test system when the possibilities for errors in such assays are taken into account. It is of interest to note that the relative affinity of SC for IgA and IgM is reversed in the two species. It is

TABLE 2

APPARENT ASSOCIATION CONSTANT (K_a) AND NUMBER OF SC-BINDING SITES (n) DETERMINED FROM SCATCHARD PLOTS OBTAINED BY BINDING ASSAYS WITH HUMAN AND RABBIT Ig PREPARATIONS

Ig-preparations	$K_a (M^{-1} \times 10^{-8})$	n	Authors
Human test system:			
polyclonal IgA dimers	0.16	0.73	Brandtzaeg (1977a)
monoclonal IgA dimers	0.10	0.64	
monoclonal IgM pentamers	0.86	0.61	
monoclonal IgA dimers	0.45	0.67	Socken and Underdown (1978)
monoclonal IgM pentamers	1.50	1.13	
Rabbit test system:			
polyclonal IgA dimers	0.47	0.34	
polyclonal IgM dimers	0.07	1.29	
polyclonal IgA dimers obtained from secretory IgA	1.21	0.70	Kühn and Kraehenbuhl (1979a)

possible that the evolution has resulted in a favourable SC-IgM
interaction in the human; this may have biological consequences
by enhancing the epithelial reception and transmission of IgM,
whose local synthesis normally is inferior to that of dimeric
IgA.

In the SC-binding studies on which the data on Table 2 are
based, it has been assumed (but not proven) that the Ig polymers
contain a homogeneous set of binding sites; the site number has
approximated one per dimeric IgA and pentameric IgM in both the
human and rabbit test system. It remains to be clarified if the
different properties of the SC-binding sites in the two types of
human polymers, as expressed by better affinity and stronger non-
covalent interactions with IgM (Brandtzaeg, 1977a), reflects a
'bonus' effect of a higher molar J-chain content. Recent
immunochemical quantitations (Brandtzaeg, 1975c; Grubb, 1978) have
challenged the concept that there is only one J chain per Ig
polymer regardless of its size (Koshland, 1975).

As shown in Table 2, three independent research groups
have now determined the affinity (K_a) of SC for Ig polymers
to be about $10^8 M^{-1}$, which is similar to values obtained for
a variety of antigen-antibody reactions. Nevertheless,
$10^8 M^{-1}$ is probably an underestimate when it comes to interactions with SC present in epithelial plasma membranes. Schiff
et al. (1980) recently reported that SC-binding experiments
in dilute solution, and kinetic measurements with anti-Ig
Sepharose to separate SC complexes, indicated a $K_a \geq 10^{10} M^{-1}$. In
experiments with binding of dimeric IgA to dispersed rabbit
mammary cells, Kühn and Kraehenbuhl (1979b) likewise found that
the association and dissociation rates were faster and K_a higher
($10^9 M^{-1}$) than that obtained with SC in solution ($10^8 M^{-1}$). These
studies suggested that membrane-bound SC is modified, probably
by a configurational change favouring its interaction with Ig
polymers.

Compared with disulphide exchange reactions *in vitro*
(Brandtzaeg, 1977a), the covalent stabilisation of SC-IgA

complexes taking place during glandular transport must be very
efficient. This process is probably enzymatically catalysed in
the secretory epithelial cells. A disulphide-exchange enzyme
obtained from rat liver microsomes has been found to promote
the binding of human SC to dimeric IgA and also to induce some
covalent stabilisation of SC-IgM complexes (Murkofsky and Lamm,
1979). The proneness for covalent stabilisation of SC-IgA
complexes probably contributes to the functional advantage on
secretory IgA compared with secretory IgM (Haneburg, 1974a,b);
but it is nevertheless the primary non-covalent interactions
with SC that reflect the potential receptor function of this
epithelial glycoprotein. The superior affinity of pentameric
IgM for SC may thus confer a secretory advantage on this Ig,
which may be of benefit in the newborn and in selectively IgA-
deficient subjects whose local IgM responses are prominent in
the intestinal mucosa (for review, see Brandtzaeg, 1981).

CHARACTERISTICS OF THE IMMUNOGLOBULIN PRODUCTS OF GLAND-
ASSOCIATED IMMUNOCYTES

All glandular sites investigated so far in man have
contained a striking preponderance of IgA-producing plasma
cells. We have calculated that almost 10^{10} such immunocytes
occur per metre of small bowel (Brandtzaeg and Baklien, 1976).
Absolute figures are difficult to obtain for other tissue sites
where the cells are much more heterogeneously distributed
throughout a glandular stroma than they are in the intestinal
lamina propria. However, it seems indisputable that the major
part of the gland-associated Ig-producing immunocyte population
is located in the gut. While IgM-producing cells constitute a
substantial proportion of the intestinal immunocytes, the
upper aero-digestive glands contain in addition a signigicant
complement of IgG- and IgD-producing cells (Brandtzaeg et al.,
1979). The reason for this discrepancy is unknown, but most
likely different antigenic and mitogenic stimulation by the
microbial flora in the intestinal and respiratory tracts may
influence the development of the regional gland-associated
immunocyte populations. The precursor populations of cells

homing to the various glandular sites may, moreover, differ to some extent for the two regions (for review, see Brandtzaeg, 1981).

The first direct evidence that IgA immunocytes in glandular sites produce mainly dimers was obtained by an SC-binding test performed on tissue sections (Brandtzaeg, 1973b). This finding was subsequently supported by our immunohistochemical localisation of J chain in the cytoplasm of 80 - 100% of IgA immunocytes in normal glandular sites (Brandtzaeg, 1974d; 1976b; Brandtzaeg et al., 1979; Korsrud and Brandtzaeg, 1980). These figures were obtained from tissue sections treated with acid urea (Brandtzaeg, 1976b). In the parotid gland, for example, such treatment raised the J-chain positivity of IgA cells from 54% to 93%, and the staining intensity was also increased (Korsrud and Brandtzaeg, 1980). The cytoplasmic J chains thus seemed to be partially concealed in most of the cells due to combination with IgA subunits.

This observation was confirmed at the ultrastructural level as we obtained enhancement of J-chain antigenicity in the endoplasmic reticulum of intestinal immunocytes after exposure to acid urea (Nagura et al., 1979a). Along with the previously noted diffuse cytoplasmic affinity for SC (Brandtzaeg, 1973b), these findings prove that a substantial completion of dimeric IgA normally takes place in the endoplasmic reticulum. Glandular IgM-producing cells likewise contain J chain and express cytoplasmic affinity for SC (Brandtzaeg, 1973b, 1974c; Brandtzaeg et al., 1979). Of additional interest is the fact that the non-covalent interactions between SC and cytoplasmic IgA dimers and IgM pentamers show the same relationship with regard to strength as that found when the SC-binding test is performed with the Ig polymers in solution (Brandtzaeg, 1974c).

Also about 40% of the IgG immunocytes and most IgD immunocytes in glandular sites produce J chains (Brandtzaeg, 1974c; Brandtzaeg et al., 1979; Korsrud and Brandtzaeg, 1980). However, J chains do not combine with IgG and are not secreted from the

IgG cells but become degraded intracellularly (Mosmann et al., 1978). Although not examined, the same probably holds true for J chains in IgD immunocytes. The biological significance of the striking J-chain production shown by glandular immunocytes is thus that IgA dimers and IgM pentamers with SC-binding sites are generated locally. After release from the immunocytes these Ig polymers are readily available for complexing with SC present in the plasma membranes of nearby secretory epithelial cells.

LOCALISATION OF SC AND IMMUNOGLOBULINS IN NORMAL AND NEOPLASTIC SECRETORY EPITHELIUM

Immunohistochemical observations

Many conflicting reports have appeared about the cellular origin of SC. Our studies have distinctly demonstrated SC in the intestinal columnar crypt cells, but we have been unable to find it associated with the mucinous content of goblet cells, regardless of the tissue-producing technique (Brandtzaeg, 1973a, 1974a). Only one of our apparently specific anti-SC reagents gave rise to goblet-cell staining, and absorption controls with purified SC showed that this conjugate lacked immunological specificity (Brandtzaeg, 1977b).

Our findings do not exclude that mucinous secretory cells have some capacity for SC synthesis. Occasional faint specific staining is indeed seen in mucinous acini of salivary and respiratory glands, especially related to the periphery of the cells (Brandtzaeg, 1977b). It has likewise been difficult to exclude at the ultrastructural level that small amounts of SC are present at the lateral borders of intestinal goblet cells (Brown et al., 1976). Moreover, Poger, Hirsch and Lamm (1976) reported that some well-differentiated villous colon carcinomas contained SC and mucin in the same cells. Also goblet cells of gastric epithelium with a moderate degree of intestinal metaplasia and signet-ring cells of gastric carcinomas have been reported to contain SC (Maeda, 1977).

The immunofluorescence staining patterns from our studies indicate that in respiratory glands there are high concentrations of SC both in the cytoplasm and in the plasma membrane of serous acini and duct cells; in salivary glands there is a faint cytoplasmic fluorescence and more distinct staining related to the cell borders; but in the intestinal epithelium the cytoplasm is more intensely fluorescent than the cell periphery. In the small bowel, SC is characteristically present in the columnar cells of the crypts of Lieberhühn, and decreases in concentration in the epithelium covering the villi, whereas in the large bowel it is generally present also in the columnar surface-lining cells (Brandtzaeg, 1974a,b, 1977b; Brandtzaeg and Baklien, 1977). Recent immunoelectron-microscopic studies have substantiated that not only do the intestinal columnar cells synthesise SC, as demonstrated by its localisation in the endoplasmic reticulum, but they do also clearly contain SC in the basolateral plasma membrane (Brown et al., 1976; Jos et al., 1979).

Immunohistochemical staining of mucosal and glandular tissue specimens fixed directly in cold ethanol have documented that IgG is, as expected, present in high concentrations diffusely in the connective tissue ground substance (Brandtzaeg, 1974a). Particularly bright staining is seen in basement membrane zones along epithelia and vessel walls. Glandular epithelium is virtually devoid of cytoplasmic IgG; but there may be an irregular faint fluorescence related to interstices, especially in the epithelium facing the gut lumen, indicating intercellular diffusion. In most normal mucosal specimens the lamina propria contains much less extracellular IgA than IgG, despite extensive local synthesis of the former (Brandtzaeg, 1974a). This is compatible with an efficient external transport of the locally produced dimeric IgA.

IgA can usually be revealed both in the cytoplasm and in relation to the basolateral borders of serous-type glandular epithelial cells. As described for SC, the latter staining feature is especially marked in respiratory and salivary glands. The epithelial distribution of IgM mimics that of IgA, but the staining is normally fainter and readily demonstrable only in the large bowel (Brandtzaeg, 1975a), as also noted by others in normal (Chen, 1971) and especially in IgA-deficient individuals with enhanced local synthesis of IgM (Heremans and Crabbé, 1967; Savilahti, 1973).

We have interpreted the fluorescence staining for IgA and IgM appearing at the lateral cell borders as related to the plasma membrane (Brandtzaeg, 1974a,b), and subsequent ultra-structural studies have confirmed such a localisation in intestinal columnar cells (Brown et al., 1976; Jos et al., 1979). Specific staining for IgD and IgE in glandular epithelia has never been seen in our laboratory (Brandtzaeg and Baklien, 1976a).

Although the epithelial distributions of SC and IgA in normal adults are very similar, the detailed patterns revealed by paired immunofluorescence staining are not completely congruent. A common feature is the fluorescence along the lateral borders of the cells as discussed above. Intracellularly, both SC and IgA are present in the apical portion of the cytoplasm, but SC alone is distinctly concentrated in a granular pattern corresponding to the Golgi zone (Munster, 1972; Brandtzaeg, 1973a, 1974a,b). Ultrastructural studies of rabbit mammary gland and human intestinal crypt cells have confirmed these immunofluorescence observations since SC but little or no IgA was found in the Golgi elements, whereas both components were present in more apically located vesicles (Kraehenbuhl et al., 1975; Brown et al., 1976).

Our immunohistochemical studies of neoplastic glandular cells have strongly supported the role of SC in the selective epithelial uptake of dimeric IgA and pentameric IgM. When the epithelial fluorescence for SC and IgA in 41 large bowel adenocarcinomas was scored on a semiquantitative scale, the results showed that the concentrations of both components were significantly related to the histological tumour grade (Rognum et al., 1980). Thus, the amounts of cytoplasmic SC and IgA were well correlated. We have also studied a case of infiltrative gastric carcinoma composed of signet-ring cells containing SC along with mucin and carcino-embryonic antigen (Brandtzaeg and Rognum, unpublished observations). In contrast to previous reports (Maeda, 1977; Ejeckam et al., 1979), both IgA and IgM along with J chain were clearly localised in the cytoplasm of the signet-ring cells, whereas most of them were completely devoid of IgG.

Studies of living cells

The first direct evidence that J-chain-containing dimeric IgA and pentameric IgM combine with SC on the surface of secretory epithelial cells came from studies of dispersed human colonic columnar cells (Brandtzaeg, 1978). A substantial fraction of the isolated cells contained free SC and secretory IgA in a cytoplasmic distribution that corresponded to the reported immunohistochemical and immunoelectron-microscopical results discussed above. On their surface the same cells were shown to bear SC complexed with J-chain-containing IgA, whereas only occasional traces of free SC were found. IgM was detected where the largest concentrations of IgA and SC occurred.

SC is thus normally exposed on the plasma membrane of columnar epithelial cells, and this fact strongly supports its proposed receptor function. The patchy appearance of the peripheral immunofluorescence staining observed, even for smeared cells that had not been treated with labelled antibody in the living state (Brandtzaeg, 1978), indicated that a redistribution of innate membrane SC takes place after complexing with the Ig polymers. This redistribution may reflect the initial step in the epithelial uptake of the polymers, since it is known that complexing in plasma membranes stimulates pinocytosis (Raff, 1976).

The above conclusions have been substantiated by studies carried out on an epithelial cell line (HT-29) established from a human colon carcinoma; in long term tissue culture most of these neoplastic cells express SC both in the cytoplasm and in the plasma membrane (Huang et al., 1976). J-chain-containing

polymeric IgA and IgM, but not monomeric IgA and IgG, will bind
to the surface of the cells (Crago et al., 1978). Moreover,
ultrastructural studies have shown that the bound dimeric IgA
becomes internalised by pinocytosis when the cells are incubated
at 37°C; the vesicles are subsequently transported through the
cytoplasm and are finally discharged across the apical surface
(Nagura et al., 1979b).

These observations have recently been extended in experiments with dispersed epithelial cells and plasma-membrane-
enriched fractions obtained from mammary glands of midpregnant
rabbits (Kühn and Kraehenbuhl, 1979b); it was found that
addition of ^{125}I-labelled dimeric IgA resulted in a saturable,
reversible time- and temperature-dependent binding process. The
binding capacity accorded with the density of free SC on the
plasma membranes, which were found to adsorb SC in amounts
inversely related to the degree of endogenous occupancy. Thus,
these authors postulated that the expression of SC on the
basolateral surface of the epithelial cells depends on the
combination of free SC with a specific membrane-receptor at
some stage in the secretion process or at the luminal surface.

CONCLUSIONS

The model proposed for selective epithelial Ig reception
and translocation (Figure 1) is compatible with the fluid
mosaic structure suggested for cell membranes (Singer and
Nicolson, 1972). Although our glandular transport model was
originally based mainly on test tube experiments with purified
proteins and on immunofluorescence studies of dead tissues, it
has recently gained strong support from observations made on
both normal and neoplastic living epithelial cells.

It should be pointed out, however, that despite the
attractive possibility that the J chain and the epithelial SC
represent 'the lock and key' in the selective external transport
of dimeric IgA and pentameric IgM, it has not been definitely
excluded that the epithelial cells express isotype-specific

receptors for IgA and IgM. Dimers of IgA could even in that case have a significant transport advantage over monomers owing to the double number of binding sites. Moreover, as mentioned in the Introduction, pure glandular secretions contain relatively high concentrations of monomeric IgA compared with IgG.

The possibility thus remains that complexing of dimeric IgA and pentameric IgM with SC is an epiphenomenon serving to stabilise the secretory immunoglobulins. On the other hand, it may be argued that the presence of monomeric IgA in external fluids is due to a combination of passive diffusion and degradation. Intercellular diffusion through epithelia probably includes monomeric IgA derived both from serum and from the abundant local IgA-producing immunocytes, which most likely release monomers in addition to dimers (Bull et al., 1971). Dimeric IgA is relatively unstable before covalent conjugation with SC, and may in part be converted to monomers by intraepithelia and intraluminal degradation. Some breakdown of secretory IgA is also likely, and may explain why a fraction of the monomeric IgA present in colostrum apparently is associated with SC (Mestecky et al., 1970).

Altogether, therefore, it seems justified to suggest that a 'first line' of specific defence in mucosal immunity is based on SC-mediated external translocation of dimeric IgA and pentameric IgM antibodies (Figure 2). During this transport process secretory IgA becomes highly stabilised by disulphide bonding to SC, whereas most secretory IgM depends on an excess of free SC to retain its non-covalently linked SC. A state of equilibrium probably exists between free SC and IgM-associated SC in the exocrine fluids, as indicated by the small white arrows in Figure 2. However, since the I determinant of free SC - which apparently is involved in the binding process - shows striking susceptibility to proteolytic enzymes (Brandtzaeg, 1975d), the external milieu must be quite deleterious for the SC-IgM complexes (Richman and Brown, 1977). Secretory IgM, therefore, seems to be of minor functional significance in the intestinal fluids (Haneburg, 1974a,b) except in selective IgA deficiency (Haneburg and Aarskog, 1975) and in infancy (for review, see Brandtzaeg, 1981).

The above emphasis on secretory IgA and secretory IgM should not detract from the fact that mucosal immunity in addition depends on innate immune mechanisms both for surface protection and for the defence of the internal tissue milieu. When antigen exclusion is insufficient due to a poor 'first line' of defence or a break in the epithelial barrier, a 'second line' of defence that mainly includes local production and exudation of IgG is initiated as part of an inflammatory response (Figure 2). Although this development teleologically constitutes 'pathotopic potentiation' of mucosal immunity, it may have deleterious consequences as discussed elsewhere (Brandtzaeg and Baklien, 1976b).

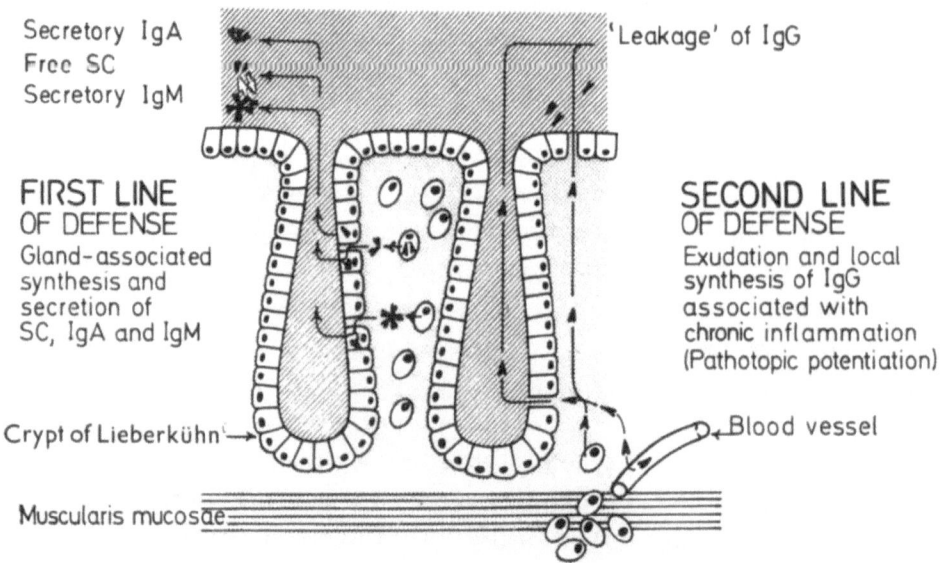

Fig. 2. Schematic representation of two types of humoral immune response
in the human large bowel mucosa. A 'first line' of specific mucosal
defence is afforded by secretory IgA and secretory IgM antibodies.
While the conjugation of dimeric IgA with SC gives rise to about
80% disulphide-bonded complexes, most of the SC-IgM complexes are
merely non-covalently stabilised and a complete association depends
on an excess of free SC in the secretion (state of equilibrium
indicated by small white arrows). The 'second line' of defence
is represented by 'pathotopic potentiation' of mucosal immunity
associated with chronic inflammation. In this process complement-
fixing IgG antibodies are supplied to the local site by exudation
from serum and by local synthesis in immunocytes whose precursors
probably are derived at random from the recirculating lymphocyte
pool and perhaps from local lymphoid follicles. Although IgG-
antibodies may reach the lumen by passive 'leakage' between
epithelial cells, their main biological effect is probably
localised to the internal tissue milieu, with both beneficial and
deleterious consequences.

REFERENCES

Bourne, F.J., 1974. Structural features of pig IgA. Immunol. Commun. <u>3</u>, 157

Brandtzaeg, P., 1968. Glandular secretion of immunoglobulins. Acta pathol. microbiol. scand. <u>74</u>, 624.

Brandtzaeg, P., 1971a. Human secretory immunoglobulins. II. Salivary secretions from individuals with selectively excessive or defective synthesis of serum immunoglobulins. Clin. exp. Immunol. <u>8</u>, 69.

Brandtzaeg, P., 1971b. Human secretory immunoglobulins. III. Immunochemical and physicochemical studies of secretory IgA and free secretory piece. Acta path. microbiol. scand. Section B <u>79</u>, 165.

Brandtzaeg, P., 1971c. Human secretory immunoglobulins. VII. Concentrations of parotid IgA and other secretory proteins in relation to the rate of flow and duration of secretory stimulus. Arch. oral Biol. <u>16</u>, 1295.

Brandtzaeg, P., 1973a. Structure, synthesis and external transfer of mucosal immunoglobulins. Ann. Immunol. (Inst. Pasteur). <u>124C</u>, 417.

Brandtzaeg, P., 1973b. Two types of IgA immunocytes in man. Nature New Biol. (Lond.) <u>243</u>, 142.

Brandtzaeg, P., 1974a. Mucosal and glandular distribution of immunoglobulin components. Immunohistochemistry with a cold ethanol fixation technique. Immunology. <u>26</u>, 1101.

Brandtzaeg, P., 1974b. Mucosal and glandular distribution of immunoglobulin components. Differential localisation of free and bound SC in secretory epithelial cells. J. Immunol. <u>112</u>, 1553.

Brandtzaeg, P., 1974c. Characteristics of SC-Ig complexes formed *in vitro*, In: The Immunoglobulin A System (ed. by J. Mestecky and A.R. Lawton) (Adv. exp. Med. Biol. <u>45</u>), pp. 87-97, Plenum Press, New York.

Brandtzaeg, P., 1974d. Presence of J chain in human immunocytes containing various immunoglobulin classes. Nature (Lond.) <u>252</u>, 418.

Brandtzaeg, P., 1975a. Human secretory immunoglobulin M. An immunochemical and immunohistochemical study. Immunology <u>29</u>, 559.

Brandtzaeg, P., 1975b. Blocking effect of J chain and J-chain antibody on the binding of secretory component to human IgA and IgM. Scand. J. Immunol. <u>4</u>, 837.

Brandtzaeg, P., 1975c. Immunochemical studies on free and bound J chain of human IgA and IgM. Scand. J. Immunol. <u>4</u>, 439.

Brandtzaeg, P., 1975d. Human secretory component. IV. Aggregation and fragmentation of free secretory component. Immunochemistry <u>12</u>, 877.

Brandtzaeg, P., 1976a. Complex formation between secretory component and
    human immunoglobulins related to their content of J chain. Scand. J.
    Immunol. 5, 411.

Brandtzaeg, P., 1976b. Studies on J chain and binding site for secretory
    component in circulating human B cells. II. The cytoplasm. Clin.
    exp. Immunol. 25, 59.

Brandtzaeg, P., 1977a. Human secretory component. VI. Immunoglobulin-
    binding properties. Immunochemistry. 14, 178.

Brandtzaeg, P., 1977b. Immunohistochemical studies on various aspects of
    glandular immunoglobulin transport in man. Histochem. J. 9, 553.

Brandtzaeg, P., 1978. Polymeric IgA is complexed with secretory component
    (SC) on the surface of human intestinal epithelial cells. Scand. J.
    Immunol. 8, 39.

Brandtzaeg, P., 1981. Development of systemic and local gut immune responses.
    In: International Conference on Infant Nutrition and Diarrhoeal Disease
    (ed. by N. Iyngkaran) in press, Kuala Lumpur.

Brandtzaeg, P. and Baklien, K., 1976a. Inconclusive immunohistochemistry of
    human IgE in mucosal pathology. Lancet. 1, 1297.

Brandtzaeg, P. and Baklien, K., 1976b. Immunohistochemical studies of the
    formation and epithelial transport of immunoglobulins in normal and
    diseased human intestinal mucosa. Scand. J. Gastroenterol. 11, Suppl.
    36, pp. 1-45.

Brandtzaeg, P. and Baklien, K., 1977. Intestinal secretion of IgA and IgM:
    a hypothetical model. In: Immunology of the Gut, Ciba Found. Symp.
    46, pp. 77-108. Elsevier/Excerpta Medica/North-Holland, Amsterdam.

Brandtzaeg, P., Fjellanger, I. and Gjeruldsen, S.T., 1968. Immunoglobulin
    M: local synthesis and selective secretion in patients with
    immunoglobulin A deficiency. Science (Wash. DC). 160, 789.

Brandtzaeg, P., Fjellanger, I. and Gjeruldsen, S.T., 1970. Human secretory
    immunoglobulins. I. Salivary secretions from individuals with normal
    or low levels of serum immunoglobulins. Scand. J. Haematol. Suppl.
    12, pp. 1-83.

Brandtzaeg, P., Gjeruldsen, S.T., Korsrud, F., Baklien, K., Berdal, P. and
    Ek, J., 1979. The human secretory immune system shows striking
    heterogeneity with regard to involvement of J-chain-positive IgD
    immunocytes. J. Immunol. 122, 503.

Brown, W.R., Isobe, Y. and Nakane, P.K., 1976. Studies on translocation of
    immunoglobulins across intestinal epithelium. II. Immuncelectron-

microscopic localisation of immunoglobulins and secretory component
in human intestinal mucosa. Gastroenterology. 71, 985.

Bull, D.M., Bienenstock, J. and Tomasi, T.B., 1971. Studies on human
intestinal immunoglobulin A. Gastroenterology. 60, 370.

Chen, S.-T., 1971. Cellular sites of immunoglobulins. II. The relative
proportions of mucosal cells containing IgG, IgA and IgM, and light
polypeptide chains of kappa and lamda immunoglobulin in human
appendices. Acta Pathol. Jap. 21, 67.

Crago, S.S., Kuhhavy, R., Prince, S.J. and Mestecky, J., 1978. Secretory
component on epithelial cells is a surface receptor for polymeric
immunoglobulins. J. exp. Med. 147, 1832.

Ejeckam, G.C., Huang, S.N., McCaughey, W.T.E. and Gold, P., 1979. Immuno-
histopathologic study on carcinoembryonic antigen (CEA)-like
material and immunoglobulin A in gastric malignancies. Cancer. 44,
1606.

Eskeland, T. and Brandtzaeg, P., 1974. Does J chain mediate the combination
of 19S IgM and dimeric IgA with the secretory component rather than
being necessary for their polymerisation? Immunochemistry. 11, 161.

Grubb, A.O., 1978. Quantitation of J chain in human biological fluids
by a simple immunochemical procedure. Acta med. scand. 204, 453.

Haneburg, B., 1974a. Human faecal agglutinins to rabbit erythrocytes
Scand. J. Immunol. 3, 71.

Haneburg, B., 1974b. Immunoglobulins in faeces from infants fed human or
bovine milk. Scand. J. Immunol. 3, 191.

Haneburg, B. and Aarskog, D., 1975. Human faecal immunoglobulins in
healthy infants and children, and in some with diseases affecting the
intestinal tract or the immune system. Clin. exp. Immunol. 22, 210.

Hanson, L.Å. and Brandtzaeg, P., 1980. The mucosal defense system. In:
Immunological disorders in Infants and Children, Ed. 2 (ed. by
R.E. Stiehm and V.A. Fulginiti) pp. 137-164. W.B. Saunders Co.,
London.

Heremans, J.F. and Crabbé, P.A., 1967. Immunohistochemical studies on
exocrine IgA. In: Gammaglobulins (ed. by J. Killander) pp. 129-139.
Almqvist and Wiksell, Uppsala.

Huang, S.W., Fogh, J. and Hong, R., 1976. Synthesis of secretory component
by colon cancer cells. Scand. J. Immunol. 5, 263.

Jerry, L.M., Kunkel, H.G. and Adams, L., 1972. Stabilisation of dis-sociable
IgA$_2$ proteins by secretory component. J. Immunol. 109, 275.

Jos, J., Labbe, F., Geny, B. and Griscelli, C., 1979. Immunoelectron-
microscopic localisation of immunoglobulin A and secretory component
in jejunal mucosa from children with coeliac disease. Scand. J.
Immunol. 9, 441.

Kemler, R., Mossman, H., Strohmaier, K., Kickhöfen, B. and Hammer, D.K.,
1975. *In vitro* studies on the selective binding of IgG from
different species to tissue sections of the bovine mammary gland.
Eur. J. Immunol. 5, 603.

Knight, K.L., Vetter, M.L. and Malek, T.R., 1975. Distribution of covalently
bound and non-covalently bound secretory component on subclasses of
rabbit secretory IgA. J. Immunol. 115, 595.

Korsrud, F.R. and Brandtzaeg, P., 1980. Quantitative immunohistochemistry
of immunoglobulin- and J-chain-producing cells in human parotid and
submandibular glands. Immunology. 39, 129.

Koshland, M.E., 1975. Structure and function of the J chain. Adv. Immunol.
20, 41.

Kraehenbuhl, J.P. and Kühn, L., 1978. Transport of immunoglobulins across
epithelia. In: Transport of Macromolecules in Cellular Systems (ed.
by S.C. Silverstein) pp. 213-228. Life Science Research Report 11.

Kraehenbuhl, J.P., Racine, L. and Galardy, R.E., 1975. Localisation of
secretory IgA, secretory component, and α heavy chain in the mammary
gland of lactating rabbits by immunoelectron microscopy. Ann. N.Y.
Acad. Sci. 254, 190.

Kühn, L. and Kraehenbuhl, J.P., 1979a. Interaction of rabbit secretory
component with rabbit IgA dimer. J. biol. Chem. 254, 11066.

Kühn, L.C. and Kraehenbuhl, J.P., 1979b. Role of secretory component, a
secreted glycoprotein, in the specific uptake of IgA dimer by
epithelial cells. J. biol. Chem. 254, 11072.

Lamm, M.E., 1976. Cellular aspects of immunoglobulin A. Adv. Immunol. 22,
223.

Lindh, E., 1974. Increased resistance of immunoglobulin A dimers to
proteolytic degradation after binding of secretory component. J.
Immunol. 114, 284.

Lindh, E. and Björk, I., 1976a. Binding of secretory component to human
immunoglobulin M. Europ. J. Biochem. 62, 271.

Lindh, E. and Björk, I., 1976b. Binding of secretory component to dimers
of immunoglobulin A *in vitro*. Mechanism of the covalent bond formation.
Eur. J. Biochem. 62, 263.

Lindh, E. and Björk, I., 1977. Relative rates of the non-covalent and covalent binding of secretory component to an IgA dimer. Acta path. mirobiol. scand. Sect. C. 85, 449.

Mach, J.P., 1970. *In vitro* combination of human and bovine free secretory component with IgA of various species. Nature (Lond.) 228, 1278.

Maeda, S., 1977. Studies of immunoglobulins in gastric juice and gastric mucosa. IV. Studies on secretory component in gastric mucosa. Sappora med. J. 46, 409.

Mestecky, J., Kraus, F.W. and Voight, S.A., 1970. Proportion of human colostral immunoglobulin A molecules containing the secretory determinant. Immunology. 18, 237.

Mosmann, T.R., Gravel, Y., Williamson, A.R. and Baumal, R., 1978. Modification and fate of J chain in myeloma cells in the presence and absence of immunoglobulin secretion. Eur. J. Immunol. 8, 94.

Munster, P.J.J. van, 1972. De secretoire component. Een immunochemisch onderzoek. Isolatie, eigenschappen, uitscheiding in secreta en localisatie in jejunumbiopten. (The secretory component. An immunochemical investigation. Isolation, properties, excretion in secretions and localisation in jejunal biopsy samples.) Thesis, University of Nijmegen.

Murkofsky, N.A. and Lamm, M.E., 1979. Effect of a disulfide-exchange enzyme on the assembly of human secretory immunoglobulin A from immunoglobulin A and free secretory component. J. biol. Chem. 254, 12181.

Nagura, H., Brandtzaeg, P., Nakane, P.K. and Brown, N.R., 1979a. Ultrastructural localisation of J chain in human intestinal mucosa. J. Immunol. 123, 1044.

Nagura, H., Nakane, P.K. and Brown, W.R., 1979b. Translocation of dimeric IgA through neoplastic colon cells *in vitro*. J. Immunol. 123, 2359.

Nakajima, S., Gillespie, D.N. and Gleich, G.J., 1975. Differences between IgA and IgE as secretory proteins. Clin. exp. Immunol, 21, 306.

Newcomb, R.W. and Ishizaka, K., 1970. Physiocochemical and antigenic studies on human E in respiratory fluid. J. Immunol. 105, 85.

Newmark, P., 1979. Pathways to secretion. Nature (London). 281, 629.

O'Daly, J.A., Craig, S.W. and Cebra, J.J., 1971. Localisation of b markers, α-chain and SC of sIgA in epithelial cells lining Lieberkühn crypts. J. Immunol. 166, 286.

Poger, M.E., Hirsch, B.R. and Lamm, M.E., 1976. Synthesis of secretory component by colonic neoplasms. Am. J. Path. 82, 327.

98

Poger, M.E. and Lamm, M.E., 1974. Localization of free and bound secretory component in human intestinal epithelial cells. A model for the assembly of secretory IgA. E. exp. Med. <u>139</u>, 629.

Radl, J., Klein, F., van der Berg, P., de Bruyn, A.M. and Hijmans, W., 1971. Binding of secretory piece to polymeric IgA and IgM paraproteins *in vitro*. Immunology. <u>20</u>, 843.

Raff, M.C., 1976. Cell-surface immunology. Scient. Am. <u>234</u>, 30.

Richman, L.K. and Brown, W.R., 1977. Immunochemistry characterization of IgM in intestinal fluids. J. Immunol. <u>119</u>, 1515.

Rodewald, R., 1976. Intestinal transport of peroxidase-conjugated IgG fragments in the neonatal rat. In: Maternofoetal Transmission of Immunoglobulins. (ed. by W.A. Hemmings) p. 137-153, Cambridge University Press, London.

Rognum, T., Brandtzaeg, P., Ørjasaeter, H., Elgjo, K. and Hognestad, J., 1980. Immunohistochemical study of secretory component, secretory IgA and carcinoembryonic antigen in large bowel carcinomas. Pathol. Res. Pract. (in press).

Savilahti, E., 1973. IgA deficiency in children. Immunoglobulin-containing cells in the intestinal mucosa, immunoglobulins in secretions and serum IgA levels. Clin. exp. Immunol. <u>13</u>, 395.

Schiff, J.M., Dorrington, K.J. and Underdown, B.J., 1980. Secretory component and immunoglobulin transport. Abstract No. 7.5.29 presented at 4th International Congress of Immunology, Paris.

Singer, S.J. and Nicolson, G.L., 1972. The fluid mosaic model of the structure of cell membranes. Science (Wash DC) <u>175</u>, 720.

Socken, D.J. and Underdown, B.J., 1978. Comparison of human, bovine and rabbit secretory component-immunoglobulin interactions. Immunohisto-chemistry. <u>15</u>, 499.

South, M.A., Cooper, M.D., Wollheim, F.A., Hong, R. and Good, R.A., 1966. The IgA system. I. Studies of the transport and immunochemistry of IgA in the saliva. J. exp. Med. <u>123</u>, 615.

Tomasi, T.B. and Czerwinski, D.S., 1976. Naturally occurring polymers of IgA lacking J chain. Scand. J. Immunol. <u>5</u>, 647.

Tomasi, T.B., Tan, E.M., Solomon, A. and Prendergast, R.A., 1965. Characteristics of an immune system common to certain external secretions. J. exp. Med. <u>121</u>, 101.

Weicker, J. and Underdown, B.J., 1975. A study on the association of human secretory component with IgA and IgM proteins. J. Immunol. <u>114</u>, 1337.

DISCUSSION

W. Leibold *(FRG)*

How do you exclude that some of the SC molecules which are taken up by dimeric IgA are not passing outside of the cell into the lumen? You don't see it; you wash it away. You have evidence that it is in the cells but how do you exclude that there are also a considerable number of these molecules just passing in between the cells and onto the lumen?

P. Brandtzaeg *(Norway)*

I can't exclude it but you know that you have tight junctions. I think there is some leakage, I wouldn't question that but we don't really know whether it can slip off the membrane when it is stuck there. We don't have any experiments indicating that it can get off the membrane. Experiments have been done in neoplastic living cells in Brown's laboratory and Mestecky's laboratory in the United States, recently. They have one neoplastic cell line producing SC where SC is exposed as I have described and where you get binding of pentameric IgM and dimeric IgA to the cell membrane. Brown has followed the sequence of events after this complexing and he shows that there is a very rapid initiation of pinocytotic vesicles in the membrane. He has followed the complexes all the way through; these cells retain polarity on culture. But I don't think he has ever tried to measure bio-radioactivity, whether he can wash away IgA off the binding. That would be the first way of testing the hypothesis - to see if you can wash away something which is stuck. I don't know about that but we have an indication from immunohistochemical staining that in the respiratory tract there is not so much staining in the cytoplasm but rather a concentration along the plasma membrane. Perhaps it may slide in the plasma membrane - I would accept that as a fairly good idea - then passes the tight junction and is shed off. Of course, this is a floating structure, it is not static, it is an ocean where things can float along the membrane. I would think the patches we see on the living cells are induced by the complexing - it is a secondary thing, starting a capping.

F.J. Bourne *(UK)*

Would you propose a similar model for the mammary gland?

P. Brandtzaeg

I think so yes, although it would probably be a little different.

F.J. Bourne

The reason I raised the point is that in the pig the majority of IgA in the secretion is of the 9S dimer type. It will bind secretory component but it appears as a 9S non-secretory molecule.

P. Brandtzaeg

That is after isolation.

F.J. Bourne

Both on isolation and by quantitation.

P. Brandtzaeg

But to show that it is without secretory component you have to isolate it, don't you?

F.J. Bourne

That's right, but we have also quantitated it on the basis of quantitating total IgA.

P. Brandtzaeg

You separate it from free SC in the quantitation?

F.J. Bourne

That's right, and then use an anti SC to quantitate secretory IgA.

P. Brandtzaeg

The problem is the same with human IgM. When you isolate it, only about 50% of it retains its secretory component. The human situation is unique for IgA in the fact that you have such possibilities for disulphide exchange reactions, which you don't seem to have in IgM also you don't have it in rabbit IgA and probably perhaps not in your system. The non-covalent binding of SC to pentameric IgM depends on an excess of free SC because this is an equilibrium situation. In the secretions you will always have an excess of free SC, so it sticks all the time, but when you try to isolate it it falls off.

K. Petzoldt (FRG)

In relation to John Bourne's question, in bovine colostrum, there is evidence of a special receptor to IgG sub-class.

P. Brandtzaeg

Yes, this is one of the things which worries me. You know there is a receptor in mammary gland cells for IgG1 in the bovine species, and also on the gut epithelial cells the enterocytes in the gut taking IgG1 back to the blood in some animals, and you never find the receptors. The receptor has not been isolated; it does not stick to the transported protein.

K. Petzoldt

In addition to this, is there any evidence that the generation of SC on the surface is controlled by any regulation mechanism such as hormones?

P. Brandtzaeg

Well, there is evidence with regard to mammary glands that the transport of IgA is hormone dependent. But the whole epithelial situation in the gland is, of course, hormone dependent so whether SC is regulated directly by hormones or just follows the whole epithelial development, I can't tell you.

J.P. Vaerman *(Belgium)*

I believe the situation is even more complicated in the rabbit because it has been shown that there are allotype differences.

P. Brandtzaeg

Yes it is the sub type G which does not bind covalently with secretory component - so that is similar to IgM. I remember that Lamb used this argument against SC as a receptor, that it combines covalently with the transported protein. But that is not a valid argument because this is the unique feature of dimeric IgA, that it has this possibility for disulphide exchange reactions with SC. It is not a general phenomenon.

J.P. Vaerman

Is secretory IgA covalently bound?

F.J. Bourne

Well, a proportion of it is non-covalently bound, this was our finding.

P. Brandtzaeg

It must be, since you can isolate it. You mentioned about 50% in your paper that did not retain SC after isolation.

K.L. Morgan *(UK)*

I was pleased to hear about the receptors on the surface of mammary epithelial cells and also on hepatocytes because it helps me to explain the situation that seems to occur in the young pig. In the young pig at three days of age it appears that there is no 11 S IgA in the serum in spite of the fact that it occurs in the colostrum. This led to the logical conclusion that it wasn't absorbed, that it remained on the epithelial surface and was in some way protected there. If you look earlier than three days, you find that 11 S IgA is in the serum but it has a very short half life which leads to the suggestion that

it is resecreted onto epithelial surfaces. Having secretory
component, this would be particularly difficult to explain in
a model system like this. This was pursued in two ways: first,
we demonstrated that in young piglets where there were no plasma
cells, you could show IgA histologically in the apical glandular
cells; secondly, we fed young piglets human milk 11 S IgA which
was absorbed and the profile in the serum was the same as that
in milk. Then we took respiratory tract secretions from these
piglets at two hourly intervals after suckling. The 11 S IgA
appeared in the secretions of these animals which, once again,
was very difficult to explain although it may be that the
answer is that there is an epithelial surface receptor for
secretory component which is transporting the molecule outwards.

P. Brandtzaeg

I don't doubt that they show the receptor but I don't know
if this can be generalised for other tissues than the mammary
glands.

B. Morein *(Sweden)*

All these proteins must be transported with some sort of
membrane protein from the internal membranes to the outer membrane, to the plasma membrane anyway. So I suppose the
secretory component must have a hydrophobic end to be transported
or it must be tied to another protein before coming to the
surface.

P. Brandtzaeg

I always thought of it as an integral membrane protein.

B. Morein

That is what I wondered; if it is then you could easily
find if it is integrated a real membrane protein, when it is
on the surface.

P. Brandtzaeg

Probably I can't but a biochemist should be able to.

B. Morein

Do you know if it has been done?

P. Brandtzaeg

No, it has not been done, but it is an obvious thing to do.

There is another intriguing thing which is how does it get from the plasma cell to the epithelial cell? In patients with a deficiency in the immune system, you can have a little cluster of three or four plasma cells. You see in the crypt epithelium that only the crypt cells facing those plasma cells take up the IgA. There are people working hard on connective tissue ground substance and claiming that there is always directional fusion in the ground substance, there are rivulets directing the diffusion. So perhaps in the future, someone may show rivulets going from the plasma cells to the epithelial cells, directing the diffusion - you never know.

W. Leibold (FRG)

Since you have the possibility to measure the binding of secretory component to IgA, have you compared monomeric immune complex IgA in their binding affinity to the dimeric non-complex ones?

P. Brandtzaeg

I'm sorry I have not done those experiments, but it would be a good thing to do. That might be a crucial experiment to exclude the possibility of isotype specific receptors.

F.J. Bourne

Well, far from exnausting the subject, I think we have exhausted ourselves. Thank you Dr. Brandtzaeg, and thank you all.

SESSION II

HYPERSENSITIVITY REACTIONS IN THE GUT

Chairmen : J. Soothill and Anne Ferguson

INDUCTION AND EXPRESSION OF MUCOSAL
CELL MEDIATED IMMUNITY

A.M. Mowat and Anne Ferguson

The Gastro-Intestinal Unit, Western General Hospital
and University of Edinburgh, Edinburgh, UK.

ABSTRACT

Direct identification and measurement of cell mediated immune (CMI) reactions in the intestinal mucosa are difficult, perhaps impossible. Our previous studies on the effector limb of mucosal CMI have identified an increase in the rate of epithelial cell mitosis (crypt cell production rate, CCPR) and intraepithelial lymphocyte (IEL) count as sensitive markers of local CMI. We have proposed that enteropathic lymphokines are responsible for the mucosal changes observed.

By analogy with induction of systemic CMI, elucidation of the induction phase of mucosal CMI will require information on antigen handling in the mucosa, and on factors which control the triggering and subsequent migration of effector T cells. Feeding of a protein antigen results in reduced humoral and CMI responses when that antigen is subsequently presented, and also causes activation of suppressor cells in the gut associated lymphoid tissues (GALT). This oral tolerance may be reversed by pretreating animals with cyclophosphamide, probably as a result of suppressor cell inhibition. Factors which influence antigen processing by the GALT may also modify the response to oral antigen.

Our work on the effects on the intestinal mucosa of a graft-versus-host reaction (GvHR) suggests that T cell activation occurs in Peyer's patches, with migration of these cells to the mucosa and subsequent intestinal damage. This reaction is influenced by many external factors and it is apparent that CMI response to oral or gut associated antigen is controlled by a complex interaction of immune and non-immune events.

INTRODUCTION

Investigations of mucosal T cells, and of cell mediated immune reactions in the gut, have proceeded more slowly than the studies of secretory antibodies. We have directed our attention to the induction of cell mediated immunity to fed antigen, and to the effects on the intestinal mucosa of local cell mediated immune reactions. In this paper we briefly review recent information on the nature of mucosal T cells and their traffic, present results of some recent experiments, and outline a hypothesis as to the several roles which mucosal T cells may play in gastrointestinal physiology and pathology.

T LYMPHOCYTES IN THE INTESTINE

There are T lymphocytes in the organised gut-associated lymphoid tissues, such as Peyer's patches and mesenteric lymph nodes, and many T cells are scattered within the mucosae of the gastrointestinal tract.

Peyer's patch lymphocytes

The majority of Peyer's patch T cells are present in the thymus dependent areas under the epithelium and around the post-capillary venules. Studies of lymphocyte traffic, which involved tracing of isotope labelled lymphocytes by autoradiography and liquid scintillation counting, showed that there was a traffic of small T lymphocytes from blood to the thymus dependent areas of Peyer's patches, but that small T lymphocytes did not enter the mucosae (Parrott and Ferguson, 1974). It is still not known whether or not there are two distinct pools of recirculating T lymphocytes, intestinal and peripheral. Cahill et al. (1977), working in sheep, reported that small lymphocytes derived from the gut preferentially recirculated to the gut lymphoid organs, but this work has been criticised because no account was taken of the contribution of lymphoblasts in their cell preparations, and de Freitas et al. (1977) could not confirm this phenomenon in mice.

Although, as well illustrated in other papers in this
Symposium, and by our experiments described below, separate
gut-associated immune reactions may occur independently of
systemic immune reactions, the cellular basis of this may be
the separate traffic of intestinal and peripheral activated
T lymphoblasts, rather than of small T cells.

Mucosal T cells

Lymphocytes, mainly medium sized, are found within the
epithelium (intraepithelial, IE lymphocytes) as well as in the
lamina propria of the gut (LP lymphocytes). Although the
small intestinal mucosa has been most extensively studied,
similar IE and LP lymphocytes are present, although in smaller
numbers, in gastric and colonic mucosae. The first evidence
that many of these mucosal lymphocytes are thymus dependent
came from the findings of low IE lymphocyte counts in animals
depleted of T cells in various ways (Fichtelius et al., 1968;
Ferguson and Parrott, 1972). Recent work, in rodents and in
man, using antisera directed against T cell antigenic determinants, has confirmed that most IE lymphocytes are T cells
(Guy Grand et al., 1974; Meuwissen et al., 1976; Selby et al.,
1980). Selby and his colleagues further report that by using
an antiserum directed against the T suppressor/cytotoxic sub-
group (antiserum OK T8, supplied by Dr Goldstein, Ortho
Laboratories, New York) some 80% of IE T lymphocytes have been
found to be of this suppressor group, whereas only 30 - 40% of
LP lymphocytes were of the suppressor phenotype.

Studies of lymphocyte traffic have shown that, just as
is the case for B cells, T immunoblasts derived from lymph or
from mesenteric lymph nodes home to the gut mucosa where most
can later be identified as intraepithelial cells (Guy Grand
et al., 1974; Rose et al., 1976a; McWilliams et al., 1975).
Further, elegant experiments involving local irradiation of
Peyer's patches or mesenteric lymph nodes, have confirmed that
the route of T cell traffic is from Peyer's patches via
mesenteric lymph node and lymph back to the intraepithelial
site in the small intestinal mucosa (Guy Grand et al., 1978).

An important additional source of T cells in the gut has been demonstrated by Rose et al., 1976b in their studies of T immunoblast migration. They found that in normal animals mesenteric T immunoblasts migrated back to the intestine, and peripheral T immunoblasts migrated to inflamed peripheral tissues. However peripheral T immunoblasts were also found to home to the gut, but only if it was the site of inflammation, for example as a result of infection with a nematode. In inflammatory intestinal disease, many components of the systemic immune apparatus, such as serum proteins, may gain access to mucosal tissue. Rose and her colleagues have now shown that, in addition to producing changes in the number and the activation of gut associated T and B immunoblasts, local disease may result in the recruitment of systemic T cells into the gut.

ANIMAL MODELS OF INTESTINAL MUCOSAL CMI

The small intestinal mucosa is a continuously changing organ, and in addition to the considerable amounts of fluid which cross the epithelium in both directions, the epithelial and connective tissue cells are regularly renewed by cell division in the crypts, and exfoliation from the surface. Since CMI reactions take a day or more to evolve, it could be argued that conditions will rarely be appropriate for a CMI reaction to occur in this organ. However, we and others have success-fully produced mucosal CMI reactions in a number of experimental situations, including graft-versus-host disease, rejection of transplanted allografts of intestine, parasite infections (comparing normal and T cell depleted hosts) and, recently, mucosal challenge with antigen in animals immunised orally or systemically.

The primary objective of our series of experiments in animals has been to establish the features of intestinal pathology and/or changes in function which mark the presence of a local CMI reaction, and which can allow measurement of the magnitude of a CMI reaction in experimental conditions and in man.

Effects of allograft rejection on small intestinal mucosa

The models which we have studied most thoroughly have
been rejection of heterotransplanted grafts of foetal intestine
in mice, and graft-versus-host disease in adult and neonatal
Fl mice. Experiments with mice which have been thymectomised,
irradiated and bone marrow reconstituted (Ferguson and Parrott,
1973) and studies of the humoral immune response to allografts
of foetal small intestine (Elves and Ferguson, 1975) confirmed
that the tissue damage in allograft rejection was thymus-
dependent and cell mediated. The effects of allograft
rejection was thymus-dependent and cell mediated. The effects
of allograft rejection on the small intestinal mucosa have
been studied by conventional histopathology with subjective
grading of the abnormality, by morphometry of paraffin sections
and counts of intraepithelial lymphocytes. We have also used
a stathmokinetic technique to measure crypt cell production
rate and scanning and transmission electron microscopy to
study epithelial changes (Ferguson and Parrott, 1973;
MacDonald and Ferguson, 1976, 1977; Ferguson et al., 1978).

The sequence of events observed in small intestinal
allograft rejection were infiltration of the lamina propria by
lymphocytes, which were also found within the epithelium;
greatly increased mitotic activity in the epithelial cells of
the crypts of Lieberkuhn with, later, flattening of the villi,
exfoliation of surface enterocytes and finally ulceration and
destruction of the mucosa. The pathology of allograft
rejection was very similar to that of the jejunal mucosa in
coeliac disease, and in helminth parasite infections of man
and animals.

By using various strain combinations, and neonatal and
adult hosts, a spectrum of intestinal pathology (as assessed
subjectively) has been demonstrated, ranging from apparently
completely normal histology, to subtotal villous atrophy with
crypt hyperplasia (Table 1). However studies of the
cytokinetics of the absorptive epithelium (the technique used

involves injection of colchicine to block mitosis in metaphase, microdissection and measurements of villi and crypts and counts of crypt metaphase (MacDonald and Ferguson, 1977)) have shown that even when conventional histological appearances are normal, there is an increase in epithelial cell proliferation rate, accompanied by increased lymphocyte infiltrate of the tissue, the two features which were found in the early stages of allograft rejection (Mowat and Ferguson, 1980$_a$). Figures 1 and 2, illustrate these findings, with results of measurements of IE lymphocyte counts, in neonatal Fl CBA x Balb/c mice which have had graft-versus-host reaction induced by injection of CBA spleen cells at the age of 6 days.

TABLE 1

SUBJECTIVE GRADING OF SMALL INTESTINAL PATHOLOGY IN ANIMAL MODELS OF CMI IN THE SMALL INTESTINAL MUCOSA

Model	Strains	Pathology of SI 1 week	2 weeks
Rejection of heterotopically transplanted allograft	CBA-Balb/c	SVA	destroyed
" "	CBA-C3H	normal	PVA
Graft-versus-host disease (neonatal host)	CBA-C3H	PVA	PVA
Graft-versus-host disease (adult host)	CBA-Balb/c		normal
" "	CBA-C3H		normal

PVA - partial villous atrophy with crypt hyperplasia;
SVA - subtotal villous atrophy with crypt hyperplasia.

As a result of these and other experiments we propose that local CMI reactions have profound effects on epithelial cell kinetics in the intestinal mucosa and that these occur in two stages (Ferguson and MacDonald, 1977).

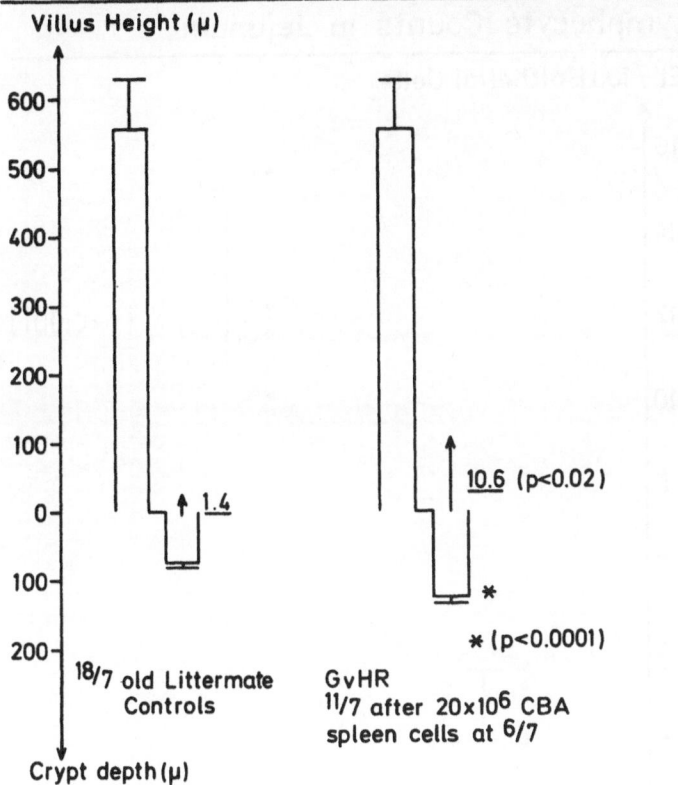

Graft-versus-Host Reaction in Neonatal F_1 (CBA×Balbc) Mice: Morphological Changes in Jejunum

Villus Height (μ)

600 —
500 —
400 —
300 —
200 —
100 —
0 —
100 —
200 —

↑ 1.4

10.6 (p<0.02)

* (p<0.0001)

^{18}/7 old Littermate Controls

GvHR
^{11}/7 after 20×10^6 CBA spleen cells at ^{6}/7

Crypt depth (μ)

Fig. 1. Measurements of villus and crypts, by a microdissection technique, and crypt cell production rate (see arrows) in neonatal mice with graft-versus-host disease; and controls.

114

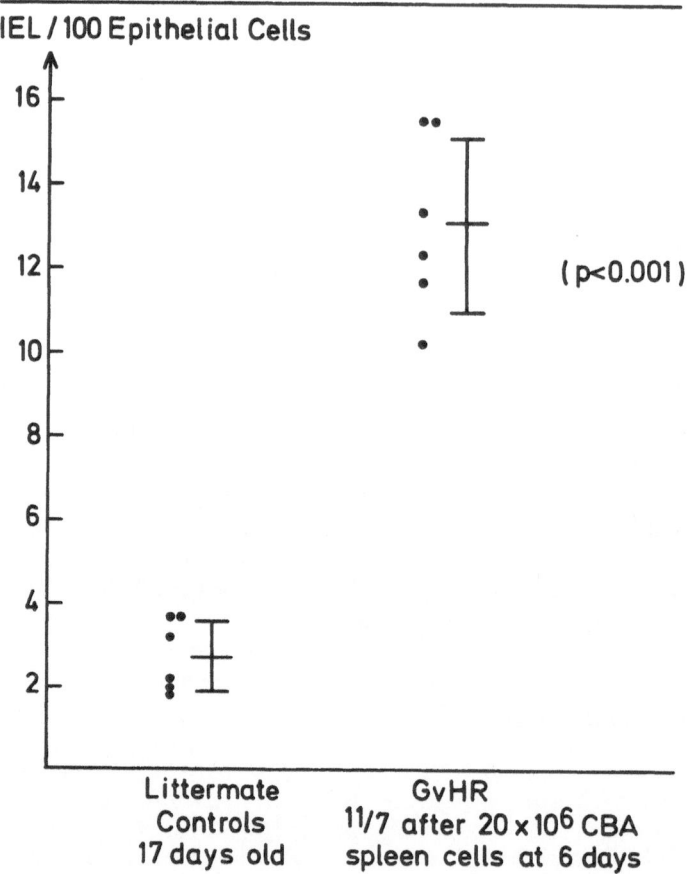

Graft-versus-Host Reaction in Neonatal (CBA x Balbc) Mice : Intraepithelial Lymphocyte Counts in Jejunum

IEL / 100 Epithelial Cells

(p<0.001)

Littermate
Controls
17 days old

GvHR
11/7 after 20 x 10^6 CBA
spleen cells at 6 days

Fig. 2.   Counts of IE lymphocytes in neonatal mice with graft-versus-host disease;   and controls.

Phase 1 appears normal to conventional histopathological examination for the villi are of normal length but there is an increase in mitotic activity of the crypts and, when compared with normals, the enterocytes move more rapidly up the sides of the villi and have a shorter lifespan.

In Phase 2 crypt hyperplasia persists with a high mitotic rate but villi are short or absent and, on the basis of electron microscopic studies of the enterocytes (Ferguson et al., 1978) it seems likely that this effect is due not to direct damage of villus enterocytes but to an effect of the underlying immune reaction on the adhesion of epithelial cells to one another and to the underlying tissues.

It is worth mentioning in passing that similar experiments were conducted on isografts and allografts of mouse colon, and changes in colonic epithelial cell kinetics were also demonstrated, during allograft rejection (Holden and Ferguson, 1976, 1979).

Mechanisms for T cell mediated damage to the intestine

The traffic of activated T cells from Peyer's patches via lymph back to the intestinal mucosa has been discussed above. Thus within a few days of the ingestion of a new antigen, or infection of the intestinal mucosa with a newly encountered agent, the potential for any of a variety of T cell mediated immune reactions will be present within the mucosa. As illustrated in Figure 3 there are a number of ways in which the presence of antigen, together with the presence of a population of antigen specific T cells, could lead to mucosal damage. These include the spectrum of antibody mediated immune reactions (including reaginic hypersensitivity and immune complex hypersensitivity) via helper T cell effects; direct cytotoxicity due to cytotoxic T cells in the lamina propria or epithelium; and/or the effect of various humoral factors secreted by activated T lymphocytes, lymphokines. Although we by no means exclude cytotoxic T cell effects, and

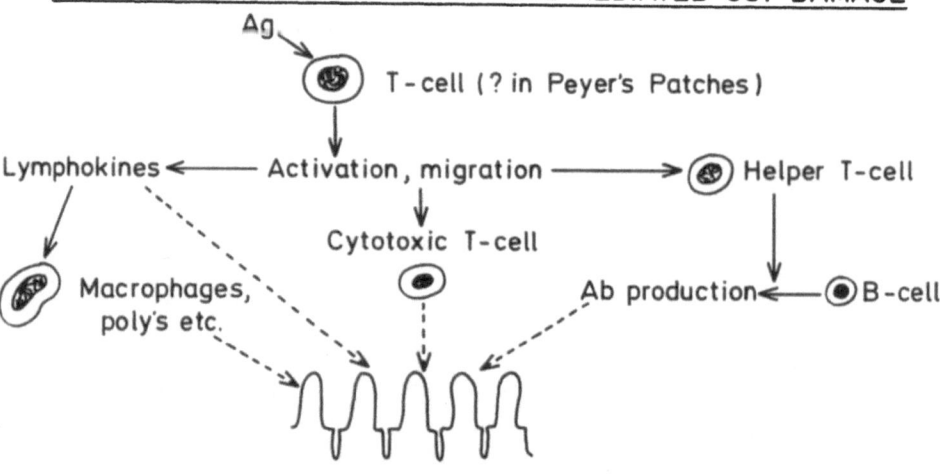

POSSIBLE MECHANISMS FOR T-CELL MEDIATED GUT DAMAGE

Fig. 3. Several possible mechanisms by which T cell mediated, or thymus dependent immune reactions, could damage the gut mucosa.

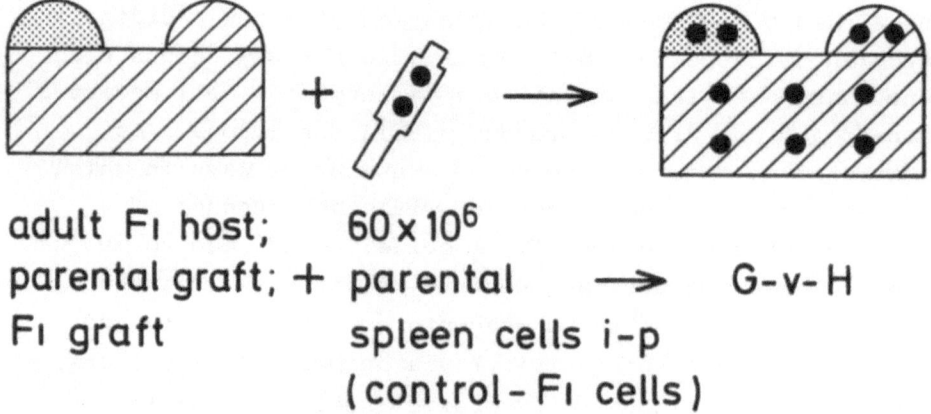

adult Fı host;   60 × 10⁶
parental graft; + parental   ⟶   G-v-H
Fı graft   spleen cells i-p
    (control- Fı cells)

Fig. 4. Protocol for experiment to study the 'innocent bystander' phenomenon in graft-versus-host disease (see text).

effects of humoral antibody, we consider that there is now good evidence that the features of intestinal mucosal damage described above are the result of secretion of lymphokines by activated T cells, rather than by direct cytotoxicity. We initially made these proposals in view of the absence of evidence of cytotoxicity by the intraepithelial lymphocytes, as assessed by electron microscopy. However, support for the existence of humoral enteropathic factors in graft-versus-host disease has been provided by the work of Elson et al., 1977. These workers produced graft-versus-host disease in mice, the animals previously having had implants of foetal small intestine. The objective of their experiments was to determine whether the intestine was injured in the graft-versus-host reaction as a direct antigenic target of immunocompetent cells or as an 'innocent bystander' to the donor host lymphoid interaction. Results of their experiments supported the latter explanation.

We tested our hypothesis, that mitotic activity of the crypts of Lieberkuhn and infiltration of the tissue with lymphocytes, were markers of the presence of CMI in the intestinal mucosa by using Elson's graft-versus-host model (Mowat and Ferguson, 1980$_b$). The protocol is outlined in Figure 4. We have examined both CBA - C3H and CBA - Balb/c strain combinations and similar results were obtained for both. Heterotopic grafts of foetal small intestine were transplanted under the kidney capsules of adult F1 foetal gut, and in the others transplanted tissue was of the parental strain CBA. Four weeks later graft-versus-host reaction was induced in the hosts by the intraperitoneal injection of 60 x 10^6 CBA spleen cells. Two weeks later the animals were injected with colchicine, killed at intervals over the next two hours and measurements of mucosal structure and epithelial cell proliferation in the crypts of Lieberkuhn, together with counts of intraepithelial lymphocytes, were made. Measurements of spleen weight confirmed the presence of graft-versus-host disease in the adult F1 hosts. Results for the CBA-Balb/c strain combination are summarised in Table 2. Although

subjective examination of intestinal histology in the host
intestine showed no difference between controls and GvH
animals, the objective measurements confirmed that villus
height was similar in the two groups but crypt cell production
rate and IE lymphocyte count were both significantly higher in
the GvH animals when compared with the controls.

TABLE 2

EFFECTS OF GRAFT-VERSUS-HOST REACTION ON INTESTINAL TISSUES OF CBA-BALB/C F1
MICE WITH HETEROTOPIC GRAFTS OF INTESTINE

Experimental group	Tissue	Villus height μm	Crypt mitoses (per hour) mean	IEL count (per 100 enterocytes) mean
Control (F1 cells)	Host jejunum	484.5	6.1	9.9
G-v-H (CBA cells)	Host jejunum	536.1	10.6 ($p < 0.02$)	16.0 ($p < 0.001$)
Control (F1 cells)	Grafted SI	288.5	3.1	3.7
G.v.H (CBA cells)	F1 graft	284.7	8.6 ($p < 0.01$)	6.9 ($p < 0.001$)
	CBA graft	290.3	6.2 ($p < 0.05$)	7.2 ($p < 0.001$)

Studies of the grafts showed that, as in previous
experiments, villus height and IE lymphocyte counts were lower
in isografts than in normally sited intestine but in both of
the types of grafts implanted in animals with GvH reaction,
crypt cell production rate and IE lymphocyte count were
significantly higher than for isografts. Thus in a GvH reaction
induced in CBA-Balb/c F1 hosts by the injection of CBA cells,
crypt hyperplasia and IE lymphocyte infiltration have been
produced in a graft of CBA foetal intestine. These results
confirm the 'innocent bystander' phenomenon in this graft-
versus-host disease model and support our hypothesis that crypt
cell production and IE lymphocyte counts are markers of this
local CMI reaction.

MUCOSAL CMI AND INTESTINAL DISEASE

On present evidence, reaginic, immune complex and T cell mediated immune reactions may all occur in the small intestine of experimental animals and various changes in intestinal structure and lymphoid cell infiltrate have been demonstrated (reviewed in Ferguson and Mowat, 1980). On present evidence, when circumstances are such that an intestinal hypersensitivity reaction to an enteric antigen is likely, and crypt hyperplasia, villus shortening and increased intraepithelial lymphocyte count are present in the intestinal biopsy, we suggest that a T cell mediated immune reaction, rather than antibody mediated hypersensitivity, is the likely mechanism of intestinal damage. Table 3 lists a number of diseases in which we would suggest that mucosal CMI is likely to be implicated as the cause of enteropathy and malabsorption.

Since in most of these intestinal hypersensitivity diseases the primary pathogenic process is induction of CMI rather than tolerance when an antigen has been fed, we have attempted to reproduce the phenomenon of mucosal CMI to a dietary antigen, in experimental animals.

TABLE 3

DISEASES IN WHICH MUCOSAL CMI CAN BE IMPLICATED AS THE CAUSE OF ENTEROPATHY AND MALABSORPTION

Coeliac disease

Cows' milk protein intolerance

Other food allergies with enteropathy

Giardiasis

Helminth infections

Tropical sprue

? autoimmune enteropathy

Graft-versus-host disease

Rejection of intestinal allograft

? vicinity of ulcer or tumour

INDUCTION OF CMI TO FED ANTIGEN

Tolerance and suppressor mechanisms

Feeding of antigen induces a secretory antibody response but little is known of the factors which will induce CMI to fed antigens. We failed in a number of previous attempts to induce CMI to fed antigens using a variety of antigen dosage, regimes, and routes of administration. In retrospect these failures can be explained by recent evidence that oral administration of antigen induces the specific immune reaction of tolerance for CMI as well as humoral immunity (Miller and Hanson, 1979). The fact that feeding of protein antigen to mice results in reduced humoral and CMI responses when that antigen is subsequently presented is probably associated with the ability of the gut associated lymphoid tissues to generate suppressor T cells in response to orally administered antigen (Ngan and Kind, 1978; Mattingly and Waksman, 1978).

We have, by using Balb/c mice, confirmed the results of others that prefeeding of mice with ovalbumin subsequently renders the mice tolerant to induction both of humoral and CMI responses to ovalbumin when given parenterally. We reasoned that if we treated animals with an agent which reduced or eliminated suppressor cell activity, it might be possible to alter the nature of the immune response to fed antigen, and thereby induce CMI. Administration of cyclophosphamide to mice in the dose of 100 mg/kg enhances CMI reactions without an appreciable effect on antibody synthesis, via suppressor cell inhibition (Askenaze et al., 1975) and so we used the following regime. Balb/c mice were treated with cyclophosphamide alone (100 mg/kg), oral ovalbumin (2 mg) alone or cyclophosphamide followed by oral ovalbumin. Four weeks later they were challenged with ovalbumin in drinking water at a dose of 0.1 mg daily for 10 days. At the end of this time the animals were killed and, in some, evidence of gut associated CMI to ovalbumin was sought by using direct migration inhibition of mesenteric lymph node cells in the presence of

TABLE 4

EFFECTS OF MUCOSAL IMMUNE REACTION TO OVALBUMIN ON INTESTINAL TISSUES

Induction	Challenge	Migration index for MLN cells*	Villus height μm	Crypt mitoses (per hour)	IEL count (per 100 enterocytes)
Cyclophosphamide		1.12	680.7	6.6	15.8
OA 2 mg	OA 0.1 mg (x 10)	1.00	638.8	8.4	14.5
Cyclophosphamide	OA 0.1 mg (x 10)	0.63 (P < 0.01)	686.5	12.0* (P = 0.025)	25.9* (P < 0.005)

* Cultured in presence of 1 mg/ml OA. As positive control popliteal and auxiliary CN cells from animals immunised by footpad injection were similarly studied; these gave MI of 0.70.

ovalbumin, and in others crypt cell production rate and IE
lymphocyte counts were made as described above. Results are
summarised in Table 4. It can be seen that, with the migration
inhibition technique, the positive control of draining lymph
nodes from mouse footpad, showed significant migration
inhibition; animals which had been fed ovalbumin alone, or
which had been given cyclophosphamide alone, had no significant
migration inhibition but the combination of cyclophosphamide
and ovalbumin resulted in the presence of lymphoid cells,
positive in the test described, in the mesenteric lymph nodes.
Furthermore, significant changes in crypt cell production rate
and IE lymphocyte counts were obtained only in the
cyclophosphamide/ovalbumin group.

These preliminary experiments indicate that there is
likely to be a spectrum in the CMI reaction to dietary antigens
which ranges from the induction of a population of sensitised
T cells on the one hand to the induction of specific tolerance,
associated with a population of suppressor cells, on the other.
This and similar animal models should allow elucidation of the
factors which influence mucosal CMI responses and may be of
value in establishing the pathogenesis of the various food
allergic diseases.

PROPOSED ROLES OF GUT MUCOSAL T CELLS

T cell subclasses and their segregation within the mucosa

In the mouse, the subclasses of T cells have been clearly
defined by using a variety of antisera, and functional tests.
For example by using the LY antisera, LY1 positive cells have
been shown to act as helpers, amplifiers, they are I restricted
and responsible for delayed hypersensitivity whereas LY23
positive cells are suppressors, have cytotoxic killer properties
and are K/D restricted in their expression. Although the
evidence is not yet conclusive, there is probably a
pluripotential stem T cell with LY1, 2 and 3 antigenic determinants. The very recently reported work, mentioned above, by
Selby et al.using human intestinal mucosa has shown that the

majority of IE lymphocytes stain with antisera to the
suppressor/cytotoxic cell marker antigens. A minority of LP
lymphocytes also stain with this antiserum and this can be
interpreted as indicating either that these also are suppressor
cells or that they are pluripotential stem T cells. The lamina
propria T cells which do not stain with the antiserum OKT8 are
probably helper cells but this remains to be proven.

Results of this experiment suggested that there is
segregation of T cells within the mucosa. Autoradiographic
studies have shown that lymphocytes enter the intestinal mucosa
from the bloodstream presumably via the vascular capillaries in
the lamina propria. A preferential accumulation of suppressor
T cells in the intraepithelial site could be produced by
preferential attraction of this subpopulation (for example by
chemotaxis) preferential retention of the T suppressor cells
within the epithelium, other T cells migrating out rapidly;
alternatively, the pluripotential T cell may migrate into the
epithelium and there further mature, in the intraepithelial
site, to the T suppressor subclass, whereas T cells further
mature to T helper cells in the lamina propria. We prefer the
first of these postulates, but, clearly, many further
experiments will be required both to confirm this single report
mentioned above, and to investigate the mechanisms for T cell
segregation within the gut.

In Figure 5 we outline our working hypothesis as to the
various roles of gut mucosal T cells.

Function of lamina propria lymphocytes

We propose that the lamina propria lymphocytes comprise
mainly pluripotential T cells, and T cells of the T helper
subclass, which secrete lymphokines after interaction with
antigen. As illustrated in Figure 5, the effects of a T cell
mediated immune reaction in the mucosa, which are likely to
be produced by soluble products of activated T cells, include
stimulation of mitosis in the crypts of Lieberkuhn, alteration

in the differentiation of epithelial cells (with increases in
the number of goblet cells, discussed by Dr. H.R.P. Miller
elsewhere in this Symposium) recruitment of lymphocytes,
macrophages and other cell types into the mucosa, and, finally,
damage to the core of the villus with exfoliation of epithelial
cells leading to villous atrophy and ultimately malabsorption.

POSTULATED ROLES OF INTESTINAL MUCOSAL T CELLS

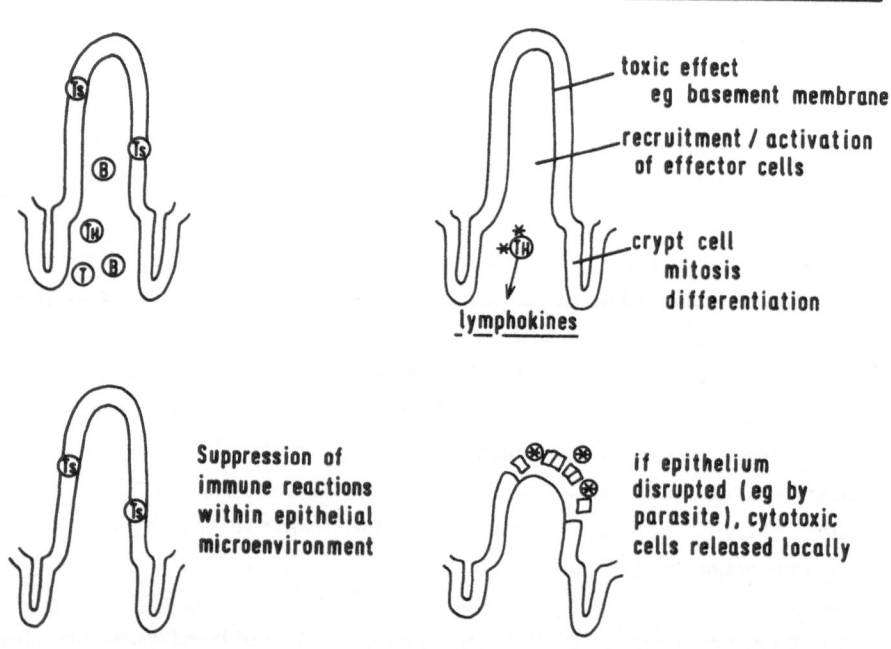

Fig. 5.   Hypothetical notes of mucosal T cells (see text). We suggest
that lamina propria T cells are mainly pluripotential T cells
and helper cells; lymphokine secretion by activated LP cells
leads to changes in intestinal mucosal structure and function.
IE T lymphocytes are of the suppressor/cytotoxic subclass;
their primary role is likely to be protection of the epithelial
microenvironment from immune mediated damage.

It is likely that mucosal CMI responses evolved as part
of the gut's mechanisms for protection against infection.
These non-specific effector mechanisms, which are initiated by
specific T cell-antigen interaction may alter the host parasite
relationship to the advantage of the host in a number of ways.
For example increased transit of enterocytes up the sides of
the villi would lead to more rapid exfoliation of adherent
bacteria, and of cells infected by intracellular parasites.
Even the damage to the lamina propria with villous atrophy
could be of value in those parasite infections where the
parasites attach to or burrow into the tissue, in that the
tissues to which the parasites are adherent would be disrupted.

Postulated function of intraepithelial lymphocytes

The columnar epithelium of the small intestine forms an
organ which is absolutely essential to life. In view of the
wealth of antigens covering its luminal surface there is the
potential for continuous antigen/antibody and antigen/cell
interactions in and around this mucosa, with all the varied
enteropathic consequences of the spectrum of local hypersensitivity. It is entirely logical, in evolutionary terms,
that a population of lymphocytes is present in the mucosa
whose principal function is to suppress immune reactions
within the 30 μm deep monolayer of the intestinal mucosal
epithelium.

Although the serologically defined subclass of T cells,
which contains cells with T suppressor properties also contains
the cytotoxic T cells (LY23 in mouse, OKT8 in man), there is no
evidence of lymphocyte mediated cytotoxicity in the normal,
intact intestinal epithelium. However it is conceivable that
when an agent (for example an enteric pathogen) destroys a
group of epithelial cells, local release of cytotoxic T cells
would provide a first line of cell mediated defence of the de-
epithelialised area, and macrophages from the lamina propria
would supplement this action.

ACKNOWLEDGEMENTS

We acknowledge the assistance of the staff of the Animal Unit, Western General Hospital, Edinburgh.

Dr. Mowat is in receipt of the Allan Fellowship of the University of Edinburgh.

REFERENCES

Askenaze, P.W., Hayden, B.J., Gershon, R.K., 1975. Augmentation of
    delayed-type hypersensitivity by doses of cyclophosphamide which
    do not affect antibody responses. J Exp Med. 141, 697.

Cahill, R.N.P., Poskitt,D.C., Frost, H., Trnka, Z., 1977. Two distinct
    pools of recirculating T lymphocytes: migratory characteristics
    of nodal and intestinal T lymphocytes. J Exp Med. 145, 420.

Elson, C.O., Reilly, R.W., Rosenberg, R.H., 1977. Small intestinal injury
    in the graft-versus-host reaction: an innocent bystander
    phenomenon. Gastroenterology. 72, 886.

Elves, M.W., Ferguson, A., 1975. The humoral immune response to allografts
    of foetal small intestine in mice. Br J Exp Pathol. 56, 454.

Ferguson, A., Carr, K.E., MacDonald, T.T., Watt, C., 1978.
    Hypersensitivity reactions in the small intestine 4 Influence of
    allograft rejection on small intestinal mucosal architecture: A
    scanning and transmission electron microscrope study. Digestion.
    18, 56.

Ferguson, A., MacDonald, T.T., 1977. Effects of local delayed
    hypersensitivity on the small intestine. In Ciba Foundation
    Symposium No 46. Elsevier North-Holland Inc 305.

Ferguson, A., Mowat, A.M., 1980. Immunological mechanisms in the small
    intestine. In: Wright R, ed. Recent advances in gastrointestinal
    pathology p. 93. WB Saunders, Eastbourne.

Ferguson, A., Parrott, D.M.V., 1972. The effect of antigen deprivation on
    thymus-dependent and thymus-independent lymphocytes in the small
    intestine of the mouse. Clin Exp Immunol. 12, 477.

Ferguson, A., Parrott, D.M.V., 1973. Histopathology and time-course of
    rejection of allografts of mouse small intestine.
    Transplantation. 15, 546.

Fichtelius, K.E., Unis, E.J., Good, R.A., 1968. Occurrence of lymphocytes
    within the gut epithelium of normal and neonatally thymectomised
    mice. Proc Soc Exp Biol. 128, 185.

De Freitas, A.A., Rose, M.L., Parrott, D.M.V., 1977. Murine mesenteric
    and peripheral lymph nodes: a common pool of small T cells.
    Nature. 270, 731.

Guy Grand, D., Griscelli, C., Vassalli, P., 1974. The gut associated
        lymphoid system: nature and properties of the large dividing
        cells. Eur J Immunol. 4, 435.

Guy Grand, D., Griscelli, C., Vassalli, P., 1978. The mouse gut T
        lymphocyte, a novel type of T cell. J Exp Med. 148, 1661.

Holden, R.J., Ferguson, A., 1979. Histopathology of a cell mediated
        immune reaction in mouse colon - allograft rejection. Gut. 17, 661.

Holden, R.J., Ferguson, A., 1979. Effects of age, antigen deprivation
        and allograft rejection on epithelial cell kinetics in mouse colon.
        Gut. 20, 234.

Mattingly, J.A., Waksman, B.H., 1978. Immunologic suppression after oral
        administration of antigen. 1 Specific suppressor cells formed in
        rat Peyer's patches after oral administration of sheep red cells,
        and their systemic migration. J Immunol. 121, 1878.

MacDonald, T.T., Ferguson, A., 1977. Hypersensitivity reactions in the
        small intestine. 2 Effects of allograft rejection on mucosal
        architecture and lymphoid cell infiltrate. Gut. 17, 81.

MacDonald, T.T., Ferguson, A., 1977. Hypersensitivity reactions in the
        small intestine. 3 The effects of allograft rejection and of
        graft-versus-host disease on epithelial cell kinetics. Cell
        Tissue Kinet. 10, 301.

McWilliams, M., Phillips-Quagliata, J.M., Lamm, L.E., 1975. Characteristics
        of mesenteric lymph node cells homing to gut associated lymphoid
        tissues in syngeneic mice. J Immunol. 115, 54.

Meuwissen, S.G.M., Feltkamp-Vroom, T.M., de la Riviere, A.B., von den
        Borne, A.E.G.K., Tytgat, G.N., 1976. Analysis of the lymphoplas-
        macytic infiltrate in Crohn's disease with special reference to
        identification of lymphocyte sub-populations. Gut. 17, 770.

Miller, S.D., Hanson, D.G., 1979. Inhibition of specific immune responses
        by feeding protein antigens. IV Evidence for tolerance and
        specific active suppression of cell mediated immune responses to
        ovalbumin. J Immunol. 123, 2344.

Mowat, A.M., Ferguson, A., 1980a. Hypersensitivity reactions in the small
        intestine 5 Induction of cell mediated immunity to a dietary
        antigen. Submitted for publication.

Mowat, A.M., Ferguson, A., 1980b. Hypersensitivity reactions in the small
        intestine 6 Pathogenesis of the graft-versus-host reaction in the
        small intestinal mucosa. Submitted for publication.

Ngan, J., Kind, L.S., 1978. Suppressor T cells for IgE and IgG in Peyer's patches of mice made tolerant by the oral administration of ovalbumin. J Immunol. 120, 861.

Parrott, D.M.V., Ferguson, A., 1974. Selective migration of lymphocytes within the mouse small intestine. Immunology. 26, 571.

Rose, M.L., Parrott, D.M.V., Bruce, R.G., 1976a. Migration of lymphoblasts to the small intestine 1 Effect of *Trichenella spiralis* infection on the migration of mesenteric lymphoblasts and mesenteric T lymphoblasts in syngeneic mice. Immunology. 31, 723.

Rose, M.L., Parrott, D.M.V., Bruce, R.G., 1976b. Migration of lymphoblasts to the small intestine 2 Divergent migration of mesenteric and peripheral immunoblasts to sites of inflammation in the mouse. Cell Immunol. 27, 36.

Selby, W.S., Janossy, G., Goldstein, G., Jewell, D.P., 1980. Suppressor T cells in human intestinal mucosa. Submitted for publication.

DISCUSSION

J. Soothill *(UK)*

I would like to make a comment on Anne Ferguson's remarks regarding a paper on chronic rotavirus infection in immuno-deficiency, with one of the patients having a marked cell mediated immunodeficiency. Dr. Levinsky has just such a child patient affected both with rotavirus and another virus - this provides support for what you are saying.

I think you are pointing to an extremely difficult concept of normality because our guts, those of you and me, are abnormal due to the hygienic circumstances in which we live, so to have quite such hygiene is probably abnormal, almost gnotobiotic. With that, let us throw it open for discussion.

J. Hall *(UK)*

Dr. Ferguson, in discussing the traffic of T lymphocytes, through the bowel, you said that Cahill et al. had not taken into account blast cells, which might have biased results. That is simply not true. The recirculation of the blasts has quite different kinetics and in any case his preparative procedures would have eliminated them, and there has also been an experiment which shows that the blasts do not contribute to that effect at all. In the sheep there is quite a genuine distinction between gut-associated, small T lymphocytes and systemic lymphocytes. Admittedly this distinction may not occur in the mouse, and it certainly does not occur in people, so it is probably something which is conditioned by antigen. It certainly does occur in sheep.

Anne Ferguson *(UK)*

I must admit I was quoting from the literature on that point. You know the literature perfectly well, because you have had an argument with that particular author.

E. Bohl *(USA)*

Could you elaborate on the mechanism whereby you obtain villus atrophy with CMI? I think you did mention that the basement membrane was disrupted and that this might result in the release or disintegration of enterocytes. There is a second aspect to this question, that of whether the mitosis or proliferation of the crypt enterocytes is a cause or effect. Normally with villus atrophy we find an extension of the crypt, which is probably due to a feedback mechanism.

Anne Ferguson

Exactly. I am sure that once there is villus atrophy, there are also feedback mechanisms. We found in our animals that around day 10 of allograft rejection, sheets of columnar epithelial cells with reasonable brush borders were exfoliated into the lumen. It was pointed out by the electron microscopist that there appeared to be separation of the epithelium from the basement membrane in the preparation of the tissues in the later stages of the rejection but not in the early stages. We suggest that there is an enteropathic effect on the structure of the villus so that epithelial cells are being formed without having a base for them to sit on, and therefore they fall off. This effect has been shown, for example, at some stages after radiation injury. Part of our reason for suggesting this is that it is healthy looking columnar epithelial cells which fall off.

To turn to the second point made by Professor Bohl, I agree that it has frequently been suggested that crypt hyperplasia is nearly always a feedback, but there is no doubt at all that it is an early phenomenon in this process and there are now quite a number of situations (some parts of the lung, gut and rotavirus infection, chronic giardiasis in mice and several diseases in man) where there are normal villi with mature enterocytes on them and yet there is crypt hyperplasia. This may be immunologically mediated but under other circumstances, for example, may be due to gut hormones or mechanical effects.

J. Bienenstock *(Canada)*

Dr. Ferguson, what is the length of a villus in a nude mouse or nude rat?

Anne Ferguson

Tom MacDonald did look at this by means of autoradiographic studies. He found no difference between clean nude mice and clean heterozygotes. I do not think that healthy, uninfected laboratory animals or most of us have active CMI reactions taking place in our normal intestines. It is only after infection that these occur, so I was not surprised that the normal nude mice had the same epithelial cells production as normal mice.

J. Bienenstock

The problem I have in interpreting some of your work and that of other people is the one to which John Soothill has already alluded, that of the concept of the norm. Most people consider the bowel as slightly infected or inflamed because of the nature of the straight morphology. That surely means that those cells which are in the bowel are interacting with their environment. If this is taken to its inevitable conclusion, the suggestion would be that the products of that lymphocyte reactivity would be involved in the regulation of the norm.

Anne Ferguson

That is one possibility, and we did think that it might be true. The lymphocytes were thought to have trophocytes, but obviously germ-free immune deficient patients are absolutely healthy and have normal absorption. I think that Dr. Bienenstock is probably being deliberately obtuse, because he himself pointed out the highly important property of the gut in induction of tolerance in dampening down immunity, and I think it is not surprising that there is not a continual enteropathic reaction in the gut. I do think that if one sees a CMI reaction as being in phases, the earliest phase being relatively low grade and not

greatly disrupting the anatomy, then that is probably
physiological, a sort of grumbling giardiasis or mild tropical
sprue which may be the human norm, but real villus atrophy
with malabsorption produces disease and one wants to avoid that
if possible.

J. Bienenstock

I am only being slightly obtuse. I think this is
important, because the real issue is what controls the norm and
the normal height, whatever you accept as being the normal
height. I am saying that you are being naive in talking about
infection versus non-infection, because I think that we are
infected all the time, and therefore the reason that we are
in the middle, as we would accept the norm, is as a result of
some of the processes to which you refer.

Anne Ferguson

We are exposed to a large number of antigens like ovalbumin, to which it is easy to make an animal mount a CMI
reaction. There is no evidence, to my knowledge, that normal
people have any evidence of T-cell mediated immune reactions to
the wealth of foodstuffs, for example, and there would be good
evidence, in several diseases of man and also, I feel sure, if
one were to look at soya allergy in animals, that in these
conditions, a part of what is new and producing the malabsorption is the development of a cell mediated immune reaction. I
would like to have the chance to prove this.

W. Leibold (FRG)

Two points. Dr. Ferguson has given such a clear concept
of T-helper, T-suppressor and T-effector cells. You mentioned
briefly that in baby mice intraepithelial cells, the lymphoid
cells, are not found before the age of three weeks. It may be
only a coincidence that the natural killer activity appears in
mice at this age. My first question, therefore, is how would
you integrate the natural killer activity into your assessment?

Secondly, we are all aware now that T-cell functions are at least highly influenced by monocytes and macrophages. How would you integrate these cells into your hypothesis?

Anne Ferguson

I think that the very fact that the intraepithelial cells are isolated from other immune cells suggests that they are certainly not involved in the induction of immunity. It is not just that lymphocytes appear in the gut of the mouse at the time other immune mechanisms evolve, because in 1972 Delphine Parrott and I published a paper showing that in grafts of intestine, the intestine only became populated with lymphocytes when the intestinal epithelial tissue of the graft was in the third week of life. Clearly, there is some environmental change in baby mice intestine that leads to it either attracting or holding lymphocytes only when it has reached the post-weaning stage. This happens in most other species before birth, and in the rat, I think, it occurs about a day or two before birth. As to the natural killer function, this could well be one of the first lines of defence, but this remains to be proven.

P. Brandtzaeg (Norway)

It has now been shown in guinea pigs, mice and man that there are Ia antigens on the enterocytes on the small intestine. I wonder how Dr. Ferguson would fit this into her hypothesis about the induction of cell mediated immunity and suppressor and T-cells.

Anne Ferguson

I do not know about that, but the hypothesis of my colleague, Alan Mowat, is that it may well be the Ia antigens on the epithelial cells which attract or hold the T-lymphocyte subclass within the epithelium, but against that it may be said that the expression of the Ia antigens is greater in the villi than in the crypts, and certainly there are more lymphocytes on the villi than on the crypts, but I understand that it is expressed better and better as the epithelial cells move up the villi whereas the distribution of lymphocytes is fairly even throughout the whole of the intestine. This would suggest that there is relatively random migration of the lymphocytes along the length of the villus. However, I do think that this is one of the mechanisms akin to secretory component hypothesis.

P. Brandtzaeg

Would you think that would be involved in the induction of helper cells or suppressor cells?

Anne Ferguson

That is one of our options, yes, but I have not got an opinion on that.

G. Mayrhofer *(UK)*

I have been looking at Ia bearing cells in the gut, and with reference to the experiment of Elson which Dr. Ferguson mentioned where parental gut was put into F_1 hybrid hosts suggesting that a humoral factor was involved in graft versus host disease affecting the parental graft. In the gut there is Ia antigen, as Dr. Brantzaeg said, on the epithelial cells but there are also vast quantities of Ia bearing cells in the *lamina propria*. The question I have recently asked is what is the origin of these cells. Are they a kind of reticular cell which is at home in the gut, produced locally in the gut, or is it part of a migratory system perhaps akin to that of macrophages? Maybe it is the same system as putting foetal parental grafts under the kidney capsule in the F_1 hybrid. The parental tissue was from hooded rats and the F_1 hybrid was a hooded typed AO. I should explain that we have two monoclonal antibodies, OX4 which recognises Ia of all rat strains and OX3 which is polymorphic and recognises the AO of hooded. When the hooded graft was put into the F_1 recipient, the hooded graft received Ia bearing *lamina propria* cells of the AO type. Perhaps this casts a slightly different light on Dr. Ferguson's interpretation of that particular experiment, because we now have a graft which is hooded in terms of epithelium but is recipient in terms of the

Ia that it bears. Ia is clearly important in graft versus host disease, so that it is possible that there is a local graft versus host reaction taking place in the Fl recipient, which perhaps had not been anticipated.

J. Soothill

Would you clarify whether the recipient of Ia in the graft is on the epithelial cells?

G. Mayrhofer

I'm sorry. I can only talk about the *lamina propria* cells.

Anne Ferguson

You are saying that the recipient cells home in to the *lamina propria*? Dr. Bazin has conducted some experiments, as I did, showing that plasma cells derived from the host infiltrate these grafts and the cell traffic studies show host cells going in to the Peyer's patches and into the mucosa, so it would be interesting if macrophages are similar in this respect.

J. Soothill

Yes, but you are not talking about the Ia on the mucosal cells. With that, I think we must close this discussion.

137

STIMULATION AND SUPPRESSION OF IgE ANTIBODIES BY ANTIGENS PRESENTED TO MUCOSAL SURFACES

Ellen Jarrett

Department of Veterinary Parasitology,
University of Glasgow, UK.

ABSTRACT

Experiments in rats and mice have shown that antigens absorbed across mucous membranes may give rise to an IgE response, or alternatively to the suppression of IgE responsiveness through the activation of immunoregulatory mechanisms. Which of these alternatives occurs seems to depend on an interaction of extrinsic factors including dose and form of antigen presentation with the intrinsic immune reactivity of the animal, which may in itself be influenced by previous events. The available evidence for these statements will be reviewed.

INTRODUCTION

Antigens are presented to mucosal surfaces in endless variety - food antigens in large amount, inhalant antigens in smaller quantities, antigens of the normal bacterial flora and of pathogenic bacteria, antigens produced by helminth parasites, drugs - all with the potential for evoking an IgE response and a state of hypersensitivity. In some individuals these antigens in fact do just that. But in the majority, IgE antibodies are not produced in detectable amounts, helminth infection excepted. We now know of course that absence of an immune response does not necessarily imply a failure of sensitisation; that it may be the expression of an immune capability to suppress that response. Therefore, when an animal does not produce IgE as a result of what might appear to be an immunogenic stimulus we must ask the question whether there has been a failure of antigen entry or alternatively whether the stimulus has induced a state of specific suppression of IgE responsiveness. Whatever the underlying mechanisms, it is axiomatic that to understand the allergic response of the minority we must understand the reasons for the failure of response in the majority. It is from this angle that I intend to examine the topic.

I shall first review the experiments which have been conducted using laboratory animals with an eye to formulating rules about the manipulations which favour an IgE response or which alternatively lead to suppression of response. Then, I shall consider to what natural circumstances these experimental results might apply and what is their relevance.

As there is not yet a very large literature on the subject I have thought it useful to list the articles (of which I am aware) and to summarise the main characteristics of the response. The list (Table 1) shows the various permutations of oral, inhalant and parenteral antigen which have been used to evoke and demonstrate the phenomena we are discussing. I include results using the guinea-pig because although the

antibodies involved are predominantly IgG1, they have the same
biological effect of mediating immediate anaphylactic reactions.

SENSITISATION FOR EXPERIMENTAL IgE OR ANAPHYLACTIC RESPONSES BY ANTIGENS PRESENTED TO THE MUCOSAE

An appraisal of the results allows one to make some broad
generalisations. When antigen is administered as a single dose
to a mucosal surface, and assuming the animal is capable of
responding to the antigen in question, the production of a
detectable IgE response would seem to depend on an adequacy of
antigen dose, and an accompaniment by some form of adjuvant
treatment.

Thus Hof and colleagues (1975) described the occurrence
of anaphylactic sensitivity to bovine serum albumin (BSA) in
mice which had been given this antigen together with *Bordetella
pertussis* (Bp) adjuvant by stomach tube. Jarrett and colleagues
(1976) and Bazin and Platteau (1976) showed that detectable
IgE antibody responses could be evoked by orally administered
egg-albumin (EA) with Bp given by the oral or intraperitoneal
routes. Rat IgE synthesis following aerosol administration of
EA with intraperitoneal Bp has been demonstrated by Van Hout
and Johnson (1972) and Gerbrandy and Bienenstock (1976) have
induced IgE tetanus antibody in mice by placing the antigen
and Bp into the trachea.

The facilitating effect of adjuvant in the induction of
IgE antibodies is not limited to mucosal presentation of
antigen. The same is true of antigen presented parenterally.

Anaphylactic sensitisation to ingested antigen may also
develop without the aid of adjuvant if the antigenic stimulus
is more prolonged. This appears to be especially true of
guinea-pigs in which sensitisation to a variety of ingested
antigens has been demonstrated (Wells and Osborne, 1911;
Ratner and Gruehl, 1933; Devey et al., 1976). Perelmutter and
Liakopoulou demonstrated a similar phenomenon in rats which

TABLE 1

STIMULATION AND SUPPRESSION OF EXPERIMENTAL IgE AND ANAPHYLACTIC RESPONSES TO ANTIGENS PRESENTED TO MUCOSAL SURFACES

Authors	Species	Antigen and route	Characteristics of response
Wells & Osborne, 1911	Guinea pigs	Corn meal by mouth	Refractoriness to anaphylactic sensitisation to injection of zein following protracted feeding of corn.
Ratner & Gruehl, 1933	Guinea-pigs	Cows milk horse serum by mouth	Sensitisation and anaphylactic shock in young and old guinea pigs.
Van Hout & Johnson, 1972	Rat. Spraque-Dawley	1% EA aerosol + Bp. i.p.	Primary and booster IgE responses. Ag found in respiratory and gastrointestinal tract.
Hof et al., 1975	Mouse. NMRl	4 mg BSA + Bp. i.g.	Anaphylactic sensitivity to 7 mg i.v. BSA
Perelmutter & Liakopoulou, 1975	Rat	Penicillin G in drinking water 0.1 - 1 μ/ml for 1-3 mo.	IgE response as detected by *in vitro* rat mast cell degranulation technique.
Jarrett et al., 1976	Rat. Hooded Lister	EA 1μg - 100 mg. i.g. Bp. i.p.	Primary IgE response after 100 μg-10 μg oral EA + Bp. i.p. Booster response after oral challenge with 100 μg - 1 μg EA but suppression of IgE booster response if primary dose > 100 μg.

TABLE 1 (CONTINUED)

STIMULATION AND SUPPRESSION OF EXPERIMENTAL IgE AND ANAPHYLACTIC RESPONSES TO ANTIGENS PRESENTED TO MUCOSAL SURFACES

Authors	Species	Antigen and route	Characteristics of response
Bazin & Platteau, 1976	Rat. Lou M/Wsl	EA 1 - 100 mg. i.g. Bp. i.p. or i.g.	Primary IgE response after 10 - 100 mg EA + Bp. i.p. or oral. Booster response after oral challenge with 100 μg - 50 mg EA.
Gerbrandy & Bienenstock, 1976	Mouse. C57BL/6 xDBA/2.F1	Tetanus toxoid - 2L + Bp. intra tracheally	Primary and booster IgE response. IgE producing cells in bronchial nodes.
Bazin & Platteau, 1977	Rat. Hooded Lister	EA 1% in food 5-45d.	Suppressed IgE response to EA and to DNP on challenge with 5 μg EA - DNP + Bp. i.p. after 5-15 days EA in food.
David, 1977	Rat. DA & Sprague - Dawley	Giant ragweed extract 0.45 mg protein. Horse serum 40 mg protein i.g. for 5d/wk for 1-20 weeks	Suppressed IgE response to subsequent immunisation (with Ag + Bp. i.p.) and protection from anaphylactic response. Best results when feeding started at 1 mo. Small frequent doses of antigen best suppression.
Devey et al., 1976	Guinea-pigs	Cows milk ad lib by mouth	Susceptibility to cows milk on i.v. challenge 13 d. after starting oral cows milk.

TABLE 1 (CONTINUED)

STIMULATION AND SUPPRESSION OF EXPERIMENTAL IgE AND ANAPHYLACTIC RESPONSES TO ANTIGENS PRESENTED TO MUCOSAL SURFACES

Authors	Species	Antigen and route	Characteristics of response
Coombs et al., 1977	Guinea-pigs	Cows milk ad lib by mouth	As above, but refractiveness to fatal anaphylactics developed after 71-86 days on milk diet. Antibody involved IgGla.
Vaz et al., 1977	Mouse C57Bl(6J xDBA/2J.Fl	EA i.g.	Suppressed IgE and IgGl response to 1 μg EA & AL(OH)3 i.p. in mice pretreated with 1.25 - 20 mg EA 1 or 8 weeks before. Waning suppression could be reinforced by further oral exposure to EA.
Hanson et al., 1977	"	"	"
Ngan & Kind, 1978	Mouse SWR C57Bl/6	EA in drinking water on alternate days for 2 weeks. Total 100 μg - 20 mg EA	Long lasting suppression of IgE response adoptively transferable with Peyers patch or spleen cells. Generation of suppressor cells required 8 feedings over 2 weeks.
Hanson et al., 1979a	Mouse C57Bl/6 X DBA/s Fl.	EA i.g.	IgG booster response to oral EA in rats primed with EA & AL(OH)3 i.p. No correlation between oral dose and magnitude of booster response.
" 1979b	"	20 mg EA i.g.	Suppressed IgE response in pre-fed mice to immunisation with 1 μg EA + EA + A(OH)3. Suppressed mice could not be reconstituted with normal or immune spleen cells.

developed reaginic antibodies to Penicillin G after prolonged feeding of this antigen.

The amount of antigen which requires to be administered by these routes to elicit a response would appear, from the evidence available, to depend on the innate IgE responsiveness of the strain of animals used. Thus 10 mg EA was the lowest effective dose in LouM/WSL rats (Bazin and Platteau, 1976), while in Hooded Lister rats which are sensitive to IgE stimulation with very small amounts of antigen (Jarrett and Stewart, 1974) oral immunisation could be achieved with as little as 10 µg of this antigen (Jarrett et al., 1976).

Whether local mucosal factors, such as a possible difference in absorptive capacity among the various strains of laboratory animal, or at different times in the same animal, may play a role in IgE responsiveness and is a subject which has not yet been explored. I should mention that in our own oral antigen experiments (Jarrett et al., 1976) we noticed a considerable between experiment variation in that quite frequently whole groups of rats failed to become sensitised for IgE production to a known immunogenic stimulus. This variability contrasted markedly with the very consistent responses achieved by parenteral immunisation, but the reasons underlying it were not discovered.

SUPPRESSION OF IgE RESPONSE AFTER ANTIGEN FEEDING

Regardless of whether or not an IgE response occurs as a result of presenting antigen to a mucosal surface a mechanism for the suppression of IgE responsiveness may have been activated as detected by a diminished or absent response to a subsequent immunising stimulus. Thus in the case where an IgE response has been induced by oral antigen and adjuvant, immunisation precedes suppression: where oral antigen is administered without adjuvant, suppression may predominate from the outset.

Let us first examine the second situation. Wells and
Osborne (1911) found that guinea-pigs which had been fed corn
meal for several weeks became refractory to anaphylactic
sensitisation by subsequent injections of zein, a corn protein.
Coombs and his colleagues demonstrated that guinea-pigs became
refractory to anaphylactic shock induced by an intravenous
milk injection, after an extended period on a milk diet.
David (1977) conducted extensive experiments to show that rats
could be specifically suppressed for the IgE response to giant
ragweed extract and horse serum by oral treatment with these
antigens and that the suppression was accompanied by protection
from anaphylactic shock. Suppression of IgE responsiveness
was more effective when oral treatment was started at one month
of age than at two or five months and small frequent doses of
antigen were more suppressive than larger exposures at longer
intervals. Vaz and colleagues (1977) found that both IgE and
IgG1 responses to a parenteral challenge of EA and adjuvant
were suppressed in mice which had previously received the
antigen without adjuvant by stomach tube. Suppression lasted
up to eight weeks after oral sensitisation but waning
suppression could be reinforced by further oral exposure to EA.
Bazin and Platteau (1977) demonstrated a similar phenomenon in
rats which had received EA in their drinking water prior to
challenge. Ngan and Kind (1978) adoptively transferred orally-
induced IgE suppression using Peyers Patch and spleen
lymphocytes. Again in their experiments frequency of antigen
exposure was found to be more important than dose for the
generation of effective suppressor cells. Hanson and associates
(1979b) in the course of an extensive study of the immune
inhibitory effects of antigen feeding also demonstrated a
suppressed IgE response to subsequent challenge in mice which
had received oral antigen.

In the above experiments the antigen was administered
orally in soluble form without adjuvant. A primary IgE response
did not occur. The subsequent challenge which tested for
responsiveness therefore had to consist of a known immunogenic
stimulus (usually antigen + adjuvant intraperitoneally) in

order to demonstrate a suppression of response in the treated
animals in comparison with previously untreated control
animals.

Turning now to the situation where antibody production
precedes suppression, this is illustrated by some experiments
which we conducted a few years ago. We found that many rats
which had been immunised by the administration of oral antigen
and adjuvant produced a circulating IgE response. A subsequent
oral challenge without adjuvant resulted in a secondary IgE
response the magnitude of which was inversely proportional to
the amount of antigen given in the priming event. In other
words animals which had been primed with a small amount of
antigen gave good booster responses while in animals primed
with a large dose, booster responses were depressed or absent
(Jarrett et al., 1976).

This is illustrated in the results reproduced below. Our
previous experience with parenteral immunisation had shown that
Hooded Lister rats could be stimulated to IgE production with
as little as 1 μg EA if given with adjuvant (Jarrett and
Stewart, 1974). In performing our first oral antigen
experiment we had assumed that a far larger dose of antigen
would require to be given by this route than by intraperitoneal
injection but, as the results in Figure 1 show, as little as
10 μg EA was sufficient to stimulate an IgE response in a
proportion of rats and most of the remainder had evidently
been primed as they produced a marked secondary response on
challenge one month later. However, as the primary dose of
antigen was increased the secondary response to the subsequent
challenge became progressively poorer, until, in most of the
rats which had received 100 mg EA on the first occasion it
failed to occur at all. Figure 2 shows the results of another
experiment which verified this phenomenon and which also
included a second challenge. Thus the immunising stimulus
which induces an IgE response can also activate a counteracting
antigen-specific suppressive mechanism which comes to
predominate with the activation of memory cells.

Oral suppression of IgE responsiveness in the rat may, or may not be accompanied by suppression of immunoglobulin of other classes depending on the tolerising protocol. Our (unpublished) experiments show that pretreatment with soluble antigen, if given in large enough amounts (e.g. 100 mg EA), leads to the suppression of both IgE and IgG responses to a subsequent immunising stimulus, while pretreatment with a much smaller amount of antigen (e.g. 1 mg EA) given with adjuvant results in the suppression of IgE responses alone.

To summarise, in common with the induction of an IgE response by parenteral immunisation, the stimulation of IgE antibodies by presenting antigens to mucosal surfaces requires attention to the strain of animal to be used, the antigen dose and the type of adjuvant. Suppression or abrogation of IgE responsiveness on the other hand is relatively easily achieved even in high IgE responder animals by the administration of a single moderately large dose of antigen or repeated stimulation with smaller amounts. The evidence available at present does not indicate any effective mechanistic difference between IgE regulation achieved by presenting antigens to the mucosae or IgE regulation by parenteral injection of antigen.

IMPLICATIONS

My own interest in the experiments I have discussed is to understand what may be going on in the normal non-allergic animal as a result of the ingestion and inhalation of potentially allergenic materials. If an IgE response is not eventually to occur, through chance conjunction of antigen and adjuvant delivery or through sheer persistence of the immunogenic stimulus, there must either be a mechanism for keeping immunogenic amounts of antigen out or the response must be actively suppressed by immune regulation. However we know that antigens are absorbed across the mucosae in amounts which in terms of the IgE system are adequate not only to stimulate but also to suppress. Therefore the second of the two mechanisms seems the most probable.

My contention then is that the absence of IgE response and the freedom of normal individuals from allergy to dietary or inhaled antigens depends on the normal absorption of amounts of antigen which are sufficient to activate the IgE suppressive mechanisms (Jarrett, 1977). In this view allergies to dietary antigens arise out of deficiencies or dysfunction of one or more components of the IgE regulatory apparatus. Although these deficiencies are genetically determined they may be overcome to a greater or lesser extent by stimulation with antigen in larger than usual amounts, or by stimulation with antigen and adjuvant.

One practical implication of the experimental results is not far to seek. At least a proportion of individuals with allergies are known to benefit from hyposensitisation therapy, in which the offending allergen in natural or modified form is injected parenterally in graded doses over a period of time. I see no reason why hyposensitising preparations should not be fed rather than injected and indeed Wortmann (1977) reports the efficacy of such treatment for paediatric allergy in a number of hospitals in Switzerland where it has apparently been carried out for some time. Further trials of oral or perhaps nasal hyposensitisation are clearly called for.

ACKNOWLEDGEMENT

The work described here was supported by grants from the Medical Research Council, the Wellcome Trust and INSERM (France). The author is a Locke Research Fellow of the Royal Society.

148

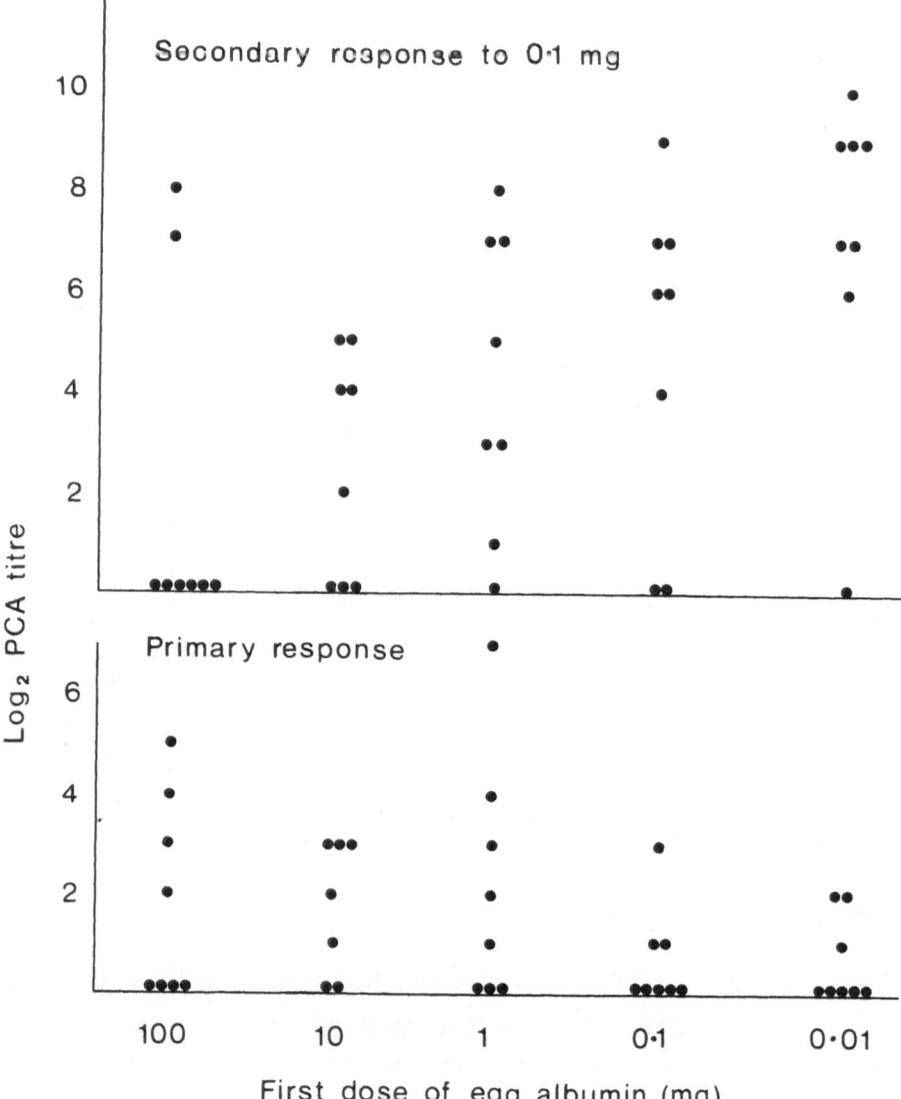

Fig. 1.   IgE response to intragastric egg-albumin. The animals were
immunised with the indicated amounts of antigen administered by
stomach tube. *Bordetella pertussis* was given by intraperitoneal
injection. One month later the rats were challenged with
intragastric antigen, but adjuvant was not given. The values
shown are for the primary IgE response on day 12 after
immunisation and the booster response on day 4 after challenge.
The values for the booster response are significantly different
(P < 0.05) (Kruskal-Wallis non parametric analysis of variance
(Siegal, 1956)). The figure depicts the results shown in Table
3 of Jarrett et al., 1976.

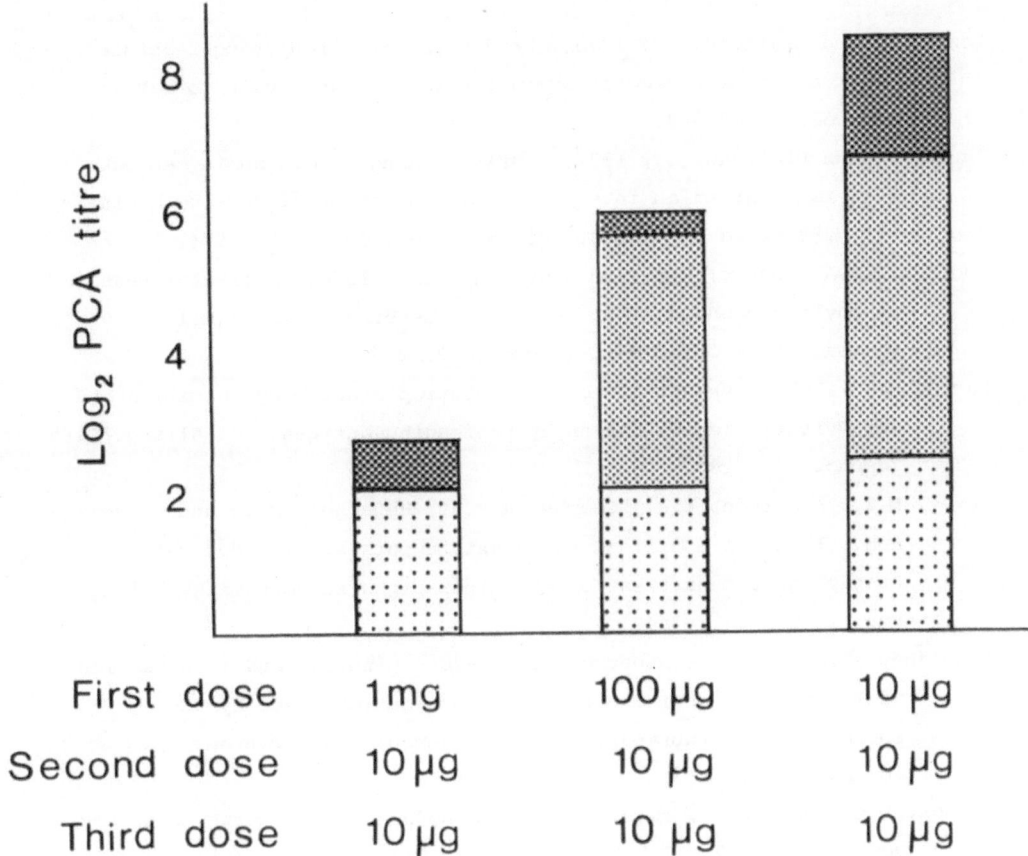

Fig. 2. IgE response to intragastric egg-albumin. The animals (6/group) were immunised with the indicated amounts of antigen as in the experiment described in Figure 1, and challenged one and two months later with 10 μg EA administered by stomach tube. Shown are the mean EA-PCA titres 12 days after initial immunisation and the increments resulting 4 days after antigen challenge. The levels of both the first and second booster responses are significantly different (P < 0.02). The figure depicts the results shown in Table 4 of Jarrett et al., 1976.

REFERENCES

Bazin, H. and Platteau, B., 1976. Production of circulating reaginic
        (IgE) antibodies by oral administration of ovalbumin to rats.
        Immunology 30, 679.

Bazin, H. and Platteau, B., 1977.   Oral feeding of ovalbumin can make
        rats tolerant to an intraperitoneal injection of DNP-ovalbumin
        and *Bordetella pertussis*. Biochem. Soc. Trans. 5, 1571.

Coombs, R.R.A., Devey, M.E. and Anderson, K.J., 1978. Refractoriness to
        anaphylactic shock after continuous feeding of cows' milk to
        guinea-pigs. Clin. Exp. Immunol. 32, 263.

David, M.F., 1977. Prevention of homocytotropic antibody formation and
        anaphylactic sensitisation by prefeeding antigen. J. Allerg. Clin.
        Immunol. 60, 180.

Devey, M.E., Anderson, K.J., Coombs, R.R.A., Henschel, M.J. and Coates,
        M.E., 1976. A modified anaphylaxis hypothesis for cot death.
        Anaphylactic sensitisation in guinea-pigs fed cows milk. Clin.
        Exp. Immunol. 26, 542.

Gerbrandy, J.L.F. and Bienenstock, J., 1976. Kinetics and localisation
        of IgE tetanus antibody response in mice immunised by the
        intratracheal, intraperitoneal and subcutaneous routes.
        Immunology 31, 913.

Hanson, D.G., Vaz, N.M., Maia, L.C.S., Hornbrook, M.M., Lynch, J.M. and
        Roy, C.A., 1977. Inhibition of specific immune responses by
        feeding protein antigens.   Int. Arch. Allergy 55, 526.

Hanson, D.G., Vaz, N.M., Rawlings, L.A. and Lynch, J.M., 1979a.
        Inhibition of specific immune responses by feeding protein antigens.
        II Effect of prior passive and active immunisation. J. Immunol.
        122, 2261.

Hanson, D.G., Vaz, N.M., Maia, L.C.S. and Lynch, J.M., 1979b. Inhibition
        of specific immune responses by feeding protein antigens. III
        Evidence against maintenance of tolerance to ovalbumin by orally
        induced antibodies. J. Immunol. 123, 2337.

Hof, H., Finger, H., Korner, C. and Milke, C., 1975. Studies on the
        immunising capacity of orally administered particulate antigen.
        I Efficacy of killed *Bordetella pertussis* cells. Zbl Bact. Hyg.
        I. Abt. Orig. A. 230, 210.

Jarrett, E.E.E. and Stewart, D.C., 1974. Rat IgE Production. I Effect
     of dose of antigen on primary and secondary reaginic antibody
     responses.   Immunology 27, 365.

Jarrett, E.E.E., Haig, D., McDougal, W. and McNulty, E., 1976. Rat IgE
     Production II. Primary and booster reaginic antibody responses
     following intradermal or oral immunisation.   Immunology 30, 671.

Jarrett, E.E.E., 1977. Activation of IgE regulatory mechanisms by
     transmucosal absorption of antigen.   Lancet ii 223.

Ngan, J. and Kind, L.S., 1978. Suppressor T cells for IgG and IgE in
     Peyers patches of mice made tolerant by oral administration of
     ovalbumin. J. Immunol. 120, 861.

Perelmutter, L. and Liakopoulou, A., 1975. Production of rat
     homocytotropic antibodies using low dose long term oral exposure
     to penicillin G. Acta Allergol. 30, 250.

Ratner, B. and Gruehl, H.L., 1933. Passage of native proteins through
     the normal gastrointestinal wall. J. Clin. Invest. 13, 517.

Siegal, S., 1956. Non parametric statistics p. 184. McGraw-Hill, Tokyo.

Van Hout, C. and Johnson, H., 1972. Synthesis of rat IgE by aerosol
     immunisation. J. Immunol. 108, 834.

Vaz, N.M., Maia, L.C.S., Hanson, D.G. and Lynch, J.M., 1977. Inhibition
     of homocytotropic antibody responses in adult inbred mice by
     previous feeding of the specific antigen. J. Allerg. Clin.
     Immunol. 60, 110.

Wells, H.G. and Osborne, T.B., 1911. The biological reactions of the
     vegetable proteins I Anaphylaxis. J. Infect. Dis. 8, 66.

Wortmann, F., 1977. Oral hyposensitisation of children with pollinosis
     or house-dust asthma. Allergol et Immunopathol. 5, 15-26.

152

DISCUSSION

<u>K. Petzoldt</u> *(FRG)*

Does the suppression which Dr. Jarrett mentioned concerning the entero-gastric application of antigen also operate if antigen is given via the respiratory tract?

<u>Ellen Jarrett</u> *(UK)*

I do not think anybody has done work on this, except perhaps John Bienenstock.

<u>J. Bienenstock</u> *(Canada)*

There is one report by John Turk, and I think he used picryl chloride.

<u>Ellen Jarrett</u>

But that was not for IgE.

<u>J. Bienenstock</u>

It was not for IgE, but that is the only report which exists of suppression via the respiratory tract, to my knowledge

<u>K. Petzoldt</u>

The reason I asked is that it is astonishing how seldom any IgE mediated reaction is seen when giving inactivated and other antigens via the respiratory tract.

<u>Ellen Jarrett</u>

I do not think that there has been any actual report of the induction of Ig suppression by giving antigens to the respiratory tract, but I would imagine that it would be very similar to giving antigens orally. If enough antigen is put in then I see no reason why it should not work in exactly the same way, but that particular experiment still remains to be done.

J. Soothill

Of course, the other problem is that of giving something to the respiratory tract without giving it to the gastro-intestinal tract. I think that is going to be a difficult question to answer, but it is clearly relevant to Dr. Bienen-stock's point.

FOOD ANTIGEN HANDLING AND IMMUNE COMPLEX FORMATION IN HEALTHY AND ALLERGIC INDIVIDUALS

R.J. Levinsky, R. Paganelli, D.M. Robertson and D.J. Atherton
Department of Immunology, Institute of Child Health,
30 Guilford Street, London WC1, UK.

ABSTRACT

Food proteins may cross the gastrointestinal mucosa antigenically intact and elicit an immune response which in most individuals is not damaging. We have investigated the levels of milk protein antigens circulating after feeding in pre-term babies, normal children and adults and compared the type of immune response elicited with that found in atopic subjects challenged with the food substance to which they react.

Very high levels of circulating B lactoglobulin (up to 100 µg/l) were found in premature infants fed a cows' milk based formula (SMA). The levels varied according to gestational age with highest levels obtained in babies of 28 - 32 weeks whereas the levels found in babies near or at full-term were akin to those of older children and adults (1 - 3 µg/l). This suggests that gut closure usually occurs in humans prior to birth.

Using an immune complex splitting assay and ones which demonstrate the immunoglobulin class involved, we have shown that in normal adults immune complexes containing β lactoglobulin and BSA circulate after drinking milk and the predominant immunoglobulin class involved is IgA. In contrast, children and adults with atopic eczema after eating milk or eggs have higher levels of circulating antigen and/or antigen containing complexes and the immunoglobulin classes involved are predominantly IgG and IgE. The complexes also react with Clq. These differences in immune response to oral antigens will be discussed in relation to mechanisms of oral tolerance in normal individuals and the immuno-pathology of the disease in patients with atopic eczema.

INTRODUCTION

The gastrointestinal tract serves two main functions; the first is as a digestive organ which actively absorbs nutrients, and the second is to provide a barrier against macromolecular antigen entry. This barrier between the gastrointestinal contents and body tissues is incomplete for there is now ample evidence that antigen entry occurs across the mucosa in all healthy individuals (reviewed by Walker and Isselbacher, 1974). The amounts which enter the circulation are insignificant nutritionally but are sufficient to immunise since antibodies to food proteins may be demonstrated to low titres in most healthy people (Peterson and Good, 1965). These antibodies are apparently not damaging and probably facilitate safe elimination of circulating food antigens. Adverse reactions do not occur in the majority of individuals in response to antigen entry; protective homeostatic mechanisms prevail and hypersensitivity reactions to food proteins are the exception.

Oral immunisation elicits a local immune response in which secretory IgA antibody (SIgA) complexes with antigen within the gut lumen thereby substantially reducing antigen entry into the circulation (Ogra and Karzon, 1970). In addition to this local immune mechanism, a state of systemic hyporesponsiveness or 'oral tolerance' is produced in which the individual is incapable of mounting an appropriate antibody response when the same antigen is subsequently given parenterally (Chase, 1946; Thomas and Parrott, 1974; Swarbrick et al, 1979). The mechanisms for maintaining this state of oral tolerance are not understood, but there is evidence from studies in mice that serum factors such as immune complexes (André et al, 1975) or IgG_1 antibody (Chalon et al, 1979) may be involved. Suppressor T cells may be generated by oral antigen administration, but as this is only transient it is unlikely to provide the entire answer (Richman et al, 1979).

Food allergy may be regarded as a major breakdown in oral tolerance. In order to understand some of the mechanisms

involved in food tolerance and how this breakdown results in
damage to food allergic patients, we have studied food antigen
handling by the gut in healthy individuals and compared their
responses to those obtained in food allergic patients.

Gut closure in man

In many species of animals the neonatal gut is initially
freely permeable to macromolecules and acquisition of maternal
immunoglobulin is derived via breast feeding. After a variable
time in different species the mucosal cells abruptly come
together to form tight junctions. This phenomenon, known as gut
closure, may be enhanced by certain factors in colostrum (Walker,
1979). Little is known about man but it is thought that gut
closure, if it occurs, must be prior to birth. Food antigen
entry has been reported in normal healthy babies as early as five
days after birth (Gruskay and Cooke, 1955), but in no greater
amounts than that absorbed by older children. In order to see
when gut closure occurs in man, we have studied food antigen
entry in premature babies. The babies' gestational age ranged
from 28 weeks to full term and each baby was studied 24 hours
after the introduction of a cows' milk based formula (SMA) given
hourly by nasogastric tube. The amounts fed were according to
birthweight. A blood sample was taken 30 minutes after the feed.
Several of the babies were initially started on breast milk but
for reasons of inadequate supply changed to the SMA formula after
the first 24 hours. The babies were also given the formula feed
before study. Using a solid phase radioimmunoassay to measure
serum levels of β lactoglobulin (Paganelli and Levinsky, 1980), a
protein which is present to a concentration of 3 mg/ml in cows'
milk, we have shown that many of the very premature infants
absorb considerably greater quantities of antigenically intact
protein that do full term babies (Table 1).

There was great variation in the levels of β lactoglobulin
absorbed but several of the very premature babies absorbed as
much as 70 - 80 ng/ml, an enormous amount in comparison to that
absorbed by healthy adults (see later). Only two premature
infants in the older gestational age group absorbed moderately

large amounts. These findings suggest that gut closure is a
pre-term event in humans, and although there is great variation,
has occurred usually by the 36th week of gestation.

TABLE 1

LEVELS OF β LACTOGLOBULIN IN PREMATURE INFANTS

Gestational age	28-35 weeks	35-40 weeks
1. SMA only	(n=12) mean 9.7 ng/ml (range 0.1-100 ng/ml)	(n=6) mean 5.0 ng/ml (range 0-25 ng/ml)
2. Breast milk for 24 hours then SMA	(n=5) mean 4.9 ng/ml (range 0-24 ng/ml)	NONE

Interestingly, those very premature infants initially
fed breast milk before going on to the cows' milk based formula
did not absorb such large amounts, indicating that some factor
in breast milk enhanced gut closure in these infants.

Antigen absorption in healthy adults

Five healthy non-atopic adults were studied by taking
sequential blood samples over a five hour period following the
ingestion of 1.2 litres of fresh cows' milk. The blood samples
were analysed for free circulating β lactoglobulin (Paganelli
and Levinsky, 1980), for immune complexes containing IgG and for
IgA (Levinsky and Soothill, 1977), for Clq binding immune complexes (Zubler et al, 1976) and for the antigen within the
immune complexes (Paganelli et al, 1979). This latter technique
involves immune complex enrichment by polyethylene glycol
precipitation; the complex is then dissociated in acid buffer
and the constituents are absorbed onto a plastic surface. After
neutral pH washing, the antigen is detected by using a
radiolabelled affinity purified specific antibody and the antibody detected by using radiolabelled antigen. Radioactive
counts bound to the plastic solid phase give an indication of

either antigen or antibody concentration within the immune complex.

After drinking 1.2 litres of milk, β lactoglobulin was found in the circulation within 30 minutes; in most of the individuals a second peak of absorption was demonstrated at 4 - 5 hours. The levels attained in all subjects were no greater than 3 ng/ml. This two peak distribution of antigen was a consistent finding and since it also occurs in animals never previously exposed to the antigen, it probably represents two different routes of absorption, the first into the portal circulation and the slower one into the lymphatics and then into the circulation.

We have previously demonstrated circulating soluble immune complexes following milk ingestion in healthy subjects (Paganelli et al, 1979). When these sera were analysed for the type of immune complex there was very little variation in the levels of IgG and Clq binding immune complexes, but all the subjects studied showed a large rise in IgA complexes again occurring within 30 minutes of ingestion and falling to baseline after approximately 90 minutes. Using the immune complex splitting technique, both β lactoglobulin and bovine serum albumin (BSA) have been demonstrated to be antigenic constituents of these complexes. A representative profile of β lactoglobulin absorption, IgA, IgG and Clq binding complexes and the two antigens within the complexes is shown in Figure 1.

These results indicate that serum IgA is involved in clearing antigens from the circulation; the fact that monomeric IgA does not activate complement or elicit other damaging reactions makes it the ideal class of immunoglobulin for safely eliminating circulating food proteins.

Route of immunisation and antibody response

It is possible that the small amounts of antigen continually entering the circulation via the gastrointestinal mucosa is a necessary prerequisite for maintaining an effective IgA antibody

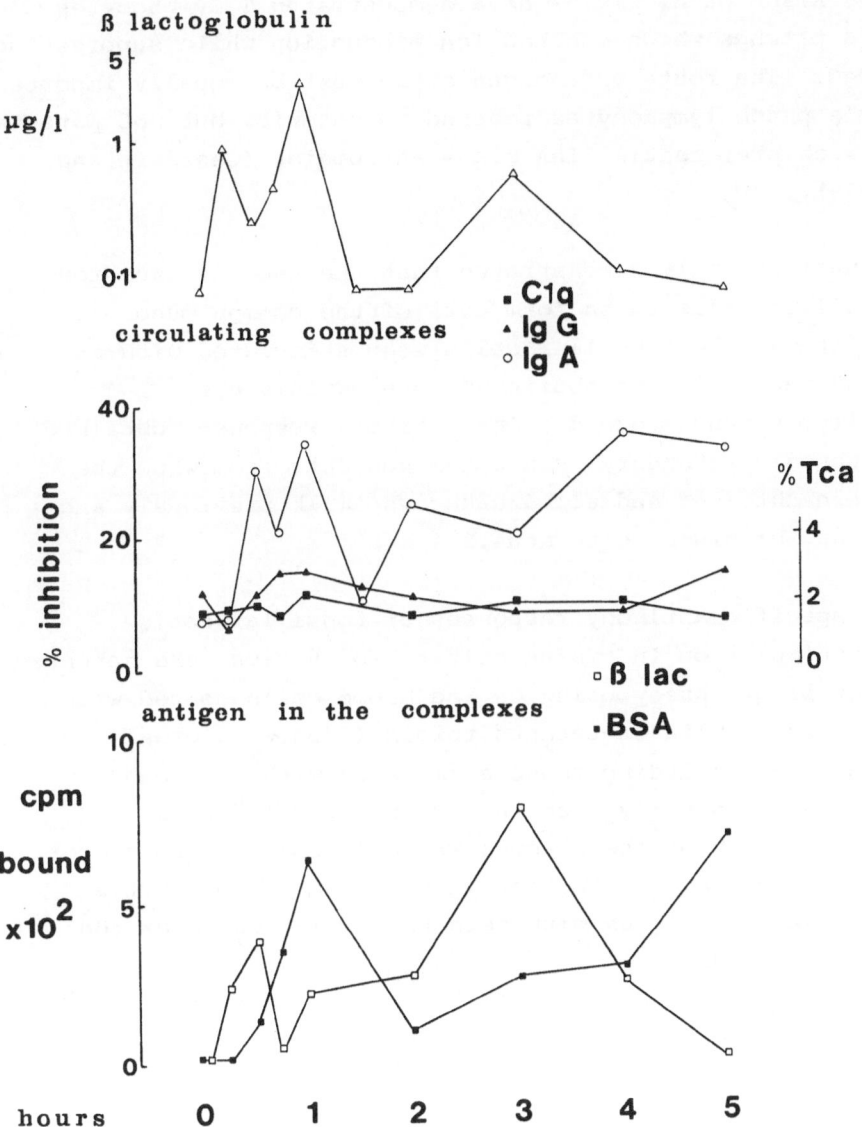

Fig. 1. Representative profile of antigen absorption (β lactoglobulin) and immune complex formation (IgG, IgA and Clq binding complexes) in a healthy non-atopic adult after drinking 1.2 litres of fresh cows' milk. Both bovine serum albumin and β lactoglobulin were shown to be antigenic constituents of the IgA immune complexes.

response. Elson et al (1979) have demonstrated T lymphocytes
in Peyer's patches which enhance IgA production while suppressing
IgM and IgG. The route of antigen entry must be equally important
for Peyer's patch lymphocytes respond to enteric, but not parenteral
antigens with preferential IgA class antibodies (Gearhart and
Cebra, 1979).

We have recently demonstrated that the same is true for
human tonsillar cells which form part of the common mucosal
immunce system. The tonsillar cells were stimulated with an
enteric antigen, β lactoglobulin and one administered
parenterally, tetanus toxoid. The antibody responses obtained
were undoubtedly secondary, since the subjects from whom the
tonsils were obtained had all drunk cows' milk previously and
had all been immunised to tetanus.

The specific antibody responses of tonsillar cells
following stimulation in tissue culture for 6 days were detected
by a direct plaque assay using ox red blood cells coated with
either β lactoglobulin or tetanus toxoid (Gronowicz et al, 1976).
Control cultures including those stimulated with pokeweed
mitogen gave consistently less than 30 plaques/10^6 cells.
Antigen specificity of the plaques was confirmed by cross-over
experiments in which β lactoglobulin stimulated lymphocytes
failed to generate plaques with tetanus toxoid coated ox red
cells and vice versa.

The reverse haemolytic plaque assay, in which ox red
cells were coated with staph. protein A and immunoglobulin class
specific antisera used to develop the plaques, was used to
determine the isotype of the immunoglobulin secreted. At
optimal doses, stimulation with tetanus toxoid produced mainly
IgG and IgM plaques, while a predominant IgA response was induced
by the food antigen β lactoglobylin (Table 2). The antigens
we used to stimulate the tonsillar lymphocytes are T dependent
and the preferential IgA antibody produced in response to
β lactoglobulin probably represents in general the type of
immune response by gut associated lymphoid tissues after initial

contact at the mucosal level. Gearhart and Cebra (1979)
suggested that the role of gut antigens may be to clonally
expand IgA precursors and perhaps to stimulate the proliferation
of less differentiated cells within the unique microenvironment
of the Peyer's patches, allowing them to develop into IgA
precursors.

TABLE 2

DIRECT PLAQUE ASSAY FOR ANTIGEN SPECIFIC PLAQUES

β lactoglobulin	mean $\pm$ SEM 117 $\pm$ 14
Tetanus toxoid	mean $\pm$ SEM 360 $\pm$ 62

INDIRECT PLAQUE ASSAY FOR IMMUNOGLOBULIN CLASS

	IgG	IgA	IgM
β lactoglobulin	253 $\pm$ 40	430 $\pm$ 77	224 $\pm$ 48
Tetanus toxoid	871 $\pm$ 30	110 $\pm$ 15	666 $\pm$ 136

Number of plaques are expressed as the mean $\pm$ SEM for three separate tonsils.
Experiments done in duplicate. Background unstimulated plaques have been
subtracted from stimulated ones.

Hence it is likely that the route of antigen entry as
well as the unique microenvironment of the gut-associated
lymphoid system is important for maintaining the IgA immune
response both at local and systemic levels and thereby
providing a safe mechanism for dealing with enteric antigens.
It is probable that the continual macromolecular absorption of
food and other antigens is a vital physiological requirement
for maintaining mucosal immunity at sites other than the
gastrointestinal tract. Lymphocytes primed by antigen entering
via the gastrointestinal mucosa home to gut-associated lymphoid
tissues such as the salivary and mammary glands where the cells
are capable of producing specific antibody to such enterically
deprived antigens. An example of this is the *E. coli*
lipopolysaccharide specific secretory IgA antibody demonstrated

in the colostrum of women fed live non-pathogenic *E. coli* bacteria during pregnancy (Goldblum et al, 1975).

The relevance of the IgA response to orally ingested antigens has yet to be established; little is known about the role of IgA apart from studies of external secretions where the immunoglobulin has been shown to have antibody activity (Turner and Rowe, 1964) and to function in immune exclusion (Stokes et al, 1975). Although our observations of IgA complexes produced, *in vivo*, in healthy adults following food ingestion suggest that serum IgA is involved in eliminating food antigens from the circulation, it does not establish the mechanism of oral tolerance. We still do not know how circulating IgA immune complexes are handled by the reticuloendothelial system or whether serum factors act in a negative feedback manner to maintain systemic hyporesponsiveness. In mice, IgG_1 antibody provides such feedback control (Chalon et al, 1979) but this is not necessarily true for man and we must retain an open mind as to whether serum IgA in complexed form plays any part in oral food tolerance.

Antigen entry in food allergic subjects

We have studied food antigen entry in children and adults with food allergy in whom the predominant symptoms were eczema, but some of the patients experienced bronchospasm after ingestion of either milk or eggs. The patients were given a cocktail of raw eggs and milk to drink; the amount administered was according to body weight. All of the patients were skin prick tested to individual milk and egg antigens and a dietary history of symptom exacerbation in response to either foodstuff obtained. Using the same techniques, we estimated free circulating antigen (β lactoglobulin and ovalbumin), IgG, IgA and Clq binding immune complexes and the antigens contained within the immune complexes. Higher levels of free circulating antigen (up to 15 ng/ml) were obtained in the food allergic patients than in the healthy non-atopic subjects fed an equivalent antigenic load. In contrast to the IgA immune complexes formed in response to food challenge in the non-atopic individuals, the food allergic individuals formed immune complexes containing IgG and IgE (Brostoff et al, 1979) as well as Clq binding ones (Paganelli et al, 1979). These immune complexes were shown to contain the food antigens β lact-oglobulin and ovalbumin by means of the immune complex splitting technique. In the majority of the patients the two peak distribution of antigen entry and immune complex formation was observed. Of interest was the observation that those patients who were skin prick test positive to the ingested food produced predominantly IgG and Clq binding complexes, whereas the skin test negative patients had higher levels of IgA complexes.

The drug Sodium Cromoglycate is thought to prevent mast cell degranulation by inhibiting the calcium influx across the cell membrane. When patients were pretreated with 1 g of oral Sodium Cromoglycate prior to ingestion of the food to which they were allergic, not only were the symptoms of skin itching and wheezing abolished, but antigen entry and immune complex formation were substantially reduced. (Figures 2 and 3).

Such clear differences in the antibody response between healthy and food allergic individuals emphasises the role of serum IgA in immune elimination. Indeed IgA deficiency is associated with food allergies (Buckley and Dees, 1969) and low levels of serum IgA have been noted in healthy infants at the age of three months who later became atopic (Taylor et al, 1973). It is unlikely that the development of food allergies is due to excessive stimulation of the immune system by large amounts of antigen crossing the gastrointestinal mucosa. The very large amounts we have demonstrated in premature babies is against this; it is more likely that the timing of antigenic exposure is critical and whether the antigen is presented together with an adjuvant. Thus, in rats, IgE responses may be elicited by a small dose of antigen when orally administered together with a powerful adjuvant (Jarrett et al, 1976). In the bottle-fed neonate, bacterial colonisation of the gut with *E. coli* could provide the necessary adjuvant, but sensitisation would only occur in the immunodeficient child. Transient IgA deficiency may be one such predisposing factor, but the association of the yeast opsonisation defect (an abnormality of the alternative complement pathway) and also heterozygous C_2 deficiency with allergy (Turner et al, 1978), suggests that others are also important.

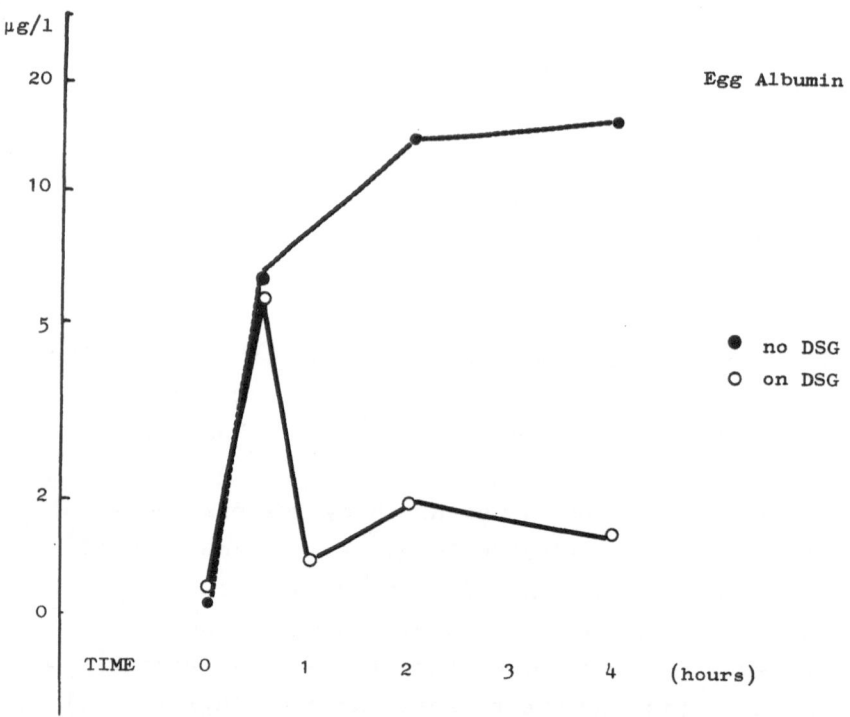

Fig. 2. Levels of circulating ovalbumin in the sera of a food allergic patient after eating 2 eggs. Prior treatment with Sodium Cromoglycate greatly reduces antigen entry but does not abolish the early 30 minute peak found in non-allergic individuals after similar antigenic challenge.

Mechanism of injury in atopic eczema

There is considerable evidence that atopic eczema is caused by allergy to ingested food (Atherton et al, 1978). We have shown that such patients absorb considerably greater quantities of food antigens into the circulation. The increase in antigen entry is facilitated when triggering of IgE sensitised mast cells occurs within the gut mucosal lining. These mast cells

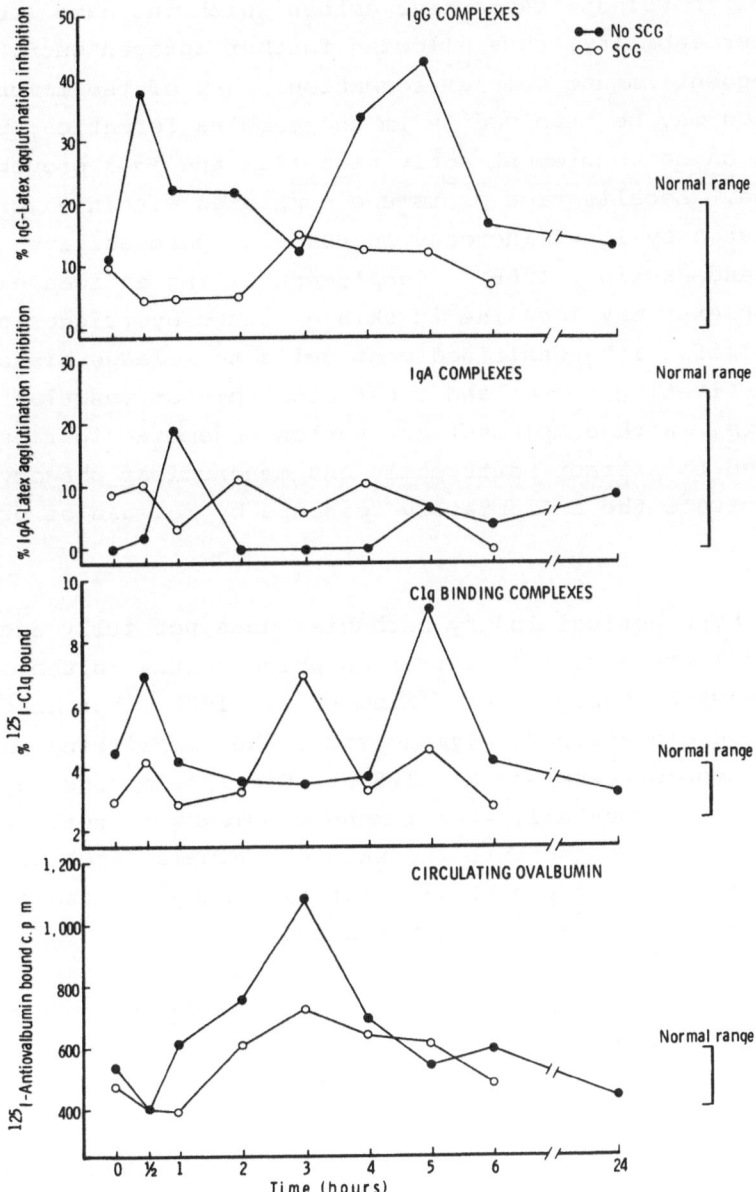

Fig. 3.   Representative profile of immune complex formation and antigen
absorption (ovalbumin) in a food allergic patient with eczema
and asthma.   The complexes following ingestion of two lightly
boiled eggs contained ovalbumin and were predominantly IgG and
Clq binding.   Prior treatment with oral Sodium Cromoglycate
blocked much of the antigen entry and immune complex formation as
well as abolishing symptoms of bronchospasm.

(Reproduced with permission Lancet i: 1270 (1979)).

degranulate to release vasoactive amines which increase local
vascular permeability, thus allowing further antigen entry
with subsequent immune complex formation. Any of the immunoglobulin classes may be involved in immune complex formation, but
those that cause complement activation (IgM and IgG) provoke
most damage. Localisation of immune complexes within an organ
is facilitated by local increase in vascular permeability
(Cochrane and Hawkins, 1968). Complement fixing antigen excess
immune complexes may localise in skin or lungs by triggering
antigen specific IgE sensitised mast cells to release histamine,
platelet activating factor and other mediators of vascular
permeability. With complement activation, chemotactic factors
are released to attract neutrophils and mononuclear phagocytes
which accentuate the inflammatory response by release of proteolytic enzymes.

This hypothetical injury mechanism does not fully account
for the small round cell infiltration which occurs in the skin
of patients with atopic eczema (Mihm et al, 1976), but histamine
may also be chemotactic for lymphocytes, thus amplifying this
mechanism (Smorgorzewska et al, 1980). Similar lesions may also
be produced experimentally when immune complexes in suitable
proportions are injected into the skin of animals (Spector and
Heeson, 1969). The lymphocyte infiltration suggests that some
of the damage may be lymphokine mediated.

These observations in food allergy provide evidence for
the inter-relationships of Type I IgE mediated and Type III immune
complex mediated hypersensitivity reactions. They may provide
the explanation for the 'late' 6 hour responses that have been
observed in a variety of clinical situations in association with
Type I hypersensitivity reactions (Solley et al, 1976; Pelikan,
1978). Sodium Cromoglycate is a poorly absorbed drug and its
effect in food allergy is probably by local inhibition of gut
mast cell degranulation, thereby reducing vascular permeability
and further antigen entry. The fact that both early and late
reactions were blocked by this drug further emphasises the close
inter-relationship of hypersensitivity injury mechanisms.

Relevance of food antigen entry to other diseases

The symptoms of food allergy are numerous; it may produce local gut effects such as the bleeding and diarrhoea of cows' milk allergy (Collins-Williams, 1962), systemic effects such as skin rashes, urticaria or eczema (Atherton et al, 1978), asthma (Buisseret, 1978), migraine (Monro et al, 1980) and there are even reports of patients with rheumatoid arthritis in whom joint symptoms are substantially improved by a diet free of certain foods (Catterall, 1979). There are also anecdotal reports of sensitivity to food substances causing psychiatric disturbances with the mood and behaviour changes being abolished by avoidance of the offending food (Singh and Kay, 1976; Tryphonas and Trites, 1979). The relevance of food antigen absorption in gastro-intestinal diseases such as coeliac disease (Kenrick and Walker-Smith, 1970), inflammatory bowel diseases (Jewell and Hodgson, 1976 and even children with malnutrition (Chandra, 1975), all conditions associated with a higher incidence of precipitating antifood antibodies, is as yet far from clear.

Now that techniques are available for measuring such antigen absorption in humans, it may become possible to establish whether food allergy is a major part of these and other diseases. In addition, the critical question to answer is what causes a breakdown in oral food tolerance and what can be done to restore the balance?

ACKNOWLEDGEMENTS

We are grateful to the Nuffield Foundation (RP), the MRC (DJA) and Fisons Ltd. (RJL) for financial support.

168

REFERENCES

André, C., Heremans, J.F., Vaerman, J.P. and Cambiaso, 1975. A mechanism for the induction of immunological tolerance by antigen feeding: antigen-antibody complexes. J. Exp. Med. 142: 1509.

Atherton, D.J., Soothill, J.F., Sewell, M., Wells, R.S. and Chilvers, C.E.D., 1978. A double blind crossover trial of an antigen-avoidance diet in atopic eczema. Lancet 1: 401.

Brostoff, J., Carini, C., Wraith, D.G., Paganelli, R. and Levinsky, R.J., 1979. Immune complexes in atopy. In: The Mast Cells (eds Pepys, J. and Edwards, A.M.) Pitman, London. p. 380.

Buckley, R.H. and Dees, S.C., 1969. Correlation of milk precipitins with IgA deficiency. N.E.J.M. 281: 465.

Buisseret, P.D., 1978. Common manifestations of cows' milk allergy in children. Lancet i: 304.

Catterall, W.E., 1979. Allergy and arthritis, Ann. Rheum. Dis. 36: 594.

Chalon, M.P., Milne, R.W. and Vaerman, J.P., 1979. In vitro immunosuppressive effect of serum from orally immunised mice. Eur. J. of Imm. 9: 747.

Chandra, R.K., 1975. Food antibodies in malnutrition. Arch. Dis. Child. 50: 532.

Chase, M.S., 1946. Inhibition of experimental drug allergy by prior feeding of the sensitising agent. Proc. of Soc. Exp. Biol. and Med. (N.Y.) 61: 257.

Cochrane, C.G. and Hawkins, D., 1968. Studies on circulating immune complexes III. Factors governing the ability of circulating complexes to localise in blood vessels. J. Exp. Med. 127: 137.

Collins-Williams, C., 1962. Cows' milk allergy in infants and children. Int. Arch. of Allergy 20: 38.

Elson, C.O., Heck, J.A. and Strober, W., 1979. T cell regulation of murine IgA synthesis. J. Exp. Med. 149: 632.

Gearhart, P.J. and Cebra, J.J., 1979. Differentiated β lymphocytes. Potential to express particular antibody variable and constant regions depends on site of lymphoid tissue and antigen load. J. Exp. Med. 149: 216.

Goldblum, R.M., Ahlstedt, S., Carlsson, B., Hanson, L.A., Jodal, U., Lidin-Janson, G. and Sohl-Akerlund, A., 1975. Antibody-forming cells in human colostrum after oral immunisation. Nature 257:797.

Gronowicz, E., Coutinho, A. and Melchers, F., 1976. A plaque assay for all
    cells secreting immunolgobulin of a given type or class. Eur. J.
    Immunol. 6: 588.

Grusklay, F.L. and Cooke, R.E., 1955. The gastrointestinal absorption of
    unaltered protein in normal infants and in infants recovering from
    diarrhoea. Pediatrics 16: 763.

Jarrett, E.E.E., Haig, D.M., McDougall, W. and McNulty, E., 1976. Rat IgE
    production II. Primary and booster reaginic antibody responses following
    intradermal or oral immunisation. Imminology 30: 671.

Jewell, D.P. and Hodgson, H.J.F., 1976. Autoimmune and inflammatory disease
    of the gastrointestinal tract. In: Immunological Aspects of the Liver
    and Gastrointestinal Tract (ed. Ferguson, A. and McSween, R.N.M.) MTP
    Press, Lancaster, p 208.

Kenrick, R.G. and Walker-Smith, J.A., 1970. Immunoglobulins and dietary
    protein antibodies in childhood coeliac disease. Gut 11: 635.

Levinsky, R.J. and Soothill, J.F., 1977. A test for antigen-antibody
    complexes in human sera using IgM of rabbit antisera to human
    immunoglobulins. Clin. Exp. Immunol. 29: 428.

Mihm, M.C., Soter, N.A., Dvorak, H. and Austen, K.F., 1976. The structure
    of normal skin and the morphology of atopic eczema. J. Invest. Derm.
    67: 305.

Monro, J., Brostoff, J., Carini, C. and Zilka, K., 1980. Food allergy in
    migraine. Lancet ii: 1.

Ogra, P.L. and Karzon, D.T., 1970. The role of immunoglobulins in the
    mechanisms of mucosal immunity to viral infection. Ped. Clin. North
    Amer. 17: 385.

Paganelli, R. and Levinsky, R.J., 1980. A solid phase radioimmunoassay for
    detecting food proteins in the serum. J. Imm. Methods. In press.

Paganelli, R., Levinsky, R.J., Brostoff, J. and Wraith, D.G., 1979. Immune
    complexes containing food proteins in normal and atopic subjects after
    oral challenge and effect of Sodium Cromoglycate on antigen absorption.
    Lancet i: 1270.

Pelikan, E., 1978. Late and delayed responses of the nasal mucosa to allergen
    challenge. Ann. Allergy 41: 37.

Peterson, R.D.A. and Good, R.A., 1965. Antibodies to cows' milk proteins -
    their presence and significance. Pediatrics 31: 209.

Richman, L.K., Chiller, J.M., Brown, W.R., Hanson, D.G. and Vaz, N.M., 1979. Enterically induced immunological tolerance. 1 Induction of suppressor T lymphocytes by intragastric administration of soluble proteins. J. Immunol. 121: 2429.

Singh, M.M. and Kay, S.R., 1976. Wheat gluten as a pathogenic factor in schizophrenia. Science 191: 401.

Smorgorzewska, E., Layward, L. and Soothill, J.F., 1980. Effect of histamine on lymphocyte mobility. Clin. Exp. Immunol. In press.

Solley, G.O., Gleich, G.J., Jordan, R.E. and Schrocter, A.L., 1976. The late phase of the immediate weal and flare skin reactions. Its dependence upon IgE antibodies. J. Clin. Invest. 58: 408.

Spector, W.G. and Heeson, W., 1969. The production of granulomata by antigen-antibody complexes. J. Path. Bact. 98: 32.

Stokes, C.R., Soothill, J.F. and Turner, M.W., 1975. Immune exclusion is a function of IgA. Nature 255: 745.

Swarbrick, E.J., Stokes, C.R. and Soothill, J.F., 1979. Absorption of antigens after oral immunisation and the simultaneous induction of specific systemic tolerance. Gut. 20: 121.

Taylor, B., Norman, A.P., Orgel, H.A., Stokes, C.R., Turner, M.W. and Soothill, J.F., 1973. Transient IgA deficiency and pathogenesis of infantile atopy. Lancet 2: 111.

Thomas, H.C. and Parrott, D.M.V., 1974. The induction or tolerance to a soluble protein antigen by oral administration. Immunology 27: 631.

Tryphonas, H. and Trites, R., 1974. Food allergy in children with hyperactivity, learning disabilities and/or minimal brain dysfunction. Ann. Allergy 42: 22.

Turner, M.W. and Rowe, D.S., 1964. Characterisation of human antibodies to *S. typhi* by gel-filtration and antigenic analysis. Immunology 7: 639.

Turner, M.W., Mowbray, J.F., Harvey, B.A.M., Brostoff, J., Wells, R.S. and Soothill, J.F., 1978. Defective yeast opsonisation and C_2 deficiency in atopic patients. Clin. Exp. Imm. 34: 253.

Walker, W.A. and Isselbacher, K.J., 1974. Uptake and transport of macro-molecules by the intestine. Gastroenterology 67: 531.

Walker, W.A., 1979. Gastrointestinal host defence: Importance of gut closure in control of macromolecular transport. In: Development of Mammalian Absorptive Processes. Ciba Foundation Symposium 70: 201.

171

Zubler, R.H., Lange, G., Lambert, P.H. and Miescher, P.A., 1976. Detection of immune complexes by modified I^{125}Clq binding test. Effect of heating on the Clq binding by immune complexes and application of the test to systemic lupus erythematosus. J. Immunol. 116: 232.

DISCUSSION

Anne Ferguson *(UK)*

Dr. Levinsky used the term astronomic when he showed a
fascinating slide of antigen absorption by newborn infants, but
in fact even before what he called closure there are values of
10 - 100 µg/l of the blood level. I am not sure of the blood
volume of a 33 week premature infant.

R. Levinsky *(UK)*

It is 80 moles/kg. We worked it out in total volume of
total antigen absorbed, and it is about ten times the amount of
that absorbed by an older child.

Anne Ferguson

Yes, but the actual amount is less than 0.1 mg, it is
0.05 mg.

R. Levinsky

Yes they are small amounts but I used the term astronomic
in comparison to adult values.

Anne Ferguson

That is in fact a lot less than some of the values
claimed for animals, isn't it?

J. Soothill *(UK)*

I think this is an important point, because there still
seems to be a difference.

R. Levinsky

In our experimental terms, when one relates the amount
of antigen being absorbed it is in the order of 0.002% of the
administered antigen dose, which is much less than that claimed
for animal experiments which have been up to 2%.

G. Mayrhofer *(UK)*

With reference to the same slide, was that a sequential study on premature children up to forty weeks?

R. Levinsky

No, those were single points. The child had to be fed for 24 hours on that preparation and that was the first bleed after that 24 hours. We have done sequential studies on a few of the premature infants, and over a period of time a drop is shown.

J. Hall *(UK)*

Might I ask at what age the human infant can make an active IgA response?

R. Levinsky

One can detect IgA in a newborn by radioimmunoassay and by two weeks of age there is certainly a definite IgA response. However, it is quite difficult to make cord blood lymphocytes produce IgA in culture.

J. Soothill

There is an IgA immunoconglutinin-like reaction in newborn humans.

J. Seifert *(FRG)*

Did you study the absorption of antigen in atopic patients? Is it increased or decreased?

R. Levinsky

The patients with eczema were all atopic, as shown by skin tests and by RAST tests. It is very much increased.

J. Soothill

I think this is an important factual question which is difficult to understand in one aspect. Dr. Levinsky spoke of

skin test positive and skin test negative subjects. I think
that he meant that they were skin test positive to the antigen
with which he was testing them. They were all skin test positive to something, but Dr. Levinsky was studying some individuals who reacted to the antigen which he was using in his
investigations and others who were also atopic, also had eczema
but did not have evidence of sensitisation to the antigen to
which he was testing. Am I right?

R. Levinsky

That is correct.

GENERAL DISCUSSION

J. Soothill *(UK)*

Dr. Jarrett, have you any idea how adjuvants within the lumen of gastro-intestinal tract work?

Ellen Jarrett *(UK)*

Presumably by absorption of the adjuvant.

H. Miller *(UK)*

Could they perhaps be removing a mucous barrier? Some of them are polycations or of that nature, and they might be stripping off the mucous barrier.

J. Soothill

Thank you. I like that.

Ellen Jarrett

Why would they not be working in exactly the same way as adjuvants are working when they are administered parenterally?

J. Soothill

You mean that within the lumen, the concept of cells going into the gastro-intestinal tract meeting the antigen and the adjuvant within the gastro-intestinal tract, and finding their way back into the body?

Ellen Jarrett

The antigen and antibodies do not actually need to be combined. Yes, both of them finding their way in and then performing in exactly the same way as though they had been administered parenterally.

J. Soothill

Yes, of course. That is a possibility. I find that slighly disappointing. I liked the idea of cells being

processed within the gut and fighting their way back in, but
there is no evidence for that. Pity. I hoped you had that.
Dr. Stokes, can you tell us why there is evidence of strain
difference in the uptake of antigen?

C. Stokes (UK)

I can give a partial answer. We looked for a strain difference in the uptake of HSA and ovalbumin in different strains
of mice and we observed differences in uptake, which were up to
tenfold in different strains. We also looked in the same
strains for strain differences in the development of oral tolerance to the fed antigens and this did not correlate. The
strains which absorbed more did not become tolerant more easily.
Whether or not it is the same for the Ig response, I do not know.

J. Soothill

But there were differences in the tolerance?

C. Stokes

Yes, but they did not correlate.

J. Quinn (Ireland)

Can you comment, Dr. Levinsky, on the rate of clearance
of the immune complexes from the skin positive and the skin
negative patients in view of the receptors for IgG and C3 on
mononuclear cells and macrophages in the absence of the same
clearance mechanisms with IgA immune complexes?

R. Levinsky (UK)

Well, I am not quite sure what the clearance mechanisms
of IgA are. Certainly, the fact that we get these two peak
distributions in both the atopic and the non-atopic suggest
that clearance mechanisms are operating quite efficiently, and
one can show that the first peak has virtually gone after about
90 minutes. That is fairly rapid clearance. One always thinks
of immune-complex disease as being a constant generation of

complexes and possibly a blockade of the reticular endothelial system, such that complexes localise within tissues, but I think that is a naive and simplistic view. One has to think that complexes, whether they are generated or not, will localise within a tissue according to certain factors. One of these is size, local increase in vascular permeability is another, and specific receptors are another and I do not think that differences in rate of clearance can possibly be important in these two models. There are sufficient numbers of other differences to explain why the normals show no symptoms whereas the atopic do show symptoms in response to food ingestion.

J. Soothill

You are implying that you do not know about IgA clearance, and certainly we do not know the mechanism, but Dr. Stokes has clearly shown that it happens and I think that is one of the interests of looking at the physiological importance of the bile system, perhaps. IgA complexes are cleared, even though we do not know how.

J. Quinn

But I was inferring the IgG complexes ought perhaps to be cleared more rapidly than IgA complexes.

C. Stokes

They probably are. The clearance of the IgA complex is probably slower than the IgG ones. It is still rapid.

J. Hall (UK)

Might I just make a comment there? I do not want to go into this subject at length now, but as you say, IgA complexes are cleared by the liver and it does seem to involve the SC receptor. It is quite rapid, as rapid as the clearance made of IgA itself. This certainly can occur therefore, in experimental systems.

P. Brandtzaeg *(Norway)*

I do not think that the statement about the SC receptor refers to the human situation, because there is no evidence that there is an SC receptor on human hepatocytes.

J. Hall

One has to admit that definitive experiments have not been done but the circumstantial evidence is very compelling. That is all one can say at the moment.

P. Brandtzaeg

I think the evidence is very compelling that there is no SC receptor in human hepatocytes, but there are other IgA receptors or another IgA receptor which is different from the usual glycoprotein receptor.

J. Hall

Well, shall we just call it a receptor for IgA? We can agree on that.

R. Levinsky

Can I ask a question of Dr. André? My data in fact would support your 1975 paper on IgA complexes possibly acting as a feedback system and being partly important in oral tolerance. Do you have anything to add to this in view of what Dr. Vaerman has recently published on IgG1?

C. André *(France)*

I have nothing to add, no. It was only indirect evidence.

R. Levinsky

Does anyone have anything to add to that?

C. André

I do believe that tolerance can be induced by T-cell suppressor, but not in the system which I was using at that

time. I think this works with T-suppressor cells when one is
using a protein antigen but when one is using particulate antigens,
the suppressor hypothesis does not hold. I have often carried
out this kind of experiment, and it does not work. I do, however, believe that humoral factors play a role in this.

W. Leibold (FRG)

This is more a question than a comment. Is it feasible
that IgA, which is known to be a particularly efficient activator
in its complex form, of the alternate pathway of the complement system, might be eliminated or cleared by the alternate
activated C3b system?

R. Levinsky

I think the evidence that IgA in complex form activates
the alternate pathways is not yet clear. Certainly Ebehard and
others have shown that aggregated IgA is an activator, but heat
aggregation IgA is totally different from immune-complex IgA.
Similarly, Ishisaka showed that aggregated IgE activated the
complement pathway and yet I do not think that anyone believes
that IgE *per se* does activate the complements.

J. Soothill

Does anyone want to comment on that? Alternative pathway of complement activation by IgA is a very often repeated
story on really quite shaky evidence. Would anyone like to
be confident that there is evidence that IgA containing antigen-
antibody complexes activates the alternative pathway of
complements?

J. Bienenstock (Canada)

There is one piece of evidence for that, using a DNP MOPC
315 system. Unfortunately, the amounts used do not lead one to
be confident that it is working *in vivo* normally. It is the
same problem.

J. Soothill

Are there any more questions or comments for Drs. Jarrett and Levinsky? If not, I think we can bring this discussion to a close.

AN ANIMAL MODEL OF ANAPHYLACTIC PEPTIC ULCERATION -
A NEW APPROACH TO ULCER DISEASE IN HUMANS?

C. André, F. André, J. Gillon, M.C. Fargier and S. Perrin
Unité de Recherche de Physiopathologie Digestive - U 45 INSERM
Pav. H, Hôpital Edouard Herriot, 69374 Lyon Cedex 2, France.

ABSTRACT

Direct immunofluorescence, using an anti-epsilon chain antiserum, of the gastric mucosa of patients with varioliform gastritis or peptic ulceration has revealed increased numbers of IgE plasma cells and activated mast cells. These studies therefore provide evidence that type 1 hypersensitivity could play an important role in the pathogenesis of these diseases, though proof of this would be difficult to obtain from human studies.

We have therefore developed an animal model using the African rodent Mastomys natalensis. Intramucosal injection of ovalbumin reliably provokes gastric ulceration in animals previously sensitised by intra-peritoneal injection. Non-sensitised animals do not develop ulcers. These lesions can be prevented by prior treatment with the mast cell stabiliser disodium cromoglycate, by prior oral tolerisation with oval-bumin or by desensitisation of previously sensitised animals.

These animal studies therefore support the hypothesis that immediate hypersensitivity may play a part in the pathogenesis of peptic ulceration in humans.

INTRODUCTION

The many animal models of peptic ulceration which have
been developed have so far failed to elucidate the aetiology
of the disease in humans. In spite of vast amounts of research,
the final pathways of the mechanism of acid secretion remain
poorly understood, and in any case there is no doubt that in
the overwhelming majority of patients the disease is not a
result of gastric acid hypersecretion. Recently, therefore,
more attention has been paid to factors which alter mucosal
resistance, and to other possible mechanisms of tissue injury.

There is little doubt that histamine has a fundamental
role both in the stimulation of acid secretion and in the
pathogenesis of peptic ulceration. It is still not clear at
what point histamine acts in the chain of events leading to
acid secretion, and the origin of the histamine released after
appropriate stimulation remains unknown. It has been suggested
that enterochromaffin cells are more likely candidates than
the relatively few mast cells present in normal gastric mucosa
(Thurnberg, 1967). However, the histamine which causes acid
secretion and that which plays a part in the pathogenesis of
ulceration, whether by stimulation of acid secretion or by
direct tissue injury, do not necessarily share the same cell
of origin, and would in either case be susceptible to
antagonism from H2-receptor blocking agents such as cimetidine.

The potential for type 1 hypersensitivity and mast cell-
mediated tissue injury exists in the gastric mucosa. It has
been suggested on clinical grounds that allergic mechanisms
may underly peptic ulceration in man (Siegel, 1977), and
Brown et al. have demonstrated large numbers of IgE cells in
the bases of peptic ulcers in humans (Brown et al., 1975).
Using the rat model of aspirin- and stress-induced gastric
mucosal ulceration, Chatterjee and Roy have equally shown that
this type of lesion is accompanied by an increase in the
numbers of mast cells in the submucous layer (Chatterjee and
Roy, 1976). Furthermore, it has been shown that disodium

cromoglycate, a specific mast cell inhibitor, prevents the development of reserpine induced ulcers in rats (Ogle and Lau, 1979).

We therefore set out to look for evidence that type 1 hypersensitivity plays some part in the pathogenesis of peptic ulceration in man by studying mucosal IgE cell numbers at various sites and under various disease conditions. However, since any such evidence can at best be no more than circumstantial, we have also developed an animal model of gastric ulceration depending on type 1 anaphylaxis, based on a model first described by Shapiro and Ivy (1926).

IgE-containing cells account for approximately 2% of all Ig-containing cells in the human intestine (Brown et al., 1975). Their distribution is, however, uneven, and the greatest numbers are found in the stomach and upper small intestine. Mayrhofer et al. (1976) have shown that many of these IgE-containing cells are likely to be mast cells, the main function of which is the release of histamine and other vasoactive amines upon appropriate antigenic challenge. IgE producing plasma cells appear to be few in number in the GI-tract, but the intestinal mast cells differ from those of other tissues in having intracytoplasmic IgE (Mayrhofer et al., 1976). Differentiation between IgE plasma cells and mast cells using immunofluorescent techniques is thus extremely difficult.

STUDIES IN HUMANS

Patients

The study involved 20 patients with peptic ulceration and 25 controls, all of whom underwent an endoscopic examination (Olympus GIF-K fibre optic endoscope). In 10 patients with gastric ulcer, biopsies of the antrum and the fundus (one per patient) were performed along the greater curvature. One biopsy was also obtained from the edge of the ulcer. Immunofluorescence staining was used to identify lymphoid B

cells from these biopsies. Biopsies obtained from the edge of
the ulcer demonstrated that the ulcer was not a cancer. In 10
patients with duodenal ulcer, one biopsy was obtained from the
edge of the ulcer as well as from surrounding macroscopically
normal duodenal mucosa and from the antrum and the fundus.
Control patients consisted of 25 subjects presenting
macroscopically and histologically normal gastric mucosa,
endoscopy having been performed because of upper GI symptoms,
but with no history of peptic ulcer disease.

Immunofluorescence method

Fragments of gastric tissue were fixed in 96% ethanol
for 24 hours at $4^{\circ}C$, following a 24-hour incubation in cold
phosphate buffered saline. This procedure reduces background
by washing out interstitial proteins (Brandtzaeg, 1974a).
Serial sections of 4 µm were cut after being embedded in
paraffin. Intracellular staining was performed in one step,
five adjacent sections being used for each of the immunoglobulin classes. Rabbit anti-human immunoglobulin A, M, G, D
and E antisera were purchased (Boehringwerke) as fluorescein
conjugates and were used as whole sera diluted 1 : 20. The
specificity of the antisera was assessed by immunoelectrophoresis against plasma proteins. In particular, the
specificity of the anti-epsilon heavy chain antiserum was
controlled against a myelomatous IgE protein (kindly furnished
by Dr. J.P. Vaerman, Institut de Pathologie Cellulaire,
Département de Médecine Expérimentale, Université de Louvain,
Belgium). Differential counts were obtained by enumerating the
brightly-stained class-specific plasma cells, according to the
tissue unit method (Brandtzaeg, 1974b). In all cases, the
observer did not know the origin corresponding to the biopsy
studied.

Results

The results, shown in Table 1, give the total number of
plasma cells observed in three tissue units and the relative
proportions of immunoglobulin-containing cells with different

TABLE 1

AVERAGE NUMBERS AND CLASS DISTRIBUTION OF Ig-CONTAINING CELLS IN THREE TISSUE UNITS

Groups	Mean cell number	Class distribution in per cent				
		IgA	IgM	IgG	IgD	IgE °
Controls (n = 25)						
Antrum	23	78	7	13.5	1	0.5
Fundus	20	80.5	6	12	1	0.5
Duodenal ulcer (n = 10)						
Antrum	129	64.5	12.5	20.5	1	1.5
Fundus	59	67	12.5	16	3	1.5
Duodenum	198	70	14.5	10	3	2.5
Ulcer	159	52	15	10.5	4	18.5
Gastric ulcer (n = 10)						
Antrum	137	62	16	17	1	4
Fundus	150	58	17	17	5	3
Ulcer	141	42	14	20	4	20

(°) Plasma cells and/or activated mast cells.

heavy chain specificities. Relatively few immunoglobulin-containing cells, predominantly of the IgA class, were detected in the gastric mucosa of control subjects.

A five to seven-fold increase in the number of plasma cells was observed in the antral mucosa of patients with gastric or duodenal ulcer. A 2.5 to eight-fold increase was observed in the fundic mucosa of these patients. The gastritis observed in the stomach of ulcer-bearing patients was associated with a relative decrease of IgA plasma cells and with an increase of IgM and IgG plasma cells. The marked increase of IgE cells is a striking feature of the edge of gastric and duodenal ulcers.

STUDIES IN ANIMALS.

Animals

Both sexes of the outbred African rodent *Praomys natalensis* (mastomys) raised in the laboratory, were used when over three months old. These animals were chosen because they have large numbers of mast cells in the GI tract, and in old age spontaneously develop gastric ulcers as a complication of mastocytoma. They received water as required and were maintained on ovalbumin-free UAR mouse food (Villemoisson/Orge, France).

Methods

Antigen and sensitisation

Ovalbumin recrystallised five times was obtained from Calbiochem. Animals were sensitised by intraperitoneal injection of 3 µg of ovalbumin in a volume of 0.2 ml with 1 mg of aluminium hydroxide.

Induction and prevention of gastric ulcer

An intramucosal injection of 1 mg of ovalbumin in 0.01 ml alone or mixed with 1 mg of sodium cromoglycate (obtained from Dr. A.E. Edwards, Fisons S.A. Laboratories) or mixed with 1 mg of doxantrazole (obtained from Dr. L. Garland, Wellcome Research Laboratories) was performed in the mucosa of the fundus region of the stomach under general anaesthetic.

The protein was injected through the serosa without perforation of the mucosa. The procedure was carried out

i.   in unsensitised control animals,

ii.   in animals which had been sensitised one week earlier and

iii. in non-immune recipient animals receiving 1 ml serum i.v. from sensitised mastomys.

The effect of cimetidine on gastric ulcer induction was studied in 10 animals. They were sensitised as above, but on the day of challenge (day 7) they were given 2 intraperitoneal doses of cimetidine 5 mg and were then allowed to drink a 2% solution of cimetidine in water until sacrifice on day 10.

Passive cutaneous anaphylaxis

The test was performed in the dorsal skin of non-immune mastomys with 50 µl of reagin sera. Incubation was for 48 hours for reagin antibodies of the IgE class and for four hours for IgG1-like activity. Heated (60 minutes, 56°C) and non-heated sera were used to test their ability to induce thermostable short-latency (IgG1) and thermolabile long-latency (IgE) reactions (Prouvost-Danon et al., 1968). Like other rodents, mastomys have two types of homocytotropic antibodies, the heat-labile IgE and one heat-stable IgG1 antibody. The titres were expressed as the reciprocal of the greatest dilution giving a 3 - 4 mm spot after injection with ovalbumin and Evans Blue.

Degranulation of peritoneal mast cells

Studies were performed as previously described (Prouvost-Danon et al., 1972) using mast cells from mastomys. The cells were collected from the peritoneal cavity from sensitised and unsensitised animals. Passive sensitisation of normal mast cells *in vitro* was performed by incubation with 25 µl of heated (60 minutes, 56°C) or non-heated sera collected in animals which were immunised for seven days. Actively and passively sensitised cells were incubated with 100 µg/ml ovalbumin at 37°C for 15 minutes. Degranulation of mast cells was determined after staining with toluidine blue.

Assay of non-homocytotropic humoral response

The presence of an ovalbumin-specific antibody was assayed in the blood of immunised animals both by precipitation with Ouchterlony immunodiffusion and by agglutination using glutaraldehyde-coupled sheep red blood cells and ovalbumin (Avrameas et al., 1969).

Assay of delayed type hypersensitivity

Delayed type hypersensitivity reactions were elicited by injecting 7.5 µg of ovalbumin in 50 µl of saline solution into one footpad. The contralateral footpad was injected with 50 µl of saline. Footpad thickness was measured with vernier calipers prior to, and 24 and 48 hours after, antigen challenge. Delayed hypersensitivity was estimated by footpad swelling.

Antigen feeding before and after sensitisation

1. Antigen prefeeding. Two groups of 12 animals each received 1 mg or 10 mg ovalbumin in 0.5 ml of 0.15 M bicarbonate buffer by gastric intubation. Sensitisation was performed 15 days after the single intragastric dose of ovalbumin. Gastric ulcer induction (n = 12) and the test of peritoneal mast cell degranulation (n = 12) were performed 7 days after sensitisation.

2. Antigen feeding after sensitisation. Twenty five animals were given 2.5 mg ovalbumin daily by gastric intubation from day 7 to day 21 after intraperitoneal sensitisation. Gastric ulcer induction by intramucosal challenge (n = 15) and mast cell degranulation tests

(n = 10) were performed on day 21. Control animals
(n = 25) were sensitised but did not subsequently receive
ovalbumin, and were tested on day 21 post sensitisation.

Results

Mastomys sensitised with ovalbumin developed a high
incidence of gastric ulcers on subsequent intramucosal challenge
with this antigen (Table 2). No lesions were present one day
after intragastric challenge but 60% of the animals exhibited
an ulcer at the challenge site on day 2, and 93% did so on
day 3. A single ulcer was produced at the challenge site and
the lesion produced was similar to that seen in gastric
ulceration in man and was associated with similar complications,
including massive haemorrhage and perforation. Unsensitised
animals did not develop an ulcer after challenge. In the group
who were challenged with a mixture of sodium cromoglycate and
ovalbumin only one out of 15 (6%) developed an ulcer. A
similar reduction of ulcer incidence was observed in animals
challenged with doxantrazole. Of the 10 animals treated with
cimetidine 3 (30%) developed ulcers (Table 2).

Of 12 animals fed a single dose of either 1 mg or 10 mg
ovalbumin 15 days before sensitisation, only 3 (25%) developed
an ulcer at day 3 after intramucosal challenge. None of the
12 animals pre-fed with ovalbumin and in whom the peritoneal
mast cell test was performed had a positive result. By
comparison, all control animals (n = 15), ovalbumin-sensitised
but not pre-fed, developed an ulcer (100%) and exhibited
(n = 10) positive mast cell degranulation tests.

Of the 15 animals which received ovalbumin orally after
sensitisation, 2 (13%) developed an ulcer on day 3 after
antigen challenge, while 12 of the 15 control animals (80%)
had ulcers. Positive mast cell degranulation tests were
observed in only 1 of the 10 animals fed with ovalbumin and in
8 of the 10 controls.

190

TABLE 2

GASTRIC ULCER INCIDENCE

Animals	No.	Days after intragastric injection of ovalbumin	Associated treatment	No. ulcers	Ulcers (%)
Non immune	25	3	no	0	0
Immune for 7 days	30	1	no	0	0
Immune for 7 days	30	2	no	18	60
Immune for 7 days	30	3	no	28	93
Non immune	8	3	1 ml immune serum	6	75
Non immune	8	3	1 ml heated immune serum	2	25
Immune for 7 days	15	3	1 mg DSCG	1	6
Immune for 7 days	10	3	1 mg DOX	1	10
Immune for 7 days	10	3	Cimetidine °	3	30

DSCG : disodium cromoglycate

DOX : doxantrazole

° Cimetidine 2 x 5 mg on Day 7, then 2% in water *ad libitum*

Seventy-five per cent of unsensitised recipient animals developed ulcers when injected i.v. with unheated serum (containing IgE and/or IgG1 antibodies) from immunised animals. Only 25% of recipient animals injected with heated serum (containing IgG1 antibodies) developed ulcers.

Passive cutaneous anaphylaxis reactions showed that homocytotropic antibodies appeared in the serum of mastomys immunised with egg albumin. The responses were often erratic and the reagin antibody level was low. The reciprocal of the titre of IgE antibodies usually ranged from 2 to 4, with some animals exhibiting a higher reaction (titre of 128). In a few animals, antibodies having IgG1-like activity were also detected with a titre of 1 or 2.

Table 3 shows the effect of incubation of peritoneal mast cells with ovalbumin in animals which did not receive ovalbumin orally. Mast cells from unsensitised animals never degranulate. On the other hand, all but one sensitised animals have mast cells which release histamine in the presence of the antigen. Incubation of mast cells from unsensitised animals with ovalbumin and serum from sensitised animals results in histamine release. This was not observed when the incubation was performed with normal serum or with heated immune serum.

The assay of non-homocytotropic humoral responses by immunodiffusion and by agglutination resulted in the detection of no antibodies. The assay of delayed type hypersensitivity was also negative.

DISCUSSION

There has been sporadic interest during the past 50 years in the possibility that allergy plays an important part in the pathogenesis of peptic ulceration. That there is an environmental factor of some significance has long been suspected from the well known seasonal variation in the natural history

TABLE 3

MAST CELL DEGRANULATION

Mast cells from animals	No. experiments	Incubation of cells and ovalbumin with and without serum	Observed degranulation	Degranulation (%)
Unsensitised	12	nothing	0	0
Sensitised for 7 days	12	nothing	11	92
Unsensitised	6	normal serum	0	0
Unsensitised	12	immune serum heated	12	100
Unsensitised	6	immune serum	0	0

of the disease, with exacerbations occurring in spring and autumn, and from the tendency of the disease to recur and remit in an unpredictable fashion, before finally waning in severity after many years. Siegel (1974) has recently called attention to a possible association between peptic ulceration and various allergic conditions, and although his observations are uncontrolled and involve only a few patients, he has claimed significant therapeutic benefit from the use of exclusion diets.

The concept of mucosal anaphylaxis in response to an ingested allergen being the initial insult which alters the mucosal resistance to acid-peptic digestion, and thus leads to ulceration, is an attractive one. Current research into the pathogenesis of ulceration is concerned mainly with possible defects in the mucosal barrier to autodigestion, with little attention being paid to the initiating mechanism. Existing animal models thus depend on insults which have little bearing on the aetiology of the disease in humans, such as drugs (aspirin, reserpine) (Rees and Turnberg, 1980) or such surgical manipulations as the Mann-Williamson operation to produce jejunal anastomotic ulcers. Even the classical stress ulcers induced in rats are of limited interest, the ulcers having little resemblance to chronic peptic ulcers in humans, and the relationship of stress to human ulceration being far from clear-cut.

The therapeutic benefit obtained with the histamine H2-receptor antagonist cimetidine leaves no doubt that histamine plays a major part in the pathogenesis of ulceration. Cimetidine reduces basal and stimulated acid secretion by an average of around 80% (Richardson, 1978), a reduction comparable to that obtained following successful vagotomy, and it is thus natural to assume that it is this reduction in acid output which leads to ulcer healing.

However, it has been shown that vagotomy leads to an increase not only in mucosal histamine levels (Troidl et al., 1978), but also, in rats, to an increased number of mucosal

mast cells. Furthermore, Levy et al. (1976) have shown that
vagotomy and cholinergic blockade prevent generalised
anaphylaxis in the rat, and they conclude that an intact vagal
reflex arc is necessary if the full immunological vascular
reaction of anaphylaxis is to occur. The effect of vagotomy
is thus more complex than simple reduction of acid output, and
vagotomy could influence the course of peptic ulceration in a
variety of ways, for example by stabilising mast cell membranes
(Troidl, 1978). Similarly, the effect of cimetidine may depend
on more than a simple reduction in acid output, since anti-
histamines have been shown to protect rats from stress-induced
ulcers only if significant numbers of mucosal mast cells could
be demonstrated before treatment (Gorizontova et al., 1975).

The upper gastrointestinal tract is well endowed with the
apparatus necessary to mount a type 1 hypersensitivity response
(Brown et al., 1975). It is therefore surprising that we know
of so few circumstances in which allergy plays a part in
clinical gastrointestinal illness. We have previously shown
that patients with acute varioliform gastritis have numerous
IgE-containing cells, likely to be for the most part mast cells
(Mayrhofer et al., 1976), in close relationship to the lesions
(André et al., 1976). Similarly, large numbers of IgE-containing cells have been demonstrated near the bases of peptic
ulcers in humans (Brown et al., 1975). The results which we
present here confirm and extend these findings, and show
clearly that the IgE cell, or activated mast cell, response is
localised to the lesion itself. This response could, of course,
be a secondary event following mucosal disruption, but the
animal studies clearly demonstrate that a type 1 hypersensitivity reaction can give rise to localised ulceration closely
resembling that seen in humans. We have also shown that both
the histamine H2-blocker cimetidine and the mast cell
stabilising agents disodium cromoglycate and doxantrazole can
block this reaction.

The first animal model of anaphylactic ulceration, using
dogs, was described in 1926 (Shapiro et al., 1926), who

emphasised the similarity in the pathological features and complications between the 'model' ulcers and the disease in humans. Our model, using the mast-cell rich African rodent, Mastomys natalensis, provides exactly similar results, and our additional studies leave us in no doubt that it is an IgE-mediated type 1 hypersensitivity reaction which causes the ulceration. We have also shown that this is a true allergic reaction by preventing ulceration either by prefeeding with the antigen (tolerance induction), or by giving the antigen orally after sensitisation but prior to challenge (desensitisation). Oral feeding of antigen is known to induce immunological tolerance (Bazin et al., 1973; André et al. 1975) and to prevent homocytotropic antibody synthesis (Bazin and Platteau, 1977; David, 1977; Vaz et al., 1977).

Shapiro and Ivy (1926) later abandoned their model because they were unable to produce a truly chronic ulcer, and all the ulcers which we have induced in the mastomys have healed within 12 days. However, truly chronic peptic ulcers in humans are quite rare, the disease rather tending to sum a relapsing and remitting course, and can thus be seen as a sequence of acute ulcers with intervals of complete healing. Repeated endoscopies performed in the course of clinical trials confirm this by showing a surprisingly high incidence of healing within one month on placebo alone (Wastell, 1978). It is also worth noting that a high incidence of healing is obtained in humans simply upon removal to a hospital environment and without specific therapy. Although removal of stress may help, it may equally be the case that hospitalisation removes the patient from a hitherto undetermined allergen in his own environment.

CONCLUSIONS

The evidence suggesting that type 1 hypersensitivity plays a part in the pathogenesis of peptic ulceration in man remains indirect, and an effect secondary to mucosal disruption cannot be excluded. Animal studies, however, confirm that localised ulceration can result from an anaphylactic reaction mediated by homocytotropic IgE antibodies. This effect can be blocked by prior tolerisation or subsequent desensitisation to the specific antigen, and by both the H2 antagonist cimetidine and the mast cell stabilising agents disodium cromoglycate and doxantrazole. A trial of disodium cromoglycate in human peptic ulcer disease may now be justified.

REFERENCES

André, C., Heremans, J.F., Vaerman, J.P. and Cambiasco, C.L., 1975.
A mechanism for the induction of immunological tolerance by
antigen feeding: antigen-antibody complexes. J. Exp. Med. 142,
1509.

André, C., Moulinier, B., Lambert, R. and Bugnon, B., 1976. Gastritis
varioliformis, allergy and disodium cromoglycate. Lancet 1, 964.

Avreamas, S., Taudou, B. and Chuilon, S., 1969. Glutaraldehyde, cyanuric
chloride and tetra-azotized O-dianisidine as coupling reagents in
the passive haemagglutination test. Immunochemistry 6, 67.

Bazin, H., André, C. and Heremans, J.F., 1973. Réponses immunologiques
induites par voie orale. Ann. Immunol. (Inst. Pasteur) 124C, 253.

Bazin, H. and Platteau, B., 1977. Oral feeding of ovalbumin can make rats
tolerant to an intraperitoneal injection of dinitrophenylated
ovalbumin and Bordetella partussis vaccine. Biochem. Soc. Trans.
5, 1571.

Brandtzaeg, P., 1974a. Mucosal and glandular distribution of
immunoglobulin components. Immunohistochemistry with a cold
ethanol fixation technique. Immunology 26, 1101.

Brandtzaeg, P., Baklien, K., Fausa, O. and Hoel, P.S., 1974b. Immunohistochemical characterization of local immunoglobulin formation in
ulcerative colitis. Gastroenterology 66, 1123.

Brown, W.R., Borthistle, B.K. and Chen, S.T., 1975. Immunoglobulin E
(Ige) and IgE-containing cells in human gastrointestinal fluids
and tissues. Clin. Exp. Immunol. 20, 227.

Chatterjee, S. and Roy, P.R., 1976. Mast cell population in stomach wall
with experimentally induced peptic ulcer. Indian J. Exp. Biol.
14, 100.

David, M.F., 1977. Prevention of homocytotropic antibody formation and
anaphylactic sensitization by prefeeding antigen. J. Allergy Clin.
Immunol. 60, 180.

Gorizontova, M.P., Alekseev, O.V. and Chernukh, A.M., 1975. Role of the
mast cells in disturbances of vascular permeability in rats with
stress due to immobilisation. Bull. Exp. Biol. Med. 79, 241.

Levy, R.M., Rose, J.E. and Johnson, J.S., 1976. Effect of vagotomy on
anaphylaxis in the rat. Clin. Exp. Immunol. 24, 96.

Mayrhofer, G., Bazin H. and Gowans, J.L., 1976. Nature of cells binding anti-IgE in rats immunised with *Nippostrongylus brasiliensis*: IgE synthesis in regional nodes and concentration in mucosal mast cells. Eur. J. Immunol. 6, 537.

Ogle, C.W. and Lau, H.K., 1979. Disodium cromoglycate: a novel gastric antiulcer agent? Eur. J. Pharmacol. 55, 411.

Prouvost-Danon, A., Peixoto, J.M. and Javierre, M.Q., 1968. Antigen-induced histamine release from peritoneal mast cells of mice producing reagin-like antibody. Immunology 15, 271.

Prouvost-Danon, A., Binaghi, R., Rochas, S. and Boussac-Aron, Y., 1972. Immunochemical identification of mouse IgE. Immunology 23, 481.

Rees, W.D.W. and Turnberg, L.A., 1980. Reappraisal of the effects of aspirin on the stomach. Lancet ii, 410.

Richardson, C.T., 1978. Effect of H2-receptor antagonists on gastric acid secretion and serum gastrin concentration. A review. Gastroenterology (suppl.) 74, 366.

Shapiro, P.F. and Ivy, A.C., 1926. Gastric ulcer. IV. Experimental production of gastric ulcer by local anaphylaxis. Arch. Int. Med. 38, 237.

Siegel, J., 1974. Gastrointestinal ulcer-Arthus reaction! Annals of Allergy 32, 127.

Siegel, J., 1977. Immunologic approach to the treatment and prevention of gastrointestinal ulcers. Annals of Allergy 38, 27.

Thurnberg, R., 1967. Localisation of cells containing and forming histamine in the gastric mucosa of the rat. Exp. Cell. Res. 47, 108.

Troidl, H., Rohde, H., Lorenz, W., Hafner, G. and Hamelmann, H., 1978. Effect of selective gastric vagotomy on histamine concentration in gastric mucosa of patients with duodenal ulcer. Br. J. Surg. 65, 10.

Vaz, N.M., Maia, L.C.S., Hanson, G. and Lynch, J.M., 1977. Inhibition of homocytotropic antibody responses in adult inbred mice by previous feeding of the specific antigen. J. Allergy Clin. Immunol. 60, 110.

Wastell, C., 1978. The problem of duodenal ulcer disease and its treatment with cimetidine. Cimetidine. The Westminster Symposium, pp 3-12 Churchill Livingstone, Edinburgh.

DISCUSSION

Anne Ferguson *(UK)*

Could Dr. André clarify the cell type which he said was found at the edge of gastric and duodenal ulcers? He said, "either IgE-containing plasma cells or activated mast cells". However, from the figures, if it was a mast cell you should be able to tell from ordinary histology, because for every 100 plasma cells there would be perhaps 20 - 30 mast cells.

C. André *(France)*

The problem is in staining. I have never been able to distinguish between immunofluorescent stained plasma cells and mast cells. Dr. Bazin has succeeded in such a distinction with bone marrow in rats, but I have never found a reliable technique for human tissues. Both types of cell are probably involved, because not every cell looks the same under immuno-fluorescent staining. Some cells are larger and brighter and do not seem to contain IgE.

P. Brandtzaeg *(Norway)*

I am amazed to hear Dr. André cannot distinguish between a mast cell and a plasma cell. What sort of section was it, a cryostat section? And what sort of preparations did you use?

C. André

No, it was not a cryostat section. It was paraffin embedded.

P. Brandtzaeg

We use alcohol-fixed paraffin embedding material and with very rare exceptions, I am certain that I have a plasma cell.

C. André

I have no difficulty in demonstrating mast cells but I have not succedded in combining immunofluorescence with a specific non-immunological stain for mast cells.

P. Brandtzaeg

That is difficult, I agree.

Anne Ferguson

I think it would be possible to do that on semi-thin sections, perhaps, but it is certainly technically very demanding.

J. Seifert *(FRG)*

Dr. André told us that it is possible to desensitise the animals by giving them the antigen from day 7 to day 21. I would like to ask for how long this desensitisation lasts. Does the animal become sensitised again after one week, for example?

C. André

No, they do not become sensitised again.

J. Seifert

Is it possible to desensitise with just one injection, and is the time period critical?

C. André

I do not know. Work needs to be done on that.

Anne Ferguson

Have you stopped feeding the animals and left them for one or two weeks? Do they remain tolerised as you describe?

C. André

We have not done this yet.

J. Soothill *(UK)*

Is peptic ulceration epidemiologically related to the state of atopy?

C. André

It is very difficult to say what is atopy. When one looks
at a patient who has one or another disease, in at least 20% of
patients there is an incidence of atopy somewhere, on the skin
of the nose or anywhere else that one cares to think of, or else
they have atopy in their families. So it is rather difficult to
make this distinction.

J. Soothill

It is quite easy to do this with asthma.

Anne Ferguson

You would have to make an intensive investigation on every
one of the patients on whom your epidemiological study was being
carried out, and it would be necessary to do at least one endoscopy since it is possible to have peptic ulceration in the
absence of any symptoms or signs.

J. Soothill

Yes, but it can be done the other way round. Prick tests
can be done on the peptic ulceration patients.

Ellen Jarrett (UK)

Can Dr. André tell us anything about the pathogenesis, or
the development, of this IgE mediated ulceration?

C. André

Ulcerations only develop after two or three days. This
allowed us to make a study of the events which occur at the site
of ulceration and we were able to study, in one single animal,
the effects of the injection of ovalbumin into the gastric wall.
This was always done on the left side.

We were able to make two kinds of study. One was a mucous
production. Using forceps, we were able to take a mucosal
sample from the exact site of the ovalbumin injection and make a

comparison with a normal site. With gas chromatography, we measured the component sugars of the glycoprotein and we were then able to demonstrate that within one or two days before the ulceration appeared there was no modification of the amount of glycoprotein present, or in the ratios of fucose and galactose.

The other study was of the gastric mucosa in the pre-ulcerous phase. We did this by measuring the incorporation of tritiated thymidine into DNA in the left side of the stomach which was subjected to the injection of ovalbumin, in comparison with the right side. In the control animal, of course, the ratio of thymidine in the left and right sides goes to one, and in the control animal which was subjected to the injection there is a small variation which is not significant since it is probably related to the trauma of injection, on day 1. However, in the sensitised animal there is a marked increase of thymidine incorporation one day after the injection into the mucosa. I believe that ulceration occurs as a result of histamine liberation by the mast cells. As a matter of fact, we ought to be making a study of the mucosa of such animals that are put in organ culture, as one does for gluten in the study of coeliac disease. In fact, we are able to demonstrate that the injection of histamine in the culture medium is able to modify the turnover of the gastric cells. This is with very small doses of histamine such as are likely to be liberated in a true anaphylactic reaction. There is stimulation of the turnover but on the other hand, with large doses, there is inhibition of the turnover.

Anne Ferguson

Thank you. I think we must draw this discussion to a conclusion now. The most important point to remember is that there is more to the gastro intestinal tract than the small bowel. One might overlook this if one read the literature. I don't know of any papers yet on the immunology of the oesophagus.

GASTROINTESTINAL HYPERSENSITIVITY IN THE PRERUMINANT CALF

P.J. Kilshaw

Nutrition Department, National Institute for Research in
Dairying, Shinfield, Reading RG2 9AT, UK.

ABSTRACT

Preruminant calves given a series of feeds of heated soyabean flour (HSF) quickly developed high titres of IgG antibodies in the serum specific for the soyabean proteins glycinin and B-conglycinin, reaginic antibodies were also detected. After sensitisation by feeding with HSF, ingestion of soluble soyabean proteins caused, in a majority of animals, gross abnormalities in gastrointestinal function. The rate of flow of digesta through the small intestine was greatly increased and there was a dramatic, but transitory, rise in the permeability of the intestinal mucosa to protein molecules. Mucosal integrity was assessed by infusing into the abomasum either milk alone or milk mixed with soyabean proteins and quantitating the leakage of β-lactoglobulin into the blood. In sensitised calves intestinal permeability changed 1 - 2 h after ingestion of soyabean protein, was greatly elevated at 4 - 6 h and had almost returned to normal again by 24 h.

A progressive increase in the sensitivity of the intestine to soyabean antigens was accompanied by a rise in the titre of homologous serum antibodies.

Feeding calves with ovalbumin also led to high antibody levels and similar gastrointestinal reactions.

INTRODUCTION

There are economic advantages in rearing preruminant calves on diets containing non-milk proteins. Soyabean protein has attracted attention for this purpose because it is readily available and has a reasonably well balanced amino acid composition. Despite industrial processing to remove well known anti-nutritional factors such as haemagglutinins and trypsin inhibitors most soya preparations have proved inferior to milk for the nutrition of the young calf.

Preruminant calves receiving diets containing high levels of soyabean protein have been reported to suffer from gastrointestinal disturbances, weight loss or poor growth (Gorrill and Thomas, 1967; Colvin and Ramsey, 1968; Smith and Sissons, 1975) and to develop persistent high titres of circulating antibodies specific for soyabean antigens (Van Adrichem and Frens, 1965; Smith and Sissons, 1975; Barratt et al., 1978; Kilshaw and Sissons, 1979a). In calves given single feeds of soya protein at 2 - 5 day intervals digestive abnormalities were not detected initially but developed gradually with successive feeds (Smith and Sissons, 1975; Sissons and Smith, 1976; Kilshaw and Sissons, 1979a). This observation prompted the speculation that gastrointestinal hypersensitivity reactions could be responsible.

This paper describes experiments to investigate in more detail the relationship between the immune response to soyabean protein and the intestinal disturbances. Gastrointestinal function after feeding with heated soyabean flour (HSF) has been assessed by two criteria, namely, the rate of flow of digesta through the small intestine, and the leakage of a marker protein from the intestinal lumen into the blood. After sensitisation by a series of feeds of HSF a high proportion of calves developed a vigorous circulating antibody response and showed severe functional abnormalities in the intestine after ingestion of soya protein.

MATERIALS AND METHODS

Calves and experimental diets

Experiments were performed with Friesian bull calves. The animals received colostrum after birth and were reared on cows' milk. At one month of age all were equipped with an abomasal cannula for the administration of experimental feeds. In addition, some of the animals were fitted with re-entrant cannulae in the distal ileum for sampling digesta. Alternatively, fistulae were constructed in the duodenum and/ or jejunum to facilitate removal of mucosal biopsies. Beginning 2 - 4 weeks after surgery single liquid feeds in which HSF (Arkasoy 50, British Arcady, Manchester) was the sole source of protein were administered twice weekly for three weeks and thereafter at intervals of 1 - 4 weeks; formulation of these feeds has been described elsewhere (Sissons and Smith, 1976). After 6 - 12 feeds about 50% of calves experienced diarrhoea within 8 h of ingesting HSF. Throughout the experimental period the calves were maintained on milk.

Flow of digesta

The flow of digesta through the small intestine was determined as described by Sissons and Smith, 1978. Briefly, phenol red was incorporated into the feed as a marker and digesta was collected from the distal ileal cannula for three hours after emergence of the dye. The material was weighed and the rate of flow over the period expressed as g/h.

Antibody determinations

Antibodies to soyabean antigens were determined by passive cutaneous anaphylaxis (PCA), passive haemagglutination or an enzyme immunoassay specific for IgG, IgA and IgM (Kilshaw and Sissons, 1979[a], Kilshaw and Slade, 1980).

Leakage of a marker protein from the gut into the blood

Cows' milk β-lactoglobulin proved to be a suitable marker
protein for these studies. Calves were fed with milk (40 g/kg
body weight) and the levels of β-lactoglobulin appearing in the
serum were determined by an enzyme immunoassay (Kilshaw and
Slade, 1980). Milk was administered before and after challenge
with HSF, or alternatively, calves were fed with a mixture of
milk and HSF. (66 g HSF/kg milk).

RESULTS

Flow of digesta and antibody production with successive feeds
of soya protein

Four calves with re-entrant cannulae in the distal ileum
were given a series of HSF feeds and on each occasion the rate
of flow of digesta through the small intestine was measured.
Serum was sampled twice weekly for antibody determinations.
A number of experimental feeds containing casein instead of
HSF were administered to control for non-specific changes in
flow rate.

The results in Figure 1 show that in two animals
(530 and 540) the flow of digesta increased progressively
with successive feeds of HSF, there was also concomitant
production of haemagglutinating and reaginic antibodies
specific for soyabean antigens. Flow rates following control
feeds containing casein were normal. A third animal (531)
showed a slight increase in flow following the ninth feed of
HSF, and the fourth (539) showed no changes. All calves had
low titres of haemagglutinating antibodies before receiving
HSF and these were thought to be of maternal origin. High
flow rates were associated with a reaginic antibody response.

The ileal effluent from calves with very high flow rates
often contained blood and large numbers of epithelial cells;
occasionally tubular fibrin casts several feet in length
emerged from the ileal cannulae suggesting leakage of plasma

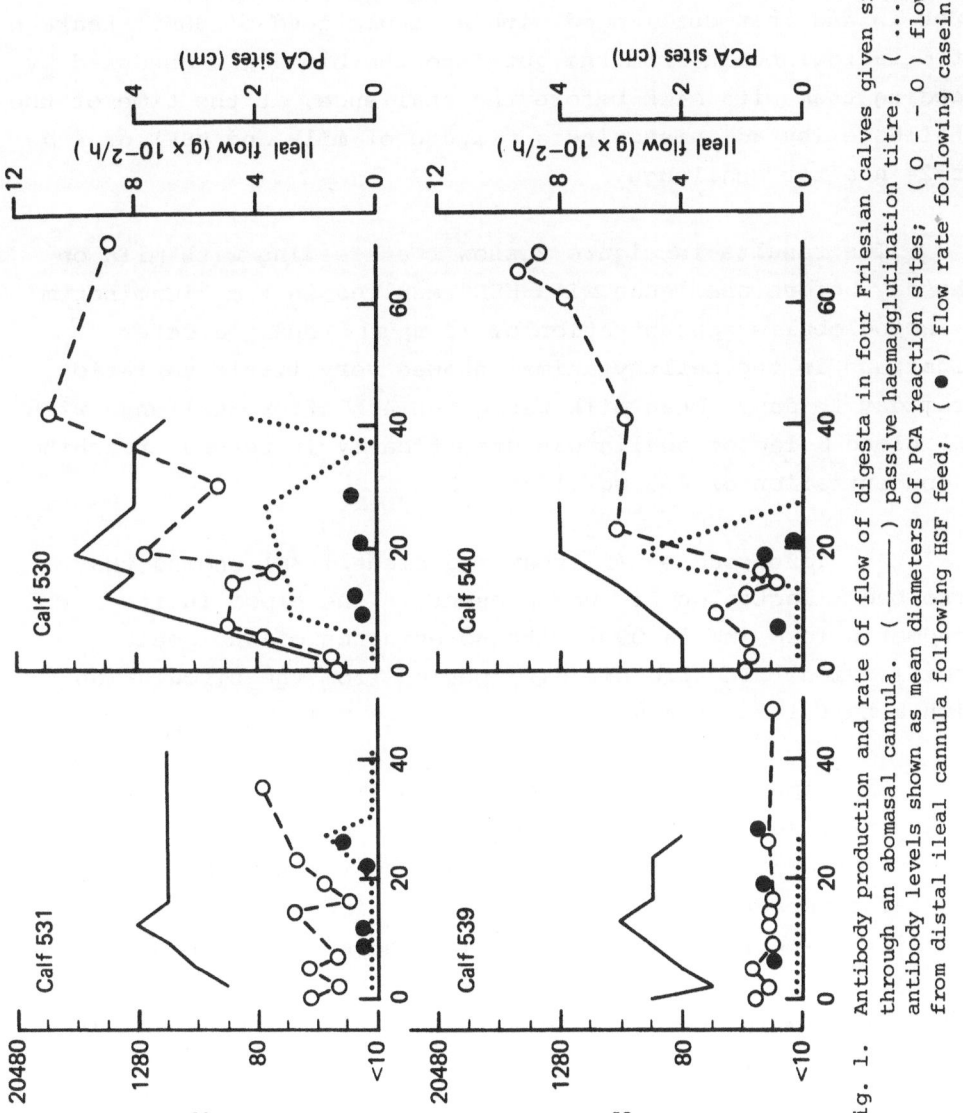

Fig. 1. Antibody production and rate of flow of digesta in four Friesian calves given single feeds of HSF through an abomasal cannula. (——) passive haemagglutination titre; (.......) reaginic antibody levels shown as mean diameters of PCA reaction sites; (O – O) flow rate of digesta from distal ileal cannula following HSF feed; (●) flow rate following casein feed.

protein into the gut lumen. There was no sign of systemic anaphylaxis or angio-oedema.

Leakage of β-lactoglobulin through the intestinal wall into the blood

Calves were sensitised with a series of feeds of soya protein and then challenged with a single feed of HSF. Leakage of β-lactoglobulin from the gut into the blood was assessed by feeding them with milk before the challenge, at the time of the challenge (by administering a mixture of milk and HSF) or 4 h or 24 h after challenge.

The results in Figure 2 show that feeding with milk on the day before challenge with HSF resulted in a maximum serum β-lactoglobulin concentration of 13 ng/ml; repeated determinations in the healthy animal showed very little variation from day to day. When milk was given 4 h after challenge with HSF blood β-lactoglobulin was dramatically increased, reaching a concentration of 433 ng/ml at 1 h.

Previous studies (Kilshaw and Slade, 1980) showed that absorbed β-lactoglobulin was present in the blood in its monomeric form (MW 18 000) with no evidence of antigenic modification. The protein disappeared from the circulation with a half life of 4 h.

Experiments in which a mixture of milk and HSF was fed to a sensitised calf showed that HSF had no effect on absorption of β-lactoglobulin during the first hour but that thereafter absorption was substantially increased (Figure 3). A similar experiment in another calf showed that serum β-lactoglobulin was still elevated 24 h after challenge but was only slightly increased by further ingestion of milk at this time (Figure 4).

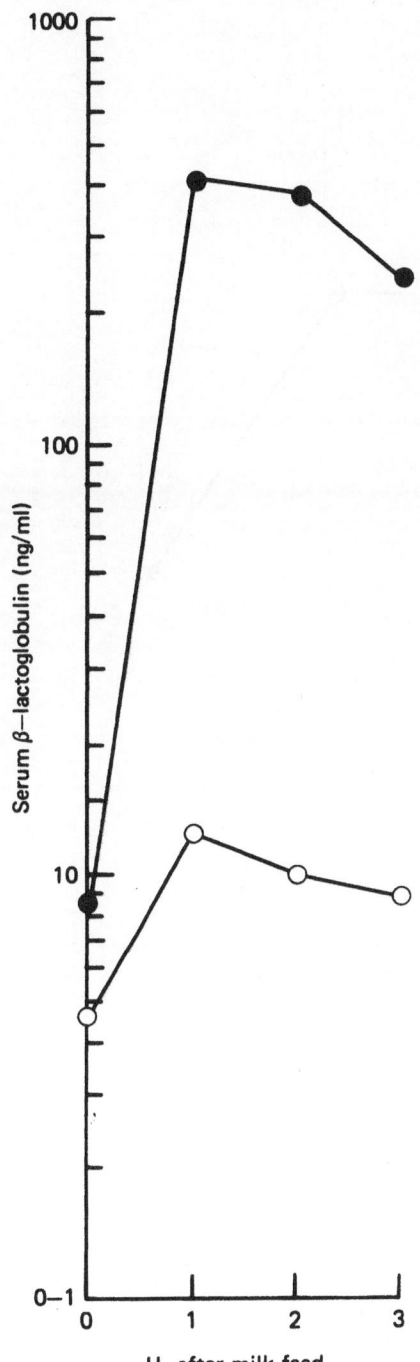

Fig. 2. Serum β-lactoglobulin levels in a sensitised calf after a milk
feed: (O —— O) before challenge with HSF; (● —— ●) 4 h after
challenge with HSF.

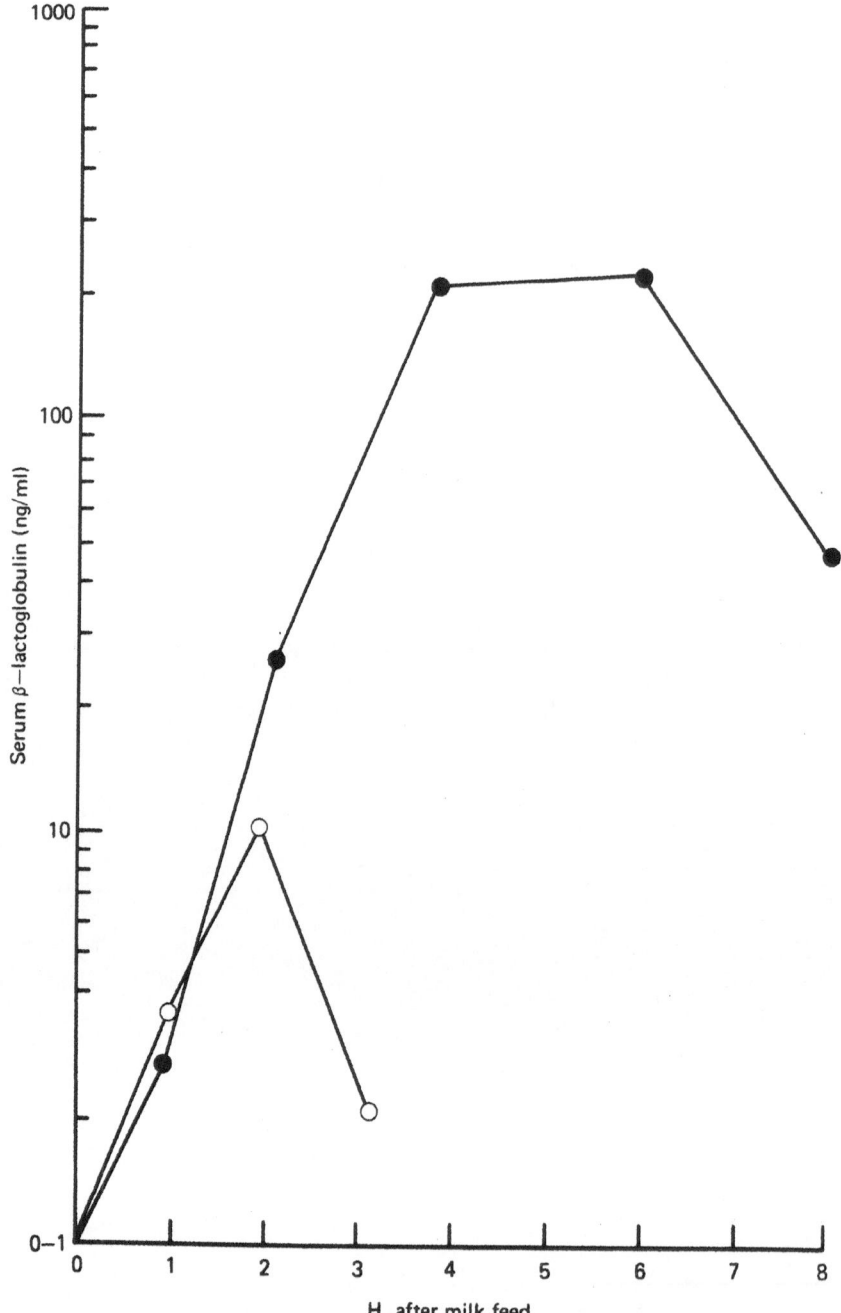

Fig. 3. Serum βᴸ-lactoglobulin levels in a sensitised calf after feeding
with: (O —— O) milk alone; (● —— ●) milk mixed with HSF.

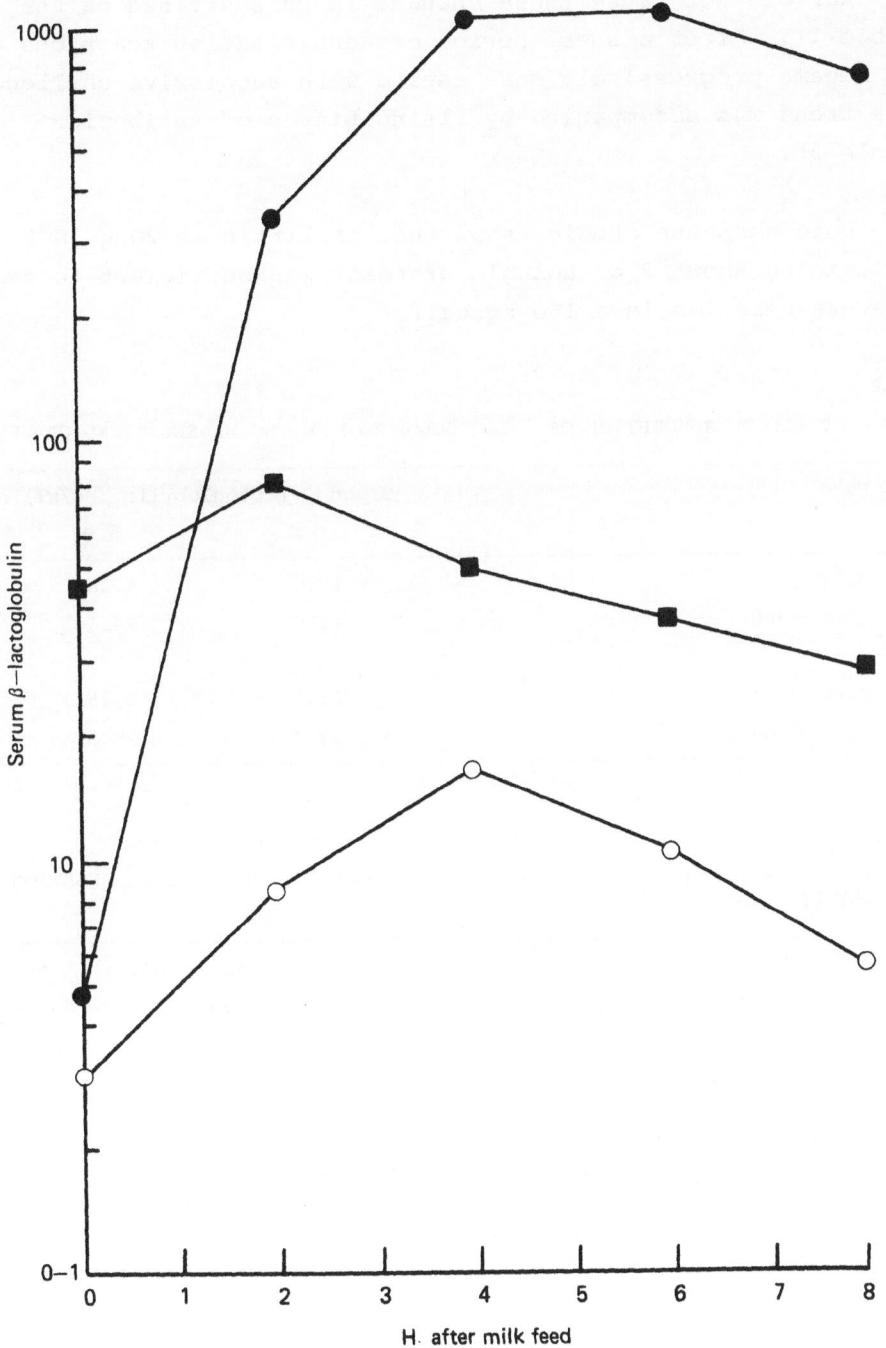

Fig. 4. Serum β-lactoglobulin levels in a sensitised calf after feeding with milk; (O —— O) 24 h before HSF; (● —— ●) mixed with HSF; (■ —— ■) 24 h after HSF.

HSF did not cause these changes in unsensitised calves
(Table 1). After a short period of sensitisation reactions to
HSF became progressively more severe with successive challenges.
This trend was accompanied by rising titres of antibodies
(Table 2).

Dose response studies show that as little as 20 g HSF
(containing about 2 g soluble protein) was sufficient to evoke
a severe reaction in a 160 kg calf.

TABLE 1

EFFECT OF HSF ON ABSORPTION OF β-LACTOGLOBULIN IN TWO UNSENSITISED CALVES

Feed	Blood β-lactoglobulin (ng/ml) at	
	2 h	4 h
Milk	12.0	12.8
Milk + HSF	14.8	14.4
Milk	26.0	23.5
Milk + HSF	30.0	28.0

TABLE 2

CHANGES IN THE SENSITIVITY OF THE INTESTINE OVER EIGHT WEEKS IN RELATION TO
ANTIBODY PRODUCTION

Blood β-lactoglobulin (ng/ml at 4 h)*	Antibodies to soya protein			Weeks after first HSF feed	Total No. HSF feeds
	IgG	IgA	IgM		
46	1 : 2560	1 : 80	1 : 80	9	12
210	1 : 2560	1 : 80	1 : 80	11	13
620	1 : 10240	1 : 160	1 : 160	13	15
1 290	1 : 40960	1 : 1280	1 : 160	17	20

* Calves were challenged with a mixture of milk and HSF.

The response to feeding with ovalbumin

To determine whether calves would develop similar responses to other food proteins two animals were given a series of experimental feeds containing ovalbumin instead of HSF. Within 2 - 3 weeks both animals had high titres of IgG antibodies to ovalbumin and experienced diarrhoea when challenged with this protein. Following the introduction of a mixture of milk and ovalbumin absorption of β-lactoglobulin was greatly increased in a sensitised compared with an unsensitised calf. (Table 3).

TABLE 3

SENSITISATION BY FEEDING WITH OVALBUMIN

| Hours after feed | Blood β-lactoglobulin after feeding: | | | |
| | Sensitised calf | | Unsensitised calf | |
	Milk	Milk + OA	Milk	Milk + OA
0	0	0	12	18
2	11	142	16	32
4	11	288	16	35

DISCUSSION

The data described here and in previous reports (Kilshaw and Sissons, 1979[a]; Kilshaw and Slade,1980) show that about 50% of calves fed soyabean protein by the regimen that has been described developed severe gastrointestinal disturbances. The belief that these were attributable to immunological mechanisms is based on the following observations. Adverse reactions to soya protein developed gradually with successive challenges and did not occur initially, neither casein nor milk provoked abnormalities in animals reacting to HSF, and the sensitivity of the gut to HSF was retained for several weeks without re-exposure to soyabean proteins.

In sensitised calves ingestion of HSF increased the rate
of flow of digesta through the distal ileum. This was partly
attributable to a decrease in transit time (Sissons and Smith,
1976) but the very large volume of fluid in the gut and the
occasional presence of fibrin suggested substantial leakage of
body fluids into the intestinal lumen.

Ingestion of milk during reactions to HSF led to blood
β-lactoglobulin levels up to 100 times greater than normal.
The magnitude of this change in absorption strongly suggests
that the permeability of the intestinal wall had increased
although it is possible that other factors such as impairment
in proteolysis of milk protein could have contributed.
Absorption increased 1 - 2 h after ingestion of HSF, was still
elevated at 4 - 6 h but had returned to normal after 24 h.
Detection of this change has provided a simple and sensitive
diagnostic test for gastrointestinal allergy in calves. It is
conceivable that a similar approach could be of value in man.

Maternal β-lactoglobulin was a suitable marker for
permeability studies because it did not evoke an antibody
response in calves and therefore its permeation through the
mucosa was not subject to immunological mechanisms for antigen
clearance and exclusion. Further, it had a suitable molecular
size for revealing permeability changes (Kingham and Loehry,
1976) and had the advantage of being quickly cleared from the
blood.

Neither free nor complexed soyabean antigens have been
detected in the serum (Kilshaw, unpublished), but their
persistence in the circulation would be unlikely in the presence
of very high antibody levels.

An increase in the sensitivity of the gut to HSF was
accompanied by rising titres of IgG, IgA and IgM antibodies in
the serum. It is not clear whether IgG antibodies were
important in causing the reactions to HSF or were merely a
consequence of increased penetration of soya antigens through

the mucosa. Low levels of reagins were detected, however, the
sensitivity of the PCA test in calves was variable and serum
from sensitised animals sometimes gave negative results.
Calves reacting severely to HSF showed immediate wheal and
flare reactions to intradermal injection of soyabean proteins.
A similar antibody response to ingested HSF occurred in calves
that had not undergone intestinal surgery (Kilshaw and Sissons,
1979a).

The immunological mechanisms responsible for the intestinal
disturbances are uncertain. Hypersensitivity in the calf gut
has been attributed to complement fixing IgGl (Barratt et al.,
1978) and to IgE (Barratt and Porter,1979). In the present
experiments and in previous studies (Smith and Sissons,1975)
functional changes in the intestine were detected 1 - 2 h after
challenge with HSF. These kinetics are consistent with Type 1
hypersensitivity.

Histological examination of mucosal biopsies removed
before, during and after,reactions to HSF have revealed neither
cellular infiltration of the lamina propria nor villous atrophy
(Kilshaw, unpublished).

A previous report established that the principal antigens
evoking the antibody response to HSF were the storage globulins
glycinin and β-conglycinin (Kilshaw and Sissons,1979b). The
present studies show that ovalbumin too induced antibody
production and gastrointestinal hypersensitivity.

Daily as well as occasional feeding with HSF evoked
vigorous and sustained antibody production (Kilshaw and
Sissons,1979a, Barratt et al., 1978). This contrasts with
observations in other experimental animals in which antigen
given orally has usually induced tolerance or a weak or short-
lived serum antibody response (Wells and Osborne,1911; Thomas
and Parrott,1974; Newby et al., 1979). Our results therefore
suggest some inadequacy in the immunological control mechanisms
of the young calf in these circumstances. The susceptibility

of ruminating animals to immunologically mediated gastro-intestinal disturbances is unknown but it is possible that degradation of foreign protein within the rumen may be an important factor in prevention.

The young calf has been shown to develop gastrointestinal hypersensitivity to dietary protein readily and without extreme immunological manipulation. This makes it an unusual and attractive experimental model for further study.

ACKNOWLEDGEMENTS

The author wishes to thank Dr. J.W. Sissons for determining the rates of flow of digesta and Mrs. H. Slade for her technical assistance.

REFERENCES

Barratt, M.E.J., Strachan, P.J. and Porter, P., 1978. Antibody mechanisms
implicated in digestive disturbances following ingestion of soya
protein in calves and piglets. Clin. exp. Immunol. 31, 305.

Barratt, M.E.J. and Porter, P., 1979. Immunoglobulin classes implicated in
intestinal disturbances of calves associated with soya protein
antigens. J. Immunol. 123, 676.

Colvin, B.M. and Ramsey, H.A., 1968. Soy flour in milk replacers for
young calves. J. Dairy. Sci. 51, 898.

Gorrill, A.D.L. and Thomas, J.W., 1967. Body weight changes, pancreas
size and enzyme activity, and proteolytic enzyme activity and
protein digestion in intestinal contents from calves fed soybean
and milk protein diets. J. Nutr. 92, 215.

Kilshaw, P.J. and Sissons, J.W., 1979a. Gastrointestinal allergy to
soyabean protein in preruminant calves. Antibody production and
digestive disturbances in calves fed heated soyabean flour.
Res. Vet. Sci. 27, 361.

Kilshaw, P.J. and Sissons, J.W., 1979b. Gastrointestinal allergy to
soyabean protein in preruminant calves. Allergenic constituents
of soyabean products. Res. Vet. Sci. 27, 366.

Kilshaw, P.J. and Slade, H., 1980. Passage of ingested protein into the
blood during gastrointestinal hypersensitivity reactions:
experiments in the preruminant calf. Clin. exp. Immunol. 41,
(in press).

Kingham, J.G.C. and Loehry, C.A., 1976. Permeability of the small
intestine after intra-arterial injection of histamine-type mediators
and irradiation. Gut. 17, 517.

Newby, T.J., Stokes, C.R., Huntley, J., Evans, P. and Bourne, F.J., 1979.
The immune response of the pig following oral immunisation with
soluble protein. Vet. Immunol. Immunopathol. 1, 37.

Sissons, J.W. and Smith, R.H., 1976. The effect of different diets
including those containing soyabean products, on digesta movement
and water and nitrogen absorption in the small intestine of the preruminant calf. Br. J. Nutr. 36, 421.

Sissons, J.W. and Smith, R.H., 1978. Measurement of flow and sampling of
digesta in the preruminant calf. J. Physiol. 283, 307.

218

Smith, R.H. and Sissons, J.W., 1975. The effect of different feeds, including those containing soya-bean products, on the passage of digesta from the abomasum of the preruminant calf. Br. J. Nutr. 33, 329.

Thomas, H.C. and Parrott, D.M.V., 1974. The induction of tolerance to a soluble protein antigen by oral administration. Immunology. 27, 631.

Van Adrichem, P.W.M. and Frens, A.M., 1965. Sojaeiwit als alimentair antigeen bij mestkalveren. Tijdschr. Diergeneesk. 90, 525.

Wells, H.G. and Osborne, T.B., 1911. The biological reactions of the vegetable proteins. J. Infectious. Dis. 8, 66.

DISCUSSION

J. Bienenstock *(Canada)*

Ellen Jarrett's work suggests that dose would make a profound difference. Do you find this?

P.J. Kilshaw *(UK)*

I have not actually tried. However, because my colleagues have been feeding very low levels of soya, less than 10%, in their milk replacer diets for some time, I suspect that low doses will not evoke this sort of response.

J. Bienenstock

The interpretation of that might be not that it does not happen but that, in fact, a regulatory system might be invoked.

My second question is what happens if you continue to feed this particular product for a prolonged period of time? Does the symptomotology go away?

P.J. Kilshaw

We have kept it up for about three months and they become progressively worse until one really has to terminate the experiment. But for this period the antibody remains high and the animals remain sensitive. However, the reaginic antibody response in most of these animals does appear to be fairly shortlived in the serum.

Anne Ferguson *(UK)*

May I just clarify a point. Did you say that your colleagues are giving small, regular doses of soya and that does not produce the effect? Are you saying that this effect occurs only with single doses once or twice a week?

P.J. Kilshaw

I don't really know; I suspect that low doses won't cause it, but I have not done the experiment myself.

Anne Ferguson

It was not so much a question of low doses as of frequent ones - several times a day, in the feed.

P.J. Kilshaw

Twice a day, yes. Certainly 30% does cause it but as regards lower levels I don't know from personal experience.

Anne Ferguson

That's 30% given every day?

P.J. Kilshaw

Yes, 30% of the protein in the feed - the remaining protein being milk protein.

H. Miller *(UK)*

Just as a point of interest, what were the calves fed on apart from the soya bean?

P.J. Kilshaw

Natural milk only; it made no difference to the response.

J. Soothill *(UK)*

The half that don't get it, and the half that do, is, I think, most interesting. You do have monovulare twins in cattle; is the response or non-response genetically determined?

P.J. Kilshaw

I don't know, but I agree this is a very good point. You probably noticed when I showed the graphs of antibody production that some of the animals had low initial titres anyway, apparently before they had been exposed, probably of maternal origin. It has been suggested by Barratt and Porter that the higher the level of the initial levels, the more likely they are to develop these disturbances. We have not found this.

Anne Ferguson

I believe Barratt and Porter introduced the idea of heating the flour and found that only unheated flour produced a proper enteropathy. Are your experiments comparable?

P.J. Kilshaw

I think that the way to avoid these problems in practice is to denature the proteins very severely. One can do this simply by treating them with hot ethanol. I believe that Barratt and Porter used ethanol-treated soya which was not treated severely enough to remove free beta-conglycinin and glycinin which they pick up by conventional techniques.

J. Soothill

There is another practical approach; if it is genetically determined you can just breed out the characteristic.

P.J. Kilshaw

Yes - but I don't think it is really a practical problem; it is an interesting model for allergy. One can get over the practical difficulties.

Anne Ferguson

The proceedings of this meeting will probably be read by people like me who don't know much about veterinary practice, except that parasitology is much more important in veterinary practice than it is in British human practice. Presumably your animals don't have parasites, or giardia or gastro intestinal infections due to virus, or am I wrong in making this assumption?

P.J. Kilshaw

I think that is correct.

Anne Ferguson

So they are also, as John Soothill pointed out this morning, 'artificially clean' compared to normal domestic animals.

P.J. Kilshaw

Well, to be frank I haven't really looked at the flora and I can't give you a straight answer to that, except that there is no excessive growth of *coli*.

Anne Ferguson

But they are kept in more or less pathogen free surroundings I suppose?

P.J. Kilshaw

Well, yes, compared with the farm.

J. Seifert *(FRG)*

There is one thing I do not understand. You told us that permeability is increased in immunised animals, but there are a lot of investigations in the literature, from André and his group and Walker, among others, which show that in immunised animals the absorption of foreign proteins is decreased. Perhaps you can explain this.

P.J. Kilshaw

Walker does believe that you can increase absorption. His recent paper on sensitisation with *Nippostrongylus* shows this. But I think that we have a reaginic type 1 reaction occurring in the gut mucosa and any protective IgA response that might be there is irrelevant.

H. Bazin *(Belgium)*

How old are your animals when your first IgE reaginic reaction occurs?

P.J. Kilshaw

All our experiments have started at about two months *post partum*. From our graph, IgE appears very quickly, within a week.

C. André *(France)*

In response to the point raised by Dr. Seifert, there are some indications in the literature that in animals immunised by the oral route there is a reduction of the absorption of the related antigen. In particular, where you are looking at Type 1 hypersensitivity, you could have a reduction of the specific antigen but an increased absorption of unrelated antigen for the reason that there is a variation of vascular phenomena.

Anne Ferguson

We must be careful not to confuse IgA and IgE. Walker has always made the point that it is IgA, and possibly IgG1 which is responsible for exclusion.

ALTERED IMMUNE FUNCTION ASSOCIATED
WITH DIETARY FACTORS

C.R. Stokes, T.J. Newby and F.J. Bourne
Department of Animal Husbandry,
University of Bristol, Langford House,
Langford, Bristol BS18 7DU, UK.

ABSTRACT

Mucosal presentation of antigens can promote both antigen specific (e.g. oral tolerance, immune exclusion) and antigen non-specific events (e.g. increased mucosal permeability to heterologous antigens). We have studied the antigen non-specific effects of two types of feeding regimes.

Firstly, the introduction of 25 mg of a new protein antigen into the diets of mice produced transient increases in macrophage function which reached a maximum 60 h after the change of diet but which had disappeared by 4 days. At the same time, the immune responsiveness to unrelated antigen given parenterally was also raised transiently, reaching a peak 5 days following the change and disappearing by 7 days. Further studies indicate that this effect may be mediated via T-cells.

Secondly, feeding B-cell mitogens (Escherichia coli lipopoly-saccharide, or dextran sulphate) to mice enhanced the tolerising effect of orally administered picryl chloride on the development of contact sensitivity to picryl chloride. Studies in the pig indicate that B-cell mitogens may similarly control immunologically induced gut damage.

INTRODUCTION

A wide variety of substances are presented via the oral route including soluble proteins and B-cell mitogens. Feeding soluble proteins promotes a number of immunological events, including immune exclusion (Walker et al., 1972; Swarbrick et al., 1979), oral tolerance (Thomas and Parrott, 1974; André et al., 1975) and cell mediated immunity (Waldmann and Henney, 1971; Huntley et al., 1979). Whilst the protective significance of the first two are clearly apparent, the functional importance of the latter is unclear. We have therefore studied the effects of lymphokines, (as generated by feeding soluble proteins) on central macrophage function *in vitro* (as measured by the rate of clearance of polyvinylpyrrolidone (PVP) (Morgan and Soothill, 1975). Since macrophages are involved in both the afferent and efferent limbs of the immune response we have further studied the effect of minor dietary change on the immune responsiveness of mice to unrelated antigens.

Feeding the contact sensitising agent picryl chloride generates the formation of both effector T-lymphocytes and suppressor B-cells (Asherson et al., 1977; Polak et al., 1975). Since Asherson et al. (1977) showed that the suppressor cells originated from the Peyer's patch we have investigated the possibility that feeding B-cell mitogens might expand the suppressor cell population and so render the animal less sensitive to subsequent challenge. Further, it has been suggested that delayed hypersensitivity reactions in the intestine may be a cause of intestinal damage (Ferguson and MacDonald, 1977) we have investigated therefore the possibility that B-cell mitogens may reduce the severity of immunologically induced gut damage.

MATERIALS AND METHODS

Experimental procedures used in the study of the effects of soluble protein antigens on polyvinylpyrrolidone (PVP) clearance and immune responsiveness have been described previously (Newby et al., 1980a). Briefly, studies were performed in CBA, A or C_3H male mice (LAC grade IV) which had been maintained upon Oxoid breeding diet which contains no ovalbumin or HSA for at least 3 weeks prior to experimentation. Soluble protein antigens, ovalbumin (ova) or human serum albumin (HSA) were either given as a 0.5% solution in the drinking water, or incorporated into the food pellets at a concentration of 1%. PVP clearance and immune responses were measured 4 days after their introduction into the diets.

Details of the experimental procedures of the mouse, B-cell mitogen study are described in Newby et al. (1980b).

EXPERIMENTS AND RESULTS

A. The effects of introducing new soluble protein antigen into the diets of mice

i) Macrophage function

The effect of the time of introduction of ovalbumin (0.5%; giving a daily dosage of 25 mg) into the diets of A strain mice, upon PVP clearance is shown in Figure 1. PVP clearance rates of control mice, maintained on a normal diet, remained constant throughout the experiment. In mice to whose drinking water from 0 h Ovalbumin had been added, the rate of clearance of PVP was significantly raised at 20 h (t = 2.59; P < 0.02) reaching a peak at approximately 70 h (t = 2.81; P < 0.01) and was no longer raised significantly at 90 h (t = 0.92; P > 0.1).

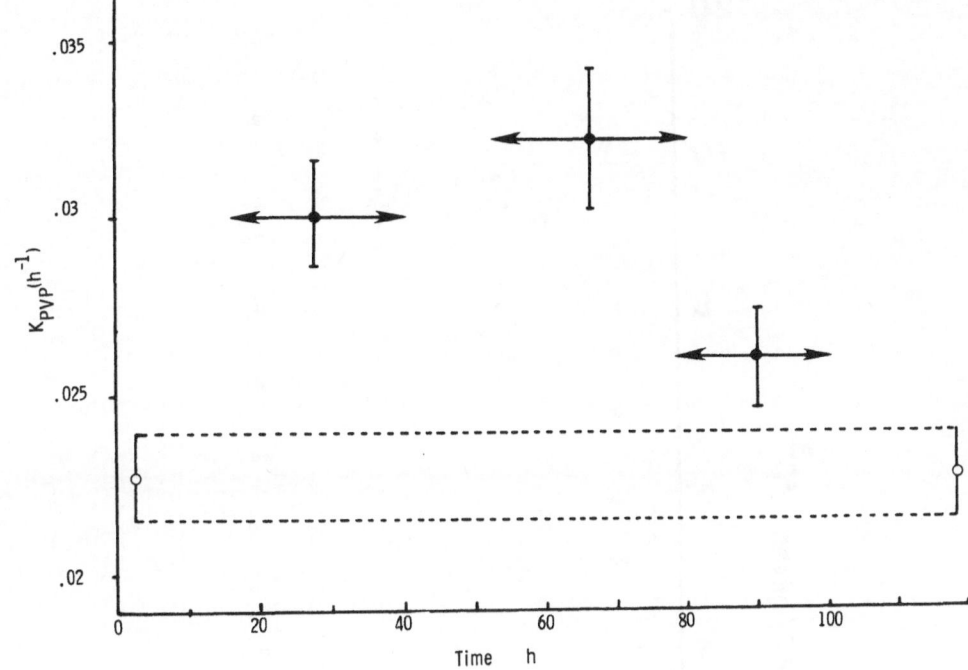

Fig. 1.   PVP clearance (K_{PVP} (h^{-1})) in A strain mice to whose drinking water
ovalbumin has been added from 0 h (Closed symbols). Control mice
(open symbols) were maintained on a normal diet and K_{PVP} (h^{-1})
remained constant during the experiment. The arrow headed
horizontal bars represent the interval between two bleeds. The
natural log of the counts of the second bleed were expressed as
a percentage of the natural log of the counts of the first and the
K_{PVP} (h^{-1}) calculated from the regression of the data from eight
animals against time. Each point represents the slope ± its
standard error (vertical bars).

ii)   Immune responsiveness

a)   Particulate antigen (SRBC)

The 4 day spleen plaque forming cell response (SPFC) to
intraperitoneal immunisation (IP) with 1 x 10^7 sheep red blood
cells (SRBC) was measured in CBA mice maintained on a normal
diet (control) and to groups of mice immunised with SRBC, 2, 5
or 7 days after the start of daily addition of HSA to the diet
(0.5% in the drinking water). The results are shown in Figure 2.
Mice fed the new antigen for days before immunisation with SRBC
showed a non-significant 2.5 fold increase in SPFC ($P < 0.1$

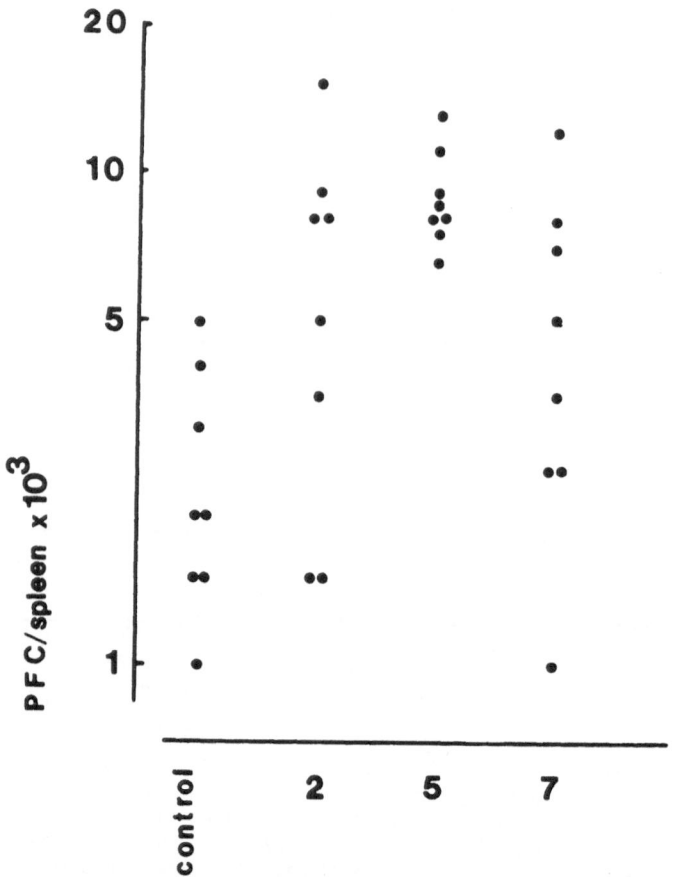

Fig. 2. Spleen plaque forming cell response to SRBC in CBA mice on a normal diet (controls) or immunised IP 2, 5 or 7 days following the introduction of HSA into the diet.

compared to controls). However, those fed the new antigen (HSA) for 5 days before the IP immunisation with SRBC showed a four fold increase, which was highly significant (P < 0.01). In contrast, 7 days feeding resulted in only a slight (2 fold) increase in the immune response (P > 0.1).

        b)   Soluble antigens (Dnp-HSA; Dnp-ficol)

The 4 day SPFC to Dnp following IP immunisation with 100 µg of either dinitrophenylated-HSA (Dnp-HSA) or dinitrophenylated ficol (Dnp-ficol) in saline was measured in CBA mice maintained on a normal diet (c) and in those to whose food pellets ovalbumin had been added for 4 days prior to the immunisation. The results are shown in Figure 3.

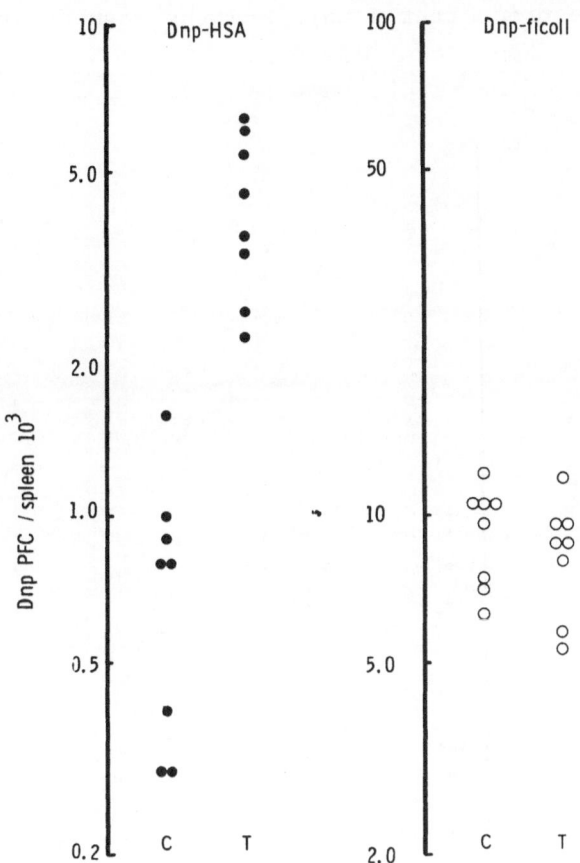

Fig. 3. Spleen plaque forming cell response to Dnp in CBA mice immunised IP with either Dnp-HSA (closed symbols) or Dnp-ficol (open symbols) whilst on a normal diet (c) or 4 days after the introduction of ovalbumin into their diet (T).

    c)   Genetic variation of altered immune responsiveness to SRBC.

Since it is known that genetic differences exist in the ability of different strains of mice to develop oral tolerance (Swarbrick and Stokes, 1979), we examined the immune response of different strains of mice 4 days after the introduction of a new dietary antigen. (The feeding regime used to induce oral tolerance).

230

Groups of eight A, C_3H and CBA mice were immunised IP.
with 1×10^7 SRBC either whilst on a normal diet or 4 days after
the introduction of ovalbumin into the food pellets. SPFC
response was measured after 4 days and the results are shown
in Figure 4.

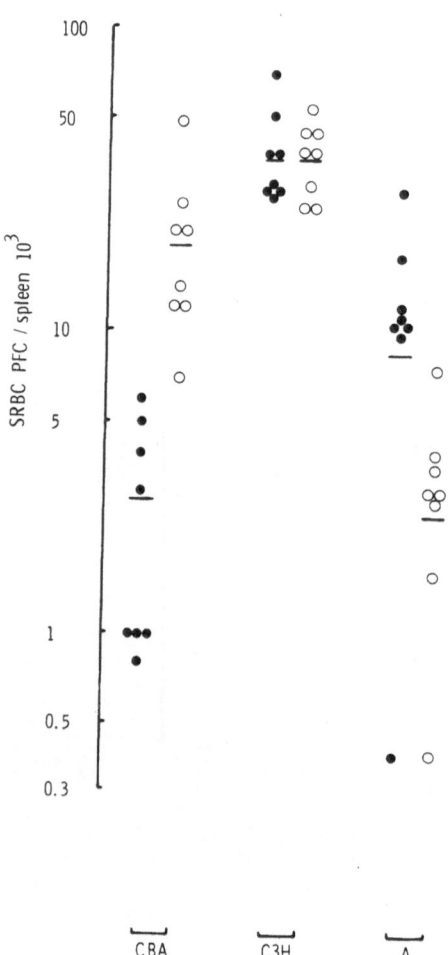

Fig. 4. Spleen plaque forming cell response to I.P. SRBC in CBA, C_3H and
A strain mice on normal diets (closed symbols) or 4 days after the
introduction of ovalbumin into their diets (open symbols).

The response in CBA mice immunised (4 days after the
introduction) was significantly greater than in those immunised
whilst on a normal diet (P < 0.01). The response in the C_3H mice

was however identical on the two feeding regimes (P > 0.1). In contrast the response in the A strain mice was significantly reduced after the addition of ovalbumin to the diet, compared to A strain mice immunised whilst on the normal diet.

iii) Low zone (T-cell) tolerance induction

The experiments in section A II b indicate a T-cell dependence for the altered immune responsiveness that occurs following the introduction of a new soluble protein into the diet. We have therefore investigated the effect of a minor dietary change on the induction to tolerance to low doses of injected deaggregated immunoglobulin, which is known to be T-cell dependent (Weigle, 1973). Figure 5 shows the 14 days serum IgG antibody response (measured by ELISA and expressed as a percentage of serum standard) in 3 groups of CBA mice to IP. immunisation with 100 µg of heat aggregated pig IgG. Two groups had 10 days earlier been injected with 60 µg of deaggregated pig IgG (tolerogen). For 4 days before and one day after tolerogen injection, one of the two groups had received ovalbumin in their diet.

Of the two groups on a stable diet the response to IgG was significantly reduced (P < 0.05) in those mice pre-treated with deaggregated IgG (tolerogen). In contrast those mice receiving the tolerogen, during the period when ovalbumin had been added to their diet, responded equally well, compared to the non-tolerogen treated controls and significantly better than those receiving the tolerogen while on a stable diet (P < 0.01).

B. The effects of feeding B-cell mitogens

i) The development of oral tolerance to contact sensitising agents

It has been shown that systemic pre-treatment with B-cell mitogens suppresses delayed hypersensitivity responses to a number of antigens (LaGrange et al., 1975). L'age-Stehr and Diamanstein (1977) and Collizzi and Bozzi, (1979) have suggested

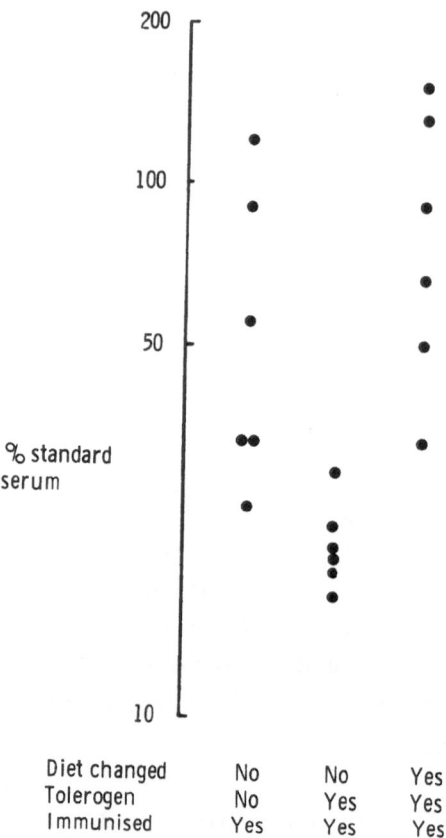

Fig. 5. Serum IgG antibody response to heat aggregated pig IgG (expressed as percentage of serum standard) in 3 groups of CBA mice. Two groups had 10 days earlier been injected 60 μg of deaggregated pig IgG (tolerogen). For 4 days before and 1 day after the tolerogen, one of the two groups had received ovalbumin in their diet.

that they act by enhancing the generation of suppressor B-cells during the induction of the immune response. Since Asherson et al. (1977) have shown that such cells originate from Peyer's patch, following feeding contact sensitising agents, we have investigated the effect of feeding *E. coli* lipopolysaccharide (LPS) (a B-cell mitogen) upon the generation of oral hyporesponsiveness to contact sensitising agents using suboptimal tolerising doses of picryl chloride.

The effect of feeding LPS on contact hypersensitivity
response was compared in four groups of mice. Group 1 mice
were painted twice with picryl chloride and served as a positive
control. Mice in group 2 were rendered hyporesponsive by
feeding picryl chloride for three days, 6 - 8 days before
topical sensitisation. Mice in groups 3 and 4 received a
single picryl chloride feed 7 days before topical sensitisation.
Mice in group 4 were also fed LPS throughout the experiment
starting 3 days before the picryl chloride feed. The regime
and results are shown in Table 1.

TABLE 1 a)   EXPERIMENTAL REGIME

Day 0	Commence daily feeding of LPS
Day 3 (2 - 4)	Picryl chloride feed
Day 10	Mice painted with picryl chloride on abdomen
Day 17	Mice painted with picryl chloride on ear
Day 18	Change in ear thickness measured

TABLE 1 b)   EFFECT OF LPS FEEDING ON ORALLY INDUCED HYPORESPONSIVENESS

Group	LPS*	Picryl Chloride	Δ Ear thickness**	% Suppression
1	–	Paint - Paint	5.9 ± 3.3	–
2	- Fed (x3)	-Paint - Paint	0.12 ± 2.06	98
3	- Fed -	Paint - Paint	5.0 ± 3.7	15
4	+ Fed	Paint - Paint	1.8 ± 0.9	75

* LPS was fed daily throughout the experiment commencing 3 days before the
picryl chloride feed.
** Mean (of 8) increment of ear thickness at 24 h in units of $10^{-3} \pm$ SD.
T statistic 1 v 4 t = 3.44 $P < 0.01$. 3 v 4 t = 2.41 $P < 0.05$
2 v 4 t = 2.30 $P < 0.05$

The results indicate that while a single picryl chloride
feed reduced the response by 15%, the group fed LPS throughout
the experiment showed a much greater reduction in response which
was significantly lower than both the non-fed group and the
group given a single picryl chloride feed, but similar to those

fed the optimal tolerising regime of three feeds. In contrast
however, feeding LPS had no effect on serum antibody levels to
Dnp.

ii)   Immunologically induced gut damage

It has been suggested that delayed hypersensitivity
reactions in the intestine may be a cause of intestinal damage
(Ferguson and MacDonald, 1977). Since the previous experiment
(B 1) has shown that feeding B-cell mitogens inhibits delayed
hypersensitivity reactions elicited at distal sites we
investigated the possibility that feeding LPS may block
immunologically induced gut damage.

Three groups of large white pigs, aged 3 - 4 weeks, which
had been exclusively fed by the sow, were studied as to their
ability to absorb Xylose and microscopically, for villous
architecture, after the following experimental regime.

Group 1, were sensitised by feeding 100 mg of ovalbumin
daily for three days. One week later they were challenged on
4 consecutive days with 2 g ovalbumin. Their ability to
absorb Xylose was measured after a further 4 days. Group 2,
acted as a specificity control, in that they were sensitised
with HSA (100 mg/day), whilst group 3 received no
sensitisation or challenge. The results (Figure 6) show that
Xylose absorption was significantly reduced in the group
challenged with ovalbumin, by comparison to the specificity
control group sensitised with HSA, and the untreated group.

Example pigs from each group were sacrificed and their
gut architecture examined, villus : crypt ratios are given in
Table 2. Compared to unsensitised controls, the mean ratio for
the pigs in group 2, sensitised with HSA, was only slightly
reduced (< 5%). In contrast, however, those sensitised and
challenged with ovalbumin showed a marked reduction (> 30%).
The gut damage (as measured by decreased Xylose absorption and
villus : crypt ratios) is thus immunologically specific. We

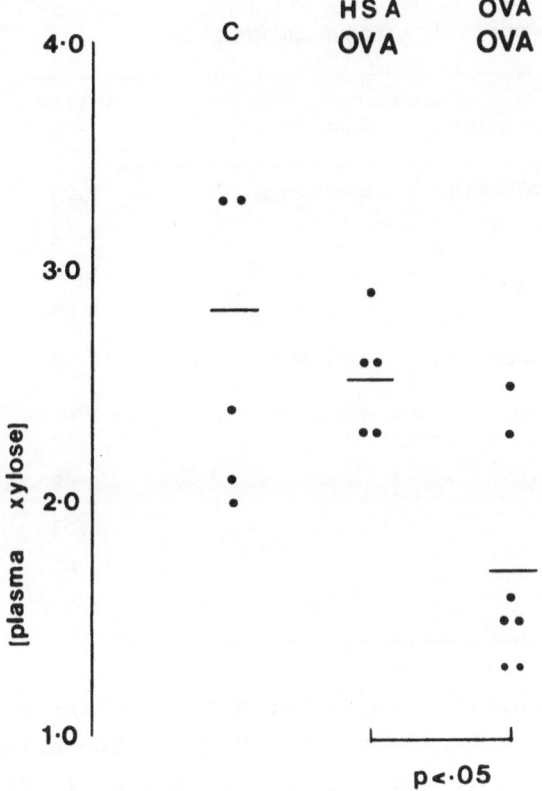

Fig. 6. Plasma Xylose concentration in three groups of pigs, 60 minutes
after Xylose feed (100 mg 1 Kg). One group had been sensitised
and challenged with ovalbumin (Ova/ova), another sensitised with
HSA and challenged with ovalbumin (HSA/ova) whilst the other was
untreated control (C).

have therefore investigated the effect of feeding a B-cell
mitogen (*E. coli* LPS) on immunologically induced gut damage.

Two groups of pigs (aged 3 - 4 weeks) were sensitised
to ovalbumin by feeding 100 mg of protein for three days.
One group also received LPS for 6 days, commencing 2 days
before the first sensitising dose of ovalbumin. After a
further week all pigs were challenged daily with 2 g ovalbumin
for 4 days. Their ability to absorb Xylose was compared
4 days later. The results are shown in Figure 7. Those
animals sensitised with ovalbumin whilst receiving LPS

TABLE 2

EFFECT OF ANTIGEN FEEDING ON VILLOUS ARCHITECTURE

Group	Treatment Sensitised	Challenged	Villus : Crypt Ratio	Mean
1	Ovalbumin	Ovalbumin	1.93	
			1.52	
			1.32	
			1.94	1.68
2	HSA	Ovalbumin	2.38	
			1.91	
			2.52	
			2.38	2.30
3	-	-	2.03	
			2.65	
			2.57	2.42

absorbed significantly more Xylose after challenge with
ovalbumin, indicating a less damaged gut. The difference
between the two groups (Figure 7) was similar to the reduction
in Xylose absorption induced by ovalbumin feeding compared to
untreated controls. (Figure 6). Thus it would appear to
prevent or at least reduce the immunologically induced gut
damage.

We have not investigated the mechanism by which LPS feeding
might reduce gut damage. However if the immunologically
induced damage involves a delayed hypersensitivity reaction it
is possible that it may act by expanding the population of
suppressor B-cells in a manner analogous to that postulated
by Collizzi and Bozzi (1979) for delayed hypersensitivity
reactions in mice.

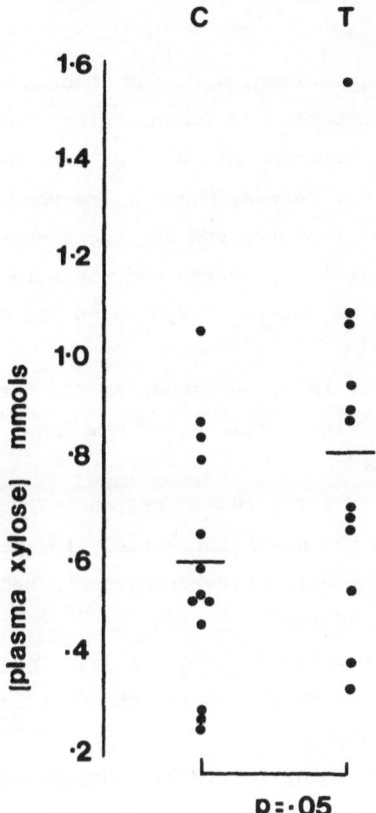

Fig. 7. Plasma Xylose concentration in two groups of pigs, 60 minutes after Xylose feed (100 mg/kg). Both groups were sensitised and challenged with ovalbumin. Test animals (T) received LPS for 6 days during the period of sensitisation.

REFERENCES

André, C., Heremans, J-F., Vaerman, J.P. and Combiaso, C.L., 1975. A
    mechanism for the induction of immunological tolerance by antigen
    feeding: antigen-antibody complexes. J. exp. Med. 142, 1509.

Asherson, G.L., Zembala, M., Perera, M.A.C.C., Mayhew, B. and Thomas, W.R.,
    1977. Production of Immunity and unresponsiveness in the mouse by
    feeding contact sensitising agents and the role of suppressor cells
    in Peyer's patches, mesenteric lymph nodes and other tissues. Cell
    Immunol. 33, 145.

Collizzi, V. and Bozzi, L., 1979. A mechanism for the depression of
    contact sensitivity with B-cell mitogens. Ann. Immunol. (Inst.
    Pasteur). 130C, 659.

Ferguson, A. and MacDonald, T.T., 1977. Effects of local delayed
    hypersensitivity on the small intestine. In: Ciba Foundation
    Symposium 46 (new series), Elsevier/Excerpta/Medica/North Holland and
    Elsevier North Holland Inc.

Huntley, J., Newby, T.J. and Bourne, F.J., 1979. The cell-mediated immune
    response of the pig to orally administered antigen. Immunology.
    37, 225.

L'age-Stehr, J. and Diamanstein, T., 1977. Suppression and potentiation
    of expression of delayed hypersensitivity by dextran sulphate.
    Immunology. 33, 179.

La Grange, P.M., Mackaness, G.B., Miller, T.E. and Pardon, P., 1975. Effect
    of bacterial lipopolysaccharide on the induction and expression of cell
    mediated immunity. 1. Depression of the efferent arc. J. Immunol.
    114, 442.

Newby, T.J., Stokes, C.R. and Bourne, F.J., 1980a. Altered
    polyvinylpyrrolidone clearance and Immune responsiveness caused by
    small dietary changes. Clin. exp. Immunol. 39, 349.

Newby, T.J., Stokes, C.R. and Bourne, F.J., 1980b. Effects of feeding
    bacterial lipopolysaccharide and dextran sulphate on the development
    of oral tolerance to contact sensitising agents. Immunology. 40.

Polak, L., Geleik, H. and Turk, J.L., 1975. Reversal by cyclophosphamide of
    tolerance in contact sensitivity. Tolerance induced by prior feeding.
    Immunology. 28, 939.

Swarbrick, E.T. and Stokes, C.R., 1979. The Immune effects of ingested
    antigens in mice; in Protein Transmission through Living Membranes
    (Ed. by W.A. Hemmings), p. 309. Elsevier/North-Holland Biomedical Press.

Swarbrick, E.T., Stokes, C.R. and Soothill, J.F., 1979. The absorption of
    antigens after oral immunisation and the simultaneous induction of
    specific systemic tolerance. Gut. 20, 121.

Thomas, H.W. and Parrott, D.M.V., 1974. The induction of tolerance to a
    soluble protein antigen by oral administration. Immunology. 27, 631.

Waldmann, R.H. and Henney, C.S., 1971. Cell mediated Immunity and antibody
    responses in the respiratory tract after local and systemic immunisation.
    J. exp. Med. 134, 482.

Walker, W.H., Isselbacher, K.J. and Bloch, K.J., 1972. Intestinal uptake of
    macromolecules : effect of oral immunisation. Science. 177, 608.

Weigle, W.O., 1973. Immunological Unresponsiveness. Adv. Immunol. 16, 61.

DISCUSSION

J. Bienenstock *(Canada)*

You are not offering explanations but perhaps I might offer a speculation and you can tell me what you think about it. One possible explanation/speculation for your dramatic inform-. ation on dietary influence and the LPS results, might come from studies I discussed previously on germ-free animals and the effects of LPS and developing flora. The possibility is that feeding the extra soluble protein changes the gut flora, which in turn is the prime influence on the regulation of the macrophages and regulation of the immune response; here you have in one the explanation of your results.

C.R. Stokes *(UK)*

We thought along those lines and we did look at gut flora very crudely in these different groups. We didn't find any difference in total gut flora. Although the organisms were similar; we didn't carry out a quantitative study. It is quite a tempting idea, I agree.

J. Bienenstock

I think it is dangerous to make the assumption that LPS acts solely as a B-cell mitogen because it is obviously capable of doing many other things, including influencing macrophages and T cells in an equally potent way.

Anne Ferguson *(UK)*

You coyly avoided mentioning the point that was in the Discussion of one of your papers which you kindly sent to me, pointing out that *E. coli* were present in large numbers in the gut.

C.R. Stokes

E. coli are present in large numbers in the lower gut but not in the small intestine.

J. Hall *(UK)*

This is a technical question. You are interpreting the clearance of RD labelled PVP as an index of macrophage function. We use PVP quite a lot for damage that is inflicted by cytotoxic agents. I just wonder if this was a gut leak caused by the same mechanism.

C.R. Stokes

I was trying to call it PVP clearance throughout and not macrophage function. Yes, there is a possibility that it is increased mucosal leakage and therefore appearing as increased macrophage function is quite a possibility. I would not like to discount it.

Anne Ferguson

When you lose protein through the gut, usually you lose a lot of lymphocytes as well which throws out the whole balance of your immune cell traffic circulation.

K. Dalsgaard *(Denmark)*

Did you take measures to exclude the presence of endotoxin?

C.R. Stokes

It was made up of sterile saline but beyond that no. But the numbers would probably be relatively low.

W. Leibold *(FRG)*

You interpret your decreased cellular immune reaction as a suppressed reaction. How do you differentiate between a lack of help and an active suppression in what you induce?

C.R. Stokes

I was just referring back to the Asherson suggestion really - well Kalitsy and Botsky's - I can't remember exactly how they demonstrated it but I would be quite happy for there to be a lack of help as well. It was a convenient line of argument originally for designing the series of experiments, but whether or not it is the actual mechanism, I don't know.

J. Soothill *(UK)*

You are looking at antibody response Dr. Stokes. As you know I feel the plaque forming cell response is a very indirect way of looking at antibody. Now that you have got antigens, have you considered measuring ABT and affinity?

C.R. Stokes

We have looked for antibody concentrations as measured by ELISA assays and the same holds true as for plaque forming cell response.

J. Soothill

Good. But it would be interesting to know whether it is a higher affinity or a higher ABT.

C.R. Stokes

Yes. We have made a preliminary study of affinity, but this showed no difference.

Anne Ferguson

Thank you Dr. Stokes. We should now move on to the general discussion.

GENERAL DISCUSSION

Anne Ferguson *(UK)*

This general discussion is intended to include not only the three papers we have just had presented but also, if it seems relevant, the work on facets of hypersensitivity which has also been presented. I would like to put forward a working hypothesis which I did mention earlier, which is that if one has hypersensitivity reactions in the intestinal mucosa which are completely IgE mediated, then villus atrophy does not occur. We do not have any evidence that malabsorption of nutrients occurs, although I think that secretion of water and electrolytes probably does. In fact, it is very difficult to measure this phenomenon; things like Dr. Kilshaw's macromolecular leak are probably the best way to measure this in animals and in people. The circumstances which lead to an enteropathy with villus atrophy may be rather different; it is interesting that clearly there are species differences, age differences, differences between results from different groups who are perhaps using slightly modified preparations of the food. Although there are quite a few medical people here I think we should recognise that we are mainly thinking about diseases of animals. It is interesting that rotavirus infection was discovered as an explanation for supposedly allergic diarrhoeas in humans and it is beginning to look as if allergic diarrhoeas are the cause of what used to be called gastro enteritis in some animals.

J. Soothill *(UK)*

I would like to ask Dr. Kilshaw to elaborate on a remark he made in passing which I think has tremendous relevance to what we are talking about in a positive sense. What is the evidence that an individual is tolerant to the proteins of the milk of his mother, and if this is so, what are the mechanisms underlying it?

P.J. Kilshaw *(UK)*

The position in my calves is that I have never been able
to detect antibody by ELISA technique specific for milk proteins.
I have never actually tried to immunise them against milk and I
believe it is known that there is a syndrome in cows in which
there is an immediate hypersensitivity to milk protein in a
small proportion of cows when they are dried off, but it is a
very small percentage. As far as the mechanism of the tolerance
is concerned, I don't know.

J. Soothill

You are suggesting that there is no background literature
so that you have to go to the basic experiments yourself?

P.J. Kilshaw

I just looked for antibody; I suppose I assumed that they
probably would be tolerant, and I failed to find antibody
against milk proteins at any stage.

J. Soothill

May I put forward a speculation that this is the function
of witch's milk (milk produced by infants immediately after
birth).

P.J. Kilshaw

I agree entirely, yes. There is one small point I would
like to add on this. In very young calves, younger than I have
been dealing with in my experiments, there is a complex in the
serum between gammaglobulin and milk protein which persists; it
has a half life of about 10 days. It has gone by the age of a
couple of months which is when I started my experiments. It
occurs to me that this might have some significance in maintaining tolerance of the young calf against maternal milk
protein - I don't know - it is a curious complex, it is not
cleared from the blood and it is not split by buffers of low pH.

J. Quinn *(Ireland)*

Campbell reported in the Cornell Veterinarian about 1970 or 1972 that certain breeds of dairy cows showed immediate hypersensitivity if left unmilked for some time. It was a significant proportion of a herd that did this.

P.J. Kilshaw

That was the paper I was referring to, but I think it was only 1% or 2%, or even fewer.

J. Quinn

I think it was more than that; he could show skin reactivity and it was passively transferable as well, I believe.

E. Bohl *(USA)*

What clinical signs did these animals show?

J. Quinn

Anaphylaxis if challenged intravenously and sometimes they showed allergic reactions in that their hair was raised and they showed patches of oedema on the skin as well. It was spontaneous. These were ordinary farm animals and the reaction was protein induced - if they were left unmilked they were apparently able to absorb their own milk proteins into their system.

K.L. Morgan *(UK)*

There were huge numbers of eosinophils in the milk of those animals that were left unmilked.

J. Bienenstock *(Canada)*

It is very dangerous to draw the conclusion that they are allergic to their own milk proteins because as far as the breast is concerned (at least in the species that have been looked at) if you give, intravenously, a variety of antigens to a variety of animals, they will be relatively selectively secreted in the

milk. You can produce tolerance via the milk as a result of
that selective secretion and as a result of the new complex
formation within the milk and the subsequent absorption, before
closure, of that antigen complex to antibody. There is a great
deal of information in the literature in this area. It would
fit better with what Dr. Quinn and others have said, to suggest
that the allergy, if such existed, was in fact due to 'foreign'
antigen that they had sequestered in their own breasts at that
particular time. If that was the case - and I throw that open
for question - then it would also be interesting to follow
that line of reasoning and ask whether that is the mechanism
whereby a certain degree of regulation or tolerance is induced
in the offspring, by the presentation of antigen through milk
that the mother has been able to control. Is there any
information in this area?

Ellen Jarrett *(UK)*

I believe Benjamin has shown tolerance to antigens in
breast milk in mice; there are one or two other reports as well.

J. Hall *(UK)*

Alec Lascelle showed some time ago in Australia that in a
very high percentage of sheep, during involution of the mammary gland, the local lymph node produced precipitating antibodies
to casein, from the milk. I don't know whether he has elaborated on that but it does look as if animals aren't tolerant
to their own milk protein.

H. Williams Smith *(UK)*

From a practical point of view it is a common phenomenon
to leave animals with milk in their mammary glands and they
never come to any harm. The point was made earlier that there
are a lot of eosinophils in these particular animals. That is
surely an abnormal situation. I feel that you are picking on
one situation here which really does not have much to do with
animal husbandry in general.

Anne Ferguson

It seems to me that it would be easy enough to prove this point by injecting a few calves with milk in complete Freund's adjuvant.

H. Williams Smith

The point I want to make is that with cows, for example, at some stage you stop milking; you do the same thing with piglets, you take them away, you want abrupt weaning. Now, for some period of time, sows immediately after weaning, are gorged with milk. It is a normal process and they never come to any harm. Going on from that, Dr. Ferguson mentioned that allergic conditions are now being seen as being responsible for gastro enteritis in animals. Would you like to enlarge on that?

Anne Ferguson

I was referring to the syndrome that we call gastro enteritis - watery diarrhoea, with or without vomiting. What I am pointing out is that you now seem to be finding out that these conditions have an allergic basis over and above the new pathogens which have been identified.

I think it is probably pointless for us to debate whether cows can or cannot make antibodies to cows milk proteins when obviously the immunological experiments have not yet been done and are not in the literature.

F.J. Bourne (UK)

In relation to the hypersensitivity state that has been referred to, namely the allergic type of diarrhoea or gastric enteritis that may occur in farm animals, I feel it might be useful if we could discuss this a little further. Following Chris Stokes' talk and work done by him and Tim Newby, an hypothesis has evolved implicating allergy to food proteins causing gut damage in pigs during the post-weaning period. This may explain the increased susceptibility to infectious enteritis

at this time. Accepting that weaning occurs between 3 and 8
weeks of age in the pig, the situation is that it is followed
within a short period by villus atrophy associated with
malabsorption, an increase in water content of the faeces, and
loss of protein into the intestinal tract. This occurs in the
absence of bacterial involvement but may nonetheless be followed
by *E. coli* proliferation. The work we have done suggests that
we can bring about similar changes by sensitising an animal to
a dietary protein. The question that must be asked is how
realistic is it for us to formulate this hypothesis, and just
how significant might this be in terms of animal production?
In the veterinary field we are on a different level when we
talk about gut enteropathy compared to the human medical situation. We really are talking about an athlete in terms of
production, we want maximum production from an animal at
maximum food conversion rate. Anything that decreases food
conversion rate decreases growth rate and decreases profit -
put another way, it increases the price of food to man.

Anne Ferguson

You have formulated an hypothesis and you are accumulating
information to support it. In fact, your ovalbumin HSA controls
do show that it does seem to be antigen specific because,
certainly, dietary alterations in themselves can influence the
epithelial cell kinetics of the gut; the amount of fibre in the
diet influences epithelial cell kinetics in small and large
bowel and certainly in mice and rats. Just because a change in
diet produces an alteration in the anatomy of the intestinal
villi and crypts it is not necessarily immunological, although
your data suggests that this maybe so. Do you suggest that
materials used to feed animals should be screened for immunogenicity? Which facet of immunogenicity is likely to be
involved, IgE or cell mediated immunity?

F.J. Bourne

A simpler approach could be the feeding of a B cell
mitogen which would have a suppressive effect rather than screen-
ing diets for their antigenicity.

Anne Ferguson

Perhaps we should consider further the experiments that have been described on endotoxin. The audience might like to know a little more about the material from which the endotoxin was prepared. Was it a mixture of different *E. coli*?

T.J. Newby *(UK)*

We have used two B cell mitogens including heat stripped *E. coli* and dextran sulphate. Both have a similar effect.

Anne Ferguson

Have you, for example, taken Peyer's patch cells and looked at the number of B cells?

T.J. Newby

No, we have not. We haven't looked at the mechanism at all; we have just produced the effect which we have so far assumed is mediated by a similar effect to that found in systemic sensitisation.

Anne Ferguson

Are there any comments on this, or any other suggestions as to ways of enhancing tolerogenic facets of the gut associated lymphoid tissues? John Bienenstock, you had a list of about ten adjuvants; you also had a list of about half a dozen tolerising factors.

J. Bienenstock

I would like to ask a question of John Bourne. The problem lies with early weaning, is that correct?

F.J. Bourne

Well, all farm animals are early weaned.

J. Bienenstock

I presume that it is the abnorm and not the norm to find those changes in the gut following weaning which occurs whenever weaning would normally occur. There must be an arbitrary cut-off point to that.

F.J. Bourne

That may be so but, of course, commercially that is not done.

J. Bienenstock

But is there a known time for weaning beyond which you don't find these GI changes, and conversely, if you wean before that time, and increasingly before that time, you find increasingly greater changes? Because if there is a cut-off point then presumably we can now deal with the two populations and see what the difference is.

F.J. Bourne

I don't know. The original observations were made by Kenworthy on pigs which were weaned between six and eight weeks of age. The observations are very similar on pigs weaned at five weeks. Commercially, the vast majority of pigs in the UK are weaned between three and six weeks. Even if I could answer your question we would still have a problem in the industry.

J. Bienenstock

We know that animals, if weaned early, are still 'athletes'; they may not be quite super-athletes in the sense you were talking about. So presumably, whatever system is invoked it is capable of self regulation at that point despite the drastic changes occurring in the gastro intestinal tract. I don't know whether there is an equivalent in man.

F.J. Bourne

This does serve to emphasise the system in which we are working. John Bienenstock suggested that the gut has tremendous reserve capacity, are we sure that this is so? However, we are looking at factors which have an influence which would probably not be recognised in the human population. In an animal population it stands out significantly. Thus a minor change in gut physiology at the time of weaning could have a very significant effect on growth rate, enteric disease and performance. May I ask Anne Ferguson what tests she would use to demonstrate malabsorption?

Anne Ferguson

If I suspected that a human patient had malabsorption, I would use five tests of absorption - a glucose tolerance test, a Zeidel's test, a Shilling test, faecal fat, a vitamin A absorption. I would certainly measure food intake and output, because immune reactions are said to influence appetite.

J. Soothill

It is a terrible habit to make multiple measurements; you get different results from each of your tests and then you choose whichever you want! I say to you gastro enterologists that your overall functional measurement of gut function is extremely bad compared, for instance, with the kidney. I think the veterinarians have some justification in not following your example!

However, I would like to give another human equivalent. I am a little bit worried about Chris Stokes talking about giving endotoxin to improve situations because John Walker-Smith has shown that the relatively immuno-deficient child with gastro enteritis (and in some cases it was fairly clear that it was of *E. coli* origin) gets a transient food allergy afterwards. So, I think you can push it either way. You have a system which pushes it one way and which is very interesting.

C.R. Stokes *(UK)*

Experiments in the mouse have shown that the timing of the endotoxin delivery is very important. Mackanes's group has shown this clearly. You can get a totally reverse effect if you give it after sensitisation. We followed their protocols and chose the timing on the basis of their results. But I am sure you could get a totally reverse effect if you fed it later.

J. Soothill

Could we underline that in the discussion?

H. Williams Smith

Could I just ask a question about this endotoxin? How many cells did you say you are giving these pigs?

C.R. Stokes

10^{10}

H. Williams Smith

I would expect to have more than that in a pig's stomach all its life.

C.R. Stokes

I can't argue against that but we have used another B cell mitogen and induced the same effect: therefore, it is tempting to suggest that it is acting by a similar mechanism.

Anne Ferguson

It has been shown in man that transient, simple, intestinal infections can produce achlorhydria I don't think this applies to rotavirus infection. Achlorhydria, more than any specific immune reaction, has been shown to influence the proximal intestinal flora in man. Dr. Webster, at Northwick Park has found bacteria colonising the proximal small intestine in immune deficient patients. When he eventually looked at their acid secretory capacity he found that it was achlorhydria that correlated with colonisation of the intestine and not IgA or IgG deficiency. That is really almost an environmental factor rather than an immunological one.

One constructive suggestion I would make is that there clearly nees to be further research on *in vitro* methods of diagnosis of allergy. Dr. Kilshaw, you impied that there are tremendous difficulties in performing the PCA reaction. Do you give the calf an intravenous injection and kill it?

P.J. Kilshaw

Yes, I give it an intravenous injection of soya protein, and it is then usually killed.

H. Bazin *(Belgium)*

Do you believe it is IgE mediated or IgG, or both?

P.J. Kilshaw

I don't know. The only evidence I have that it is IgE is that the PCA test has a 72 hour latent period and the work of Hammer suggests that it is E rather than G. But I haven't tested heat stability of the reaginic antibody or its molecular weight so I can't be sure.

H. Bazin

What percentage of animals have hypersensitivity?

P.J. Kilshaw

About half.

H. Bazin

It is enormous. I have never known of one species with such a percentage of hypersensitivity, without adjuvants or anything.

P.J. Kilshaw

It is not a natural situation at all. I am infusing large
quantities of soya protein directly into the abomasum twice
weekly. It is certainly not the type of situation which occurs
on the farm.

Anne Ferguson

I have thought that the trypsin inhibitor might be important. Hanson in Denver has published an Abstract in one of the
American journals which shows that using a trypsin inhibitor
can influence the tolerogenicity of feeding of ovalbumin to
mice. But, of course, if you can get it with ovalbumin alone
that is another good theory out of the window.

P.J. Kilshaw

Well no, that would have trypsin inhibitor in it.

Anne Ferguson

Ovalbumin?

P.J. Kilshaw

Probably, ovamucoid. It is not pure at all in those
circumstances. It would not be practical to feed purified ovalbumin to a calf. I am certain there is ovamucoid there.

Anne Ferguson

What amount of ovalbumin did you give them?

P.J. Kilshaw

To sensitise, I feed 100 g.

H. Bazin

Why are you sure that it is not a Type 3 hypersensitivity?

P.J. Kilshaw

Type 3 doesn't fit the kinetics very well. The change occurs between 1 and 2 hours after challenge. It is probably quicker than that because one has to consider the time for the digesta to leave the abomasum and enter the small intestine. So it probably occurs sooner than 1 hour; other evidence from flow studies indicates that it occurs within about half an hour. So that makes it a bit unlikely. Secondly, I would have expected a cellular infiltrate in my mucosal biopsies after the reaction had occurred. I thought probably that I would have detected some C3 activation in the serum by counter immunoelectrophoresis. The negative findings from those studies seem to suggest that a Type 1 was more likely.

Anne Ferguson

You certainly get a dramatic polymorphic infiltrate in coeliac disease 4 to 8 hours after challenge. Bellamy, working in pigs, showed lovely pictures of enormous numbers of polymorphs but, again, at four hours.

P.J. Kilshaw

I sampled throughout. I sampled at six hours after challenge and then at 24 hours. So I have got a sample at the height of the action.

J. Quinn

I would like to comment on a complement and its activation in the bovine system. There is a naturally occurring serum protein in bovine serum called conglutinin which will react with activated complement, especially with C3b. This will result in a fairly rapid clearance. Did you look for this?

P.J. Kilshaw

Actually, I did look for changes in conglutinin for slightly different reasons and I didn't detect any. But there might not be any changes in total conglutinin level despite complement activation. I know it is naturally occurring but I thought initially that if there was a lot of immune complex in the serum one might detect a reduction of conglutinin, but there wasn't any.

R. Levinsky *(UK)*

In fact, the only way you could possibly detect complement activation is to look for C3b and there are methods of doing that now.

SESSION III

IMMUNE RESPONSE TO MICRO-ORGANISMS AND PROTECTION

Chairmen : T.J. Newby and E. Bohl

PASSIVE IMMUNITY AGAINST ENTERIC VIRAL INFECTIONS OF PIGLETS

E.H. Bohl and Linda J. Saif

Department of Veterinary Science, Ohio Agricultural
Research and Development Center, Wooster, Ohio 44691, USA.

ABSTRACT

An immunologic system has evolved whereby newborn animals derive an appreciable degree of protection from enteric infections by means of passive immunity. This report explores some of the facets of this system, using infections of swine with transmissible gastroenteritis virus, rotavirus, or enterovirus as examples. In swine, and probably in most monogastric animals, passive immunity against enteric infections is dependent on the ingestion – at normal intervals for the particular species – of colostrum or milk which contain appropriate levels of specific antibodies, with those of the IgA class being most protective. In swine, and probably in most monogastric animals, antibodies of the IgA class appear to occur in mammary secretions only, or primarily, as a result of an appropriate antigenic stimulation of the intestinal tract. This type of information, and the variables involved, is of special value when attempting to design an immunisation programme which will provide passive immunity against enteric infections.

Many enteric infections occur as enzootics, wherein young animals become infected during the suckling period or shortly after weaning. Pigs are usually protected from rotaviral or enteroviral infections during the first 2 to 5 weeks of age because of passive immunity, after which time an intestinal infection usually occurs. The occurrence and possible significance of boosting lactogenic immunity by natural re-infection or by vaccination are discussed and some results given.

INTRODUCTION

From the time of birth, most animals are reared in an
environment of limited sanitary conditions and, consequently,
are generally exposed to potential pathogens. This is well
illustrated when an attempt is made to rear orphan newborn
animals. Invariably, under conventional husbandry conditions,
they become sick and often die. However, a protective
immunologic system has evolved which tends to safeguard the
newborn against those pathogens normally found in its environment. With most animals, this system depends on the ingestion
of colostrum and milk, which provides a temporary degree of
passive immunity. Fortunately, during the period of passive
immunity, the young become partially susceptible to infection
with ubiquitous pathogens; allowing for only mild, if any,
clinical signs, and for development of semi-permanent active
immunity which replaces the temporary passive immunity.

Although animal husbandrymen and scientists have long
been aware of this protective system, only recently have some
of its mechanisms and intricacies been better understood.
This is especially true as it relates to the protection of
mucosal surfaces against infectious agents.

This report will discuss some characteristics of the
passive immune system as it applies to enteric viral infections
of pigs, with emphasis on rotavirus and transmissible gastroenteritis virus (TGEV). Some of this information should be
relevant to other animal species, especially monogastric
animals.

INFLUENCE OF PASSIVE IMMUNITY ON ENZOOTIC ENTERIC INFECTIONS

As a preface to discussing passive immunity, a few
comments on the immunoglobulin system in swine are indicated.
Pigs are essentially born agammaglobulinaemic. Immunoglobulins
are absorbed from colostrum for only the first 12 to 36 hours
after birth (Payne and Marsch, 1962). IgG accounts for about

80% of the total immunoglobulin in colostrum but rapidly declines so that a 30-fold decrease occurs during the first week of lactation, and remains a minor component of milk during the remainder of lactation (Curtis and Bourne, 1971). Although the level of IgA in colostrum is only 16% of that of IgG, it declines only 3-fold and soon becomes the predominant immunoglobulin in milk (Curtis and Bourne, 1971; Porter and Allen, 1972). IgM is at low level in both colostrum and milk. In colostrum, nearly all of the IgG and 40% of IgA are derived from serum; but in milk more than 90% of IgA and IgM, and 70% of IgG are produced in the mammary gland (Bourne and Curtis, 1973). Thus, colostrum can be considered a concentrated serum transudate, while milk is a secretion. The transition from colostrum to milk occurs during the first 3 to 7 days of lactation, with the predominant change occurring during the first 24 hours. As used in this report, milk refers to mammary secretions occurring only after 72 hours post-partum.

Many enteric viral infections of swine occur at a young age when pigs have a variable degree of passive immunity acquired from nursing immune mothers. A similar situation occurs with most species of animals and to a lesser extent with man, depending on sanitary conditions. Most of these enzootic viral infections will be either subclinical or will result in clinical signs which are less severe than would usually occur in immunologically susceptible animals. Since many infections cannot be prevented, the objective is to provide satisfactory immunity, sanitation, nutrition, and environmental conditions so as to prevent or minimise disease. Thus, there is interest in how an optimal level of passive immunity can be routinely and consistently provided to young animals so as to minimise disease from enzootic enteric infections.

Two types of studies are indicated: (1) How can existing immunity in females best be boosted so as to provide passive immunity? This will be discussed later. (2) What might be the overall benefits derived from improved passive immunity to the young? In regard to the latter, little may be accomplished if

immunity provided to suckling animals is of such high degree
that infection would occur only after weaning, at a time when
animals may be more susceptible to a severe infection.
Weanling diarrhoea is often a serious problem in pigs, other
animals, and children, especially when sanitation, nutrition,
and environmental conditions are poor. An absence or decline
in lactogenic immunity - due to antibodies in milk - or humoral
immunity probably contributes to the occurrence or severity of
weanling diarrhoea.

Enzootic infections of pigs occur with enteroviruses
(Wenner et al., 1960), TGEV (Bohl, 1975; Morin et al., 1978),
and rotaviruses (Bohl et al., 1978; de Leeuw et al., 1979).
Faecal excretion of these viruses generally occurs in 3- to
9-week-old pigs during the latter part of the suckling period
or shortly after weaning. Whether faecal excretion of virus
at this time results from (1) an initial infection, or (2) a
massive viral replication from a previous low-grade or latent
gut infection is not known. Regardless, it is probably
related to a decline or interruption in lactogenic or humoral
immunity, with the former, generally, being more important.

Enteroviruses

About 11 serotypes of porcine enteroviruses have been
described (Knowles et al., 1979). Primary replication of
enteroviruses are thought to occur in the alimentary tract,
especially the ileum. However, clinical signs result from a
secondary localisation in other organs; such as, central
nervous system, lungs, or foetuses. Most young pigs become
infected with some serotypes, usually while they have some
degree of lactogenic or humoral passive immunity; and disease
is seldom observed (Wenner et al., 1960; Singh and Bohl, 1972).

TGE virus

This virus is a member of the coronavirus genus (Tajima,
1970). It causes a devastating disease in susceptible newborn
pigs, characterised by vomiting, diarrhoea, dehydration and,

generally, a 100% death loss; although swine of all ages can
be infected and show diarrhoea. Viral replication occurs in
the villous enterocytes, which accounts for the clinical signs.
There is no safe and effective vaccine, nor practical method
of treatment. Herd infections can be either enzootic or
epizootic, with losses much more severe in the latter
(Bohl, 1975). In enzootic infections, diarrhoea does not
usually occur in pigs less than 8 days old, due to lactogenic
immunity derived from the sow.

Porcine rotavirus

This virus was first reported as a cause of diarrhoea in
piglets in 1976 (Woode et al., 1976). Rotaviruses have been
associated with diarrhoea in several animal species including
man (Flewett and Woode, 1978). The pig serves as a good model
for the study of rotaviral infections. Rotavirus is most
commonly associated with 'white scours' in 2- to 4-week-old
pigs (Bohl et al., 1978; de Leeuw et al., 1979). Viral
replication occurs primarily in villous enterocytes. There
is probably more than 1 serotype of porcine rotavirus, but
precise information is lacking.

All serum samples from adult, conventionally reared
swine which we have tested contained neutralising antibodies
against porcine rotavirus. Serum and milk samples have been
sequentially collected from 5 sows during lactation and tested
for neutralising antibody against porcine rotavirus (OSU
strain). Results have been similar and those from one sow are
summarised in Table 1. Antibody titres in milk are usually
similar or often higher than those in serum, as occurred with
this sow. This information suggests that the milk antibodies
are primarily of the IgA class. Of special interest was the
marked increase in antibody titres in milk which occurred
between post-partum day 20 and 48. We think this was due to
severe viral exposure of the sow resulting from contact with
her infected pigs. Pigs in this litter began shedding rotavirus when 23 days old (Table 1). This phenomenon has been

observed in several other sows, with antibody titres increasing
more in milk than in serum. This may be due either to (1) an
increased migration of rotaviral sensitised IgA immunocytes
from the re-infected gut of the sow to the mammary gland, or
(2) a lacteal entrance of the virus from infected suckling pigs.

TABLE 1

ANTIBODY TITRES OF SOW (NO. 36-1) DURING LACTATION. FAECAL SHEDDING OF
ROTAVIRUS WAS FIRST DETECTED IN PIGS WHEN 23 DAYS OLD

Day post-partum	Rotaviral antibody titre*	
	Serum	Milk
1	98	280
13	110	125
20	150	95
34	420	460
48	480	1 400

* Reciprocal of dilution giving an 80% plaque reduction with porcine
rotavirus.

When milk whey is fractionated by gel filtration,
rotaviral antibody is primarily associated with the IgA
fractions, as previously reported (Saif and Bohl, 1979). Thus,
the IgA class of antibody is similar to that which occurs when
swine are naturally or experimentally infected with virulent
TGEV (Bohl et al., 1972).

We have followed the course of infection in about 6
litters of pigs from the same herd by obtaining rectal swabs at
various time intervals and testing for rotavirus by a cell-
culture-immunofluorescent test (Bohl, 1979). Findings were
similar in all litters, in that rotaviruses were detected when
pigs were 3 to 7 weeks of age. The findings in one litter are
summarised in Table 2. In this litter, rotaviruses were
detected in at least one rectal swab sample from all 9 pigs
between 31 to 34 days of age. In some pigs, only a very mild
diarrhoea was associated with the infection. However, pig
number 9 had severe diarrhoea and was euthanatised (Table 1).

Smears from the small intestinal mucosa revealed that a high percentage of the epithelial cells contained rotaviral antigen as determined by immunofluorescent staining.

From several pigs (numbers 3, 5, 6; Table 2) of this litter, rotavirus was again detected after several days of negative findings, suggesting either a sporadic shedding of virus or infection with a different porcine rotavirus serotype. We think the latter more probable. De Leeuw et al., 1979 have also reported similar findings.

TABLE 2

DETECTION OF ROTAVIRUS FROM RECTAL SWABS OF PIGS IN 1 LITTER (41-2), USING A CELL CULTURE-IF TEST. PIGS WERE WEANED WHEN 42 DAYS OLD.

| Pig | Days of age | | | | | | | | | | | | | |
no.	11	13	24	31	32	33	34	35	38	42	45	49	53	56
1		-	-			+	+	+		+	-	-	-	-
2	-			+	+	+			-					
3		-	-			+	-	-	-	+	-	-	-	-
4							+		-	-	-	-	-	-
5							+		-	-	+	-	-	-
6	-	-	-	-	+	+	+	+	-	-	+	-	-	-
7						-	+	-	-	-	+	-	-	-
8						-	+	+	-	-	-	-	-	-
9	-		-			+*								

* Pig no. 9 had severe diarrhoea when 33 days old, and was euthanatised. Enterocytes were IF positive for rotavirus.

VIRAL CELLULAR TROPISM AS RELATED TO IMMUNITY

With any infectious disease, the mechanism of immunity is largely determined by its pathogenesis. Thus, a few comments on cellular tropism of enteric viruses. The ability of a virus to cause diarrhoea appears to result from a massive infection of either villous enterocytes or crypt enterocytes. Because of their importance, a few relevant characteristics of enterocytes are described. Enterocytes of the small intestines proliferate in the crypts and migrate to the tips of the villi where they are sloughed. During migration, which takes from 2 to 10 days in the pig depending on many factors, the enterocytes become

more differentiated and enzymatically mature (Moon, 1971;
Lipkin, 1973). The enzymatic maturity and proliferative rate
of enterocytes appear to determine their suitability for
replicating sites by different viruses (Moon, 1978).

TGEV and rotavirus infect villous enterocytes and it is
their malfunction or destruction that results in diarrhoea.
Thus, the objective of passive immunity is to protect these
enterocytes against viral infection. This is normally
accomplished by having a constant supply of IgA antibodies in
the lumen of the gut, as occurs when pigs nurse - every 1 to 2
hours - immune sows. Haelterman (1965) has referred to this
immunologic mechanism as lactogenic immunity. Ingested IgA
antibodies apparently protect enterocytes either by
neutralising the ingested virus before cellular adsorption or
by 'coating' the luminal surface of enterocytes. Credence of
the latter is provided by the report that milk IgA binds
specifically to the luminal surfaces of villous epithelium in
the proximal small intestine of the rat (Nagura et al., 1980).
In contrast, serum antibodies have not been shown to protect
villous enterocytes against TGE viral infection.

Some parvoviruses infect crypt enterocytes, resulting in
villous atrophy and diarrhoea. Examples are the feline
panleucopaenia virus (Carlson and Scott, 1977) and canine
parvovirus (Appel et al., 1978). A porcine parvovirus has
been reported to infect lymphoid cells of the gut but not crypt
enterocytes, and there was an absence of diarrhoea (Brown et
al., 1980). We know of no reports of viruses infecting crypt
enterocytes of swine or man, but this situation could change
as it recently did in the dog. Epizootics of canine parvoviral
diarrhoea have been reported from several countries since 1978.
It appears to be a new disease, as no canine serum samples have
been found positive before June 1978 in USA (Carmichael et al.,
1980).

Immunity against viral infections of crypt enterocytes
seems to be associated with the presence of serum antibodies.

At least, these are the conclusions which can be drawn from studies on feline panleucopaenia (Davis et al., 1970). This is in marked contrast to the local or lactogenic immunity which is necessary with viral infections of villous enterocytes.

A major difference in pathogenesis between viral infections of villous enterocytes and crypt enterocytes may be the pathway by which viruses arrive at these cells. This may well be the basic characteristic which determines the effective immune mechanism. There is every indication that rotavirus and TGEV infect villous enterocytes from the luminal surface after having been ingested. In contrast, it is thought that feline panleucopaenia virus infects crypt enterocytes by a haematogenous route (Carlson and Scott, 1977). If such is the case, then it is easy to understand the role of serum anti-bodies in protecting crypt enterocytes.

The intestinal cell tropism of some enteric viruses have not been determined; such as, enteroviruses, reoviruses, and adenoviruses. It is reasonable to believe that some enteric viruses principally infect gut lymphoid tissue, without causing diarrhoea. If this situation exists, what is the immune mechanism for protecting such cells?

VACCINATION PROCEDURES FOR PROVIDING PASSIVE IMMUNITY AGAINST ENTERIC VIRAL INFECTIONS

Since TGE is such a highly fatal disease in newborn pigs, there has been much interest in development of a vaccine for use in pregnant swine, which would provide passive immunity to suckling pigs. The problem posed in developing such a vaccine has been rather unique, in that the objective is to protect villous enterocytes. TGE was apparently the first disease for which any attempt had been made to develop this type of vaccine. Interest in this area now extends to rotaviruses and other enteric coronaviruses as they also infect villous enterocytes of a number of different species. However, at this point it should be reiterated that immunity against viral infections of crypt enterocytes is probably due to circulating antibodies; thus, vaccination procedures which provide systemic immunity should suffice against parvoviral diarrhoea.

In this section, we will comment on some of the characteristics and variables associated with lactogenic immunity in newborn pigs, with emphasis on TGEV and rotavirus.

Immunoglobulin classes of antibodies in milk as related to immunity

TGE antibodies in mammary secretions occur primarily in two immunoglobulin classes, IgG and IgA (Bohl et al., 1972). In milk of sows which have been naturally or experimentally infected with virulent TGEV, antibodies are principally associated with IgA (Saif et al., 1972). When milk whey of these sows is fractionated by gel filtration on Sephadex G-200, antibody activity is mainly associated with IgA fractions (Figure 1). TGE antibody titres are usually higher in milk than in serum throughout lactation. These sows provide good immunity to their suckling pigs against TGEV.

Intramuscular or intramammary inoculations of serologically negative pregnant swine with live virulent or attenuated TGE viral preparations have resulted in milk anti-bodies which have been almost entirely of the IgG class (Bohl et al., 1972; Saif et al., 1972; Bohl and Saif, 1975). Antibody titres were highest in colostrum, less in serum, and declined rapidly in milk to low levels in 5 to 10 days post-partum. Figure 2 illustrates the gel filtration (Sephadex G-200) results conducted on a milk whey sample from a sow which had been injected intramammarily with virulent virus, 42 and 17 days pre-partum. TGE neutralising antibodies were associated primarily, if not solely, with IgG. Antibody titres were higher in serum and milk from sows inoculated intramammarily than intramuscularly, which also correlated with the ability of the intramammarily inoculated sows to provide better protection to suckling pigs. Generally, limited to poor

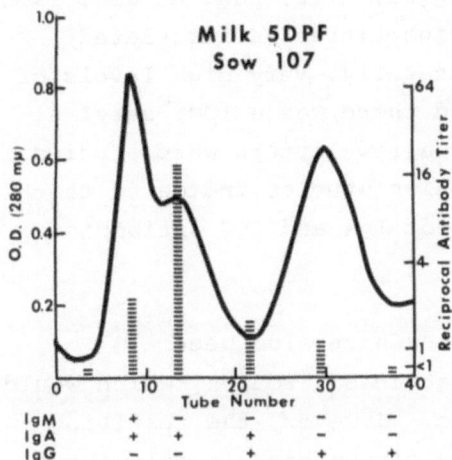

Fig. 1.   Gel filtration on Sephadex G-200 of a 5-day post-partum milk
          sample from a sow which had been infected orally with virulent
          TGE virus 32 days pre-partum. Reproduced from Bohl et al., 1974,
          with kind permission of Plenum Press, New York.

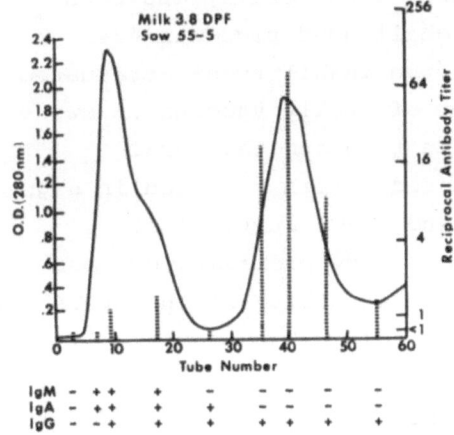

Fig. 2.   Gel filtration on Sephadex G-200 of a 3.8-day post-partum milk
          sample from a sow which had been injected intramammarily with
          virulent TGE virus 17 and 42 days pre-partum. Reproduced from
          Bohl et al., 1974, with kind permission of Plenum Press, New York.

protection has been provided to pigs nursing sows which had been intramuscularly inoculated with live attenuated TGE vaccines (Bohl et al., 1972; Tamoglia, 1972; Bohl et al., 1975). However, when a vaccine of very high titre was inoculated intramuscularly and, later, intranasally, very high levels of colostral antibodies occurred, and there was a 100% survival of challenged pigs, although only a few litters were studied (Kaji and Shimizu, 1978). Adsorption studies indicated that about equal amounts of low levels of IgA and IgG antibodies occurred in milk.

Live attenuated virus vaccines have also been administered by the oral and/or intranasal routes, which would seem to be the procedure of choice. However, the resulting TGE antibodies in milk were of low titres; and in only about 50% of the sows could IgA antibodies be detected, and then in low levels (Bohl and Saif, 1975). Protection of suckling pigs was limited or poor, but better than when vaccine was given intramuscularly. Pensaert (1979) also reported poor results when pregnant swine were vaccinated, first orally and then intramuscularly, as mortality of challenged pigs was 65%. We interpret these results as due to the inability of attenuated virus adequately to infect the gut of orally vaccinated swine. In contrast, Hess et al., 1978 have reported that oral administration of their B1 attenuated strain resulted in high levels of IgA antibodies in milk and a 90% survival of challenged pigs. These results look very promising but more work should be done to determine the stability of the avirulent state of the viral vaccine.

Leucocyte cell-cultured TGEV vaccine

This is an unique and interesting type of experimental vaccine. A small plaque variant strain of TGEV was derived from a persistently infected swine leucocyte cell line originally infected with virulent virus (Woods, 1978). The virus vaccine was avirulent for 3-day-old pigs. When administered, by a variety of routes, to pregnant swine,

relatively high levels of antibodies were detected in 3-day
post-partum milk. Challenge of 3-day old suckling pigs
resulted in fairly good protection as only 14 and 29% died in
2 studies, respectively (Woods, 1978; Woods and Pedersen, 1979).
As a result of passage in leucocyte cell cultures, the cell
tropism of the variant virus had changed so that unidentified
cells within the lamina propria of young pigs were infected
rather than villous enterocytes, as judged by immunofluorescence
(Woods et al., 1980).

Boosting of antibody in mammary secretions

Since many enteric infections are enzootic in nature,
adult females will usually have been previously infected, but
possibly only when they were young. Thus, immunisation may
more often involve a boosting effect rather than a priming,
or initiating, effect. This is especially true with rotaviral
and enteroviral infections. Only limited information is
available on the variables which are involved in boosting the
titre and immunoglobulin classes of antibodies in milk of
immunologically primed animals or humans. Parenteral
immunisation with *Vibrio cholerae* lipopolysaccharides boosted
the level of IgA antibodies in milk of primed women (Svennerholm
et al., 1977). Our studies show that colostrum and milk antibody titres can be markedly boosted by parenteral vaccination
of sero-positive pregnant or lactating swine with a rotavirus
or TGEV vaccine. For example, Table 3 summarises the antibody
responses in serum and milk of a sow which was intramuscularly
vaccinated 7 days pre-partum with a TGEV and a porcine rotavirus vaccine. Antibody titres for both viruses increased
markedly in serum, and were higher in colostrum and in milk for
the first few days post-partum than normally occurs in non-
vaccinated animals. Faecal shedding of rotavirus was first
detected in pigs of this litter when 31 days old, which is
about the normal age for faecal shedding in non-vaccinated
litters (See Table 2). We interpret the rotaviral infection
as being due either to ineffective immunisation or to a
different rotavirus serotype than the vaccine strain. Following

infection of the pigs, there was a 4-fold increase in antibody
titre in milk but only a slight increase in serum of the sow.
Similar results for a non-vaccinated animal were previously
discussed and shown in Table 1.

TABLE 3

ANTIBODY TITRES OF SOW (NO. 48-1) VACCINATED WITH PORCINE ROTAVIRUS
(OSU STRAIN) AND TGEV. LIVE CELL-CULTURED VIRUSES WERE INTRAMUSCULARLY
INJECTED 7 DAYS PRE-PARTUM. FAECAL SHEDDING OF ROTAVIRUS WAS FIRST
DETECTED IN PIGS WHEN 31 DAYS OLD.

| Day pre- or post-partum | Antibody titres* | | | |
| | TGEV | | Rotavirus | |
	Serum	Milk	Serum	Milk
-7	40		150	
0.5	400	2 000	370	4 200
7	1 800	500	1 600	340
14	740	350	1 020	270
28	520	310	450	120
42	450	210	540	520

* Reciprocal of dilution giving an 80% plaque reduction of porcine
  rotavirus or TGEV.

About 50% of the swine herds in Ohio, USA, contain TGE
serologically positive animals. Thus, some animals will need
to be immunologically primed and others boosted. Some
vaccination procedures may be better for priming, and others
for boosting, immunity. Parenterally administered TGE vaccines
can appreciably boost antibody titres in serum, colostrum and
milk of previously infected swine and, presumably, provide
increased protection to suckling pigs. This effect may be the
principal justification for using parenterally injected TGE
vaccines (Stepanek et al., 1979). We usually recommend this
procedure for helping control enzootic TGE infections but have
no precise information on its value.

It is important to know the immunoglobulin classes of
TGE viral and rotaviral antibodies in milk which result from
vaccinating previously infected animals, using a variety of

vaccination procedures. Such studies are underway in our
laboratory.

Neonatal colibacillosis

The immunologic findings with TGE prompted our research
group to try similar vaccination procedures using
enterotoxigenic *Escherichia coli* (EETC). Pregnant swine were
vaccinated with live EETC either by oral exposure with high
dosages or by intramuscular injections. When newborn pigs
from these vaccinated or non-vaccinated sows were orally
challenged with EETC, protection was much more effective in
pigs suckling the orally vaccinated sows (Kohler et al., 1975).
Kohler (1978) then took this procedure to the field and very
favourable results have been obtained; to the extent that it
is a commonly used immunising procedure in midwestern USA for
protecting newborn pigs against *E. coli* diarrhoea. By this
procedure, the previously isolated strain or strains of EETC
from the involved herd are grown in commercial pasteurised
milk, usually in quart or gallon containers. The 'cultured'
milk is then fed to pregnant swine about 4 weeks before parturition. A recent report has shown that oral immunisation of
lactating sows with EETC (08 : K88) stimulated an IgA antibody
response in mammary secretions (Evans, et al., 1980).

PROCEDURES FOR INITIATING THE PRODUCTION OF IgA ANTIBODIES IN MAMMARY SECRETIONS

We initially reported evidence for an immunologic gut-
mammary link in 1972, stating that TGE viral antibodies of the
IgA class occurred in milk of swine only as a result of a
previous infection of the gut (Bohl et al., 1972; Saif et al.,
1972). We also postulated that the most appropriate explanation
for this immunologic finding was 'a relocation of TGE viral
sensitised immunocytes from the lamina propria to the mammary
gland, possibly via lymphatic and blood vessels' (Bohl et al.,
1972). These conclusions were drawn from investigations
involving the administration of virulent or attenuated TGEV
using a variety of routes - oral, intramuscular, or intramammary.

These immunologic concepts have since been either confirmed or
elaborated upon, using a variety of antigens, in swine (Bohl
and Saif, 1975; Saif and Bohl, 1977; Hess et al., 1978; Evans
et al., 1980), rabbits (Montgomery et al., 1974), man (Goldblum
et al., 1975), rats (Michalek et al., 1976), and mice (Roux
et al., 1977). A gut-mammary link which provides high levels
of IgA antibodies in colostrum and milk is highly advantageous
for protecting the newborn against those enteric infections
which are enzootic or endemic in the parent population.

We were interested in knowing if there is an immunologic
respiratory-mamary link, similar to the gut-mammary link.
Consequently, pregnant swine were intranasally exposed to
pseudorabies virus, which causes an infection, mainly, of the
upper respiratory tract. The ensuing antibodies in milk were
primarily, if not solely, of the IgG class; and although high
titres occurred in colostrum, they declined rapidly to very
low levels in milk after 6 to 12 days' lactation (Saif and
Bohl, 1977). This suggests that such a link does not occur.
Nor do we know of any direct evidence that IgA antibodies in
milk protect the young against respiratory infections. This
information discouraged us from attempting to use a respiratory
infection as a means of stimulating the production of IgA antibodies in the mammary gland; as might occur if a modified
enteric virus were to replicate in the respiratory tract.

ACKNOWLEDGMENTS

This work was supported in part by Public Health Service
research grant AI-10735 from the National Institute of Allergy
and Infectious Diseases, and by a Special Grants Programme
No. 901-15-137, Science and Education Administration,
Cooperative Research, United States Department of Agriculture.

We thank Kathy L. Miller, Peggy Weilnau, Joyce Snyder,
and Arden Agnes for technical assistance.

REFERENCES

Appel, M.J.G., Cooper, B.J., Greisen, H. and Carmichael, L.E., 1978.
Status report: Canine viral enteritis. J. Am. Vet. Med. Assoc.
173, 1516.

Bohl, E.H., 1975. Transmissible gastroenteritis. In: Diseases of Swine,
Ed. by H.W. Dunne and A.D. Leman, p. 168. Iowa State University
Press, Ames, Iowa.

Bohl, E.H., 1979. Diagnosis of diarrhea in pigs due to transmissible
gastroenteritis virus or rotavirus. In: Viral Enteritis in Humans
and Animals. Ed. by F. Bricout and R. Scherrer. INSERM Colloq.
90, 341.

Bohl, E.H. and Saif, L.H., 1975. Passive immunity in transmissible gastroenteritis of swine: Immunoglobulin characteristics of antibodies
in milk after inoculating virus by different routes. Infect.
Immun. 11, 23.

Bohl, E.H., Gupta, R.K.P., Olquin, M.V.F. and Saif, L.J., 1972. Antibody
responses in serum, colostrum and milk of swine after infection or
vaccination with transmissible gastroenteritis virus. Infect.
Immun. 6, 289.

Bohl, E.H., Saif, L.J., Gupta, R.K.P. and Frederick, G.T., 1974. Secretory
antibodies in milk of swine against transmissible gastroenteritis
virus. Adv. Exp. Med. Biol. 45, 337.

Bohl, E.H., Frederick, G.T. and Saif, L.J., 1975. Passive immunity in
transmissible gastroenteritis of swine: Intramuscular injection
of pregnant swine with a modified live-virus vaccine. Am. J. Vet.
Res. 36, 267.

Bohl, E.H., Kohler, E.M., Saif, L.J., Cross, R.F., Agnes, A.G. and
Theil, K.W., 1978. Rotavirus as a cause of diarrhea in pigs.
J. Am. Vet. Med. Assoc. 172, 613.

Bourne, F.J. and Curtis, Jill, 1973. The transfer of immunoglobulins IgG,
IgA and IgM from serum to colostrum and milk in the sow.
Immunology 24, 157.

Brown, T.T. Jr., Paul, P.S., and Mengeling, W.L., 1980. Response of
conventionally raised weanling pigs to experimental infection with
a virulent strain of porcine parvovirus. Am. J. Vet. Res. 41, 1221.

Carmichael, L.C., Joubert, J.C. and Pollock, R.V.H., 1980. Hemagglutination by canine parvovirus: Serologic studies and diagnostic applications. Am. J. Vet. Res. 40, 784.

Carlson, J.H. and Scott, F.W., 1977. Feline panleukopenia. II. The relationship of intestinal mucosal cell proliferation rates to viral infection and development of lesions. Vet. Pathol. 14, 173.

Davis, E.V., Gregg, G.G. and Beckenhauer, W.H., 1970. Infectious feline panleukopenia (Developmental report of a tissue culture origin formalin inactivated vaccine). Vet. Med./Small Anim. Clin. 65,237.

Curtis, Jill and Bourne, F.J., 1971. Immunoglobulin quantitation in sow serum, colostrum and milk and the serum of young pigs. Biochim. Biophys. Acta. 236, 319.

de Leeuw, P.W., Ellens, G.J. and Hilbink, F.W., 1979. Rotavirus-associated recurrent diarrhoea in nursing piglets. In: Viral Enteritis in Humans and Animals. Ed. by F. Bricout and R. Scherrer. INSERM Colloq. 90, 349.

Evans, P.A., Newby, T.J., Stokes, C.R., Patel, D. and Bourne, F.J., 1980. Antibody responses of the lactating sow to oral immunisation with *Escherichia coli*. Scand. J. Immunol. 11, 419.

Flewett, T.H. and Woode, G.N., 1978. The rotaviruses. Brief review. Arch. Virol. 57, 1.

Goldblum, R.M., Ahlstedt, S., Carlsson, B., Hanson, L.A., Jodal, V., Lidin-Janson, G. and Sohl-Akerlund, A., 1975. Antibody-forming cells in human colostrum after oral immunisation. Nature 257, 797.

Haelterman, E.O., 1965. Lactogenic immunity to transmissible gastro-enteritis of swine. J. Am. Vet. Med. Assoc. 147, 1661.

Hess, R.G., Bachman, P.A. and Mayr, A., 1978. Attempts to develop an immunoprophylaxis against transmissible gastroenteritis (TGE) in pigs. III. Passive immune transfer after oral vaccination with attenuated TGE virus strain Bl. Zentralbl Veterinaermed B 25, 308.

Kaji T. and Shimizu, Y., 1978. Passive immunisation against transmissible gastroenteritis virus in piglets by ingestion of milk of sows inoculated with attenuated virus. Natl. Inst. Anim. Health Q. (Tokyo) 18, 43.

Knowles, N.J., Buckley, L.S. and Pereira, H.G., 1979. Classification of porcine enteroviruses by antigenic analysis and cytopathic effects in tissue culture: Description of 3 new serotypes. Arch. Virol. 62, 201.

Kohler, E.M., 1978. Results of 1976 field trials with oral *Escherichia coli* vaccination of sows. Vet. Med./Small Anim. Clin. <u>73</u>, 352.

Kohler, E.M., Cross, R.F. and Bohl, E.H., 1975. Protection against neonatal enteric colibacillosis in pigs suckling orally vaccinated sows. Am. J. Vet. Res. <u>36</u>, 757.

Lipkin, M., 1973. Proliferation and differentiation of gastrointestinal cells. Physiol. Rev. <u>53</u>, 891.

Michalek, S.M., McGhee, J.R., Mestecky, J., Arnold, R.R. and Bozzo, L., 1976. Ingestion of *Streptococcus mutans* induces secretory immunoglobulin A and carries immunity. Science <u>192</u>, 1238.

Montgomery, P.C., Cohn, J. and Lally, E.T., 1974. The induction and characteristics of secretory IgA antibodies. Adv. Exp. Med. Biol. <u>45</u>, 453.

Moon, H.W., 1971. Epithelial cell migration in the alimentary mucosa of the suckling pig. Proc. Soc. Exp. Biol. <u>137</u>, 151.

Moon, H.W., 1978. Mechanisms in the pathogenesis of diarrhea: A review. J. Am. Vet. Med. Assoc. <u>172</u>, 443.

Morin, M., Solorzano, R.F., Morehouse, L.G. and Olson, L.D., 1978. The postulated role of feeder swine in the perpetuation of the transmissible gastroenteritis virus. Can. J. Comp. Med. <u>42</u>, 379.

Nagura, H., Nakane, D.K. and Brown, W.R., 1978. Breast milk IgA binds to jejunal epithelial in suckling rats. J. Immunol. <u>120</u>, 1330.

Payne, L.C. and Marsch, C.L., 1962. Gamma globulin absorption in the baby pig: The nonselective absorption of heterologous globulins and factors influencing absorption time. J. Nutr. <u>76</u>, 151.

Pensaert, M.B., 1979. Immunity in TGE of swine after infection and vaccination. In: Viral Enteritis in Humans and Animals. Ed. by F. Bricout and R. Scherrer. INSERM Colloq. <u>90</u>, 281.

Porter P. and Allen, W.D., 1972. Classes of immunoglobulins related to immunity in the pig. J. Amer. Vet. Med. Assoc. <u>160</u>, 511.

Roux, M.E., McWilliams, M., Phillips-Quagliata, J.M., Weisz-Carrington, P. and Lamm, M.E., 1977. Origin of IgA-secretory plasma cells in the mammary gland. J. Exp. Med. <u>146</u>, 1311.

Saif, L.J. and Bohl, E.H., 1977. Immunoglobulin classes of antibodies in milk of swine after intranasal exposure to pseudorabies virus or transmissible gastroenteritis virus. Infect. Immun. <u>16</u>, 961.

Saif, L.J. and Bohl, E.H., 1979. Role of secretory IgA in passive immunity of swine to enteric viral infections. In: Immunology of Breast Milk. Ed. by P.L. Ogra and D. Dayton, p. 237. Raven Press, New York.

Saif, L.J., Bohl, E.H. and Gupta, R.K.P., 1972. Isolation of porcine immunoglobulins and determinations of the immunoglobulin classes of transmissible gastroenteritis viral antibodies. Infect. Immun. 6, 289.

Singh, K.V. and Bohl, E.H., 1972. The pattern of enteroviral infections in a herd of swine. Can. J. Comp. Med. 36, 243.

Stepanek, J., Mensik, J., Franz, J. and Hornich, M., 1979. Epizootiology, diagnosis and prevention of viral diarrhoea in piglets under intensive husbandry conditions. Proc. 21st World Vet. Congr. (Moscow) 6, 43.

Svennerholm, A.M., Holmgren, J., Hanson, L.A., Lindblad, B.S., Qureshi, F. and Rahimtoola, R.J., 1977. Boosting of secretory IgA antibody responses in man by parenteral cholera vaccination. Scand. J. Immunol. 6, 1345.

Tajima, M., 1970. Morphology of transmissible gastroenteritis virus of pigs. A possible member of coronaviruses. Arch. ges Virus Forsch. 29, 105.

Tamoglia, T.W., 1972. Present status of products available for use against transmissible gastroenteritis. J. Am. Vet. Med. Assoc. 160, 554.

Wenner, H.A., Beran, G.W. and Werder, A.A., 1960. Enteroviruses of swine. II. Studies on the natural history of infection and immunity. Am. J. Vet. Res. 21, 958.

Woode, G.N., Bridger, J.C., Hall, G.A., Jones, J.M. and Jackson, G., 1976. The isolation of reovirus-like agents (rotaviruses) from acute gastroenteritis of piglets. J. Med. Microbiol. 9, 203.

Woods, R.D., 1978. Small plaque variant transmissible gastroenteritis virus. J. Am. Vet. Med. Assoc. 173, 643.

Woods, R.D. and Pedersen, N.C., 1979. Cross-protection studies between feline infectious peritonitis and porcine transmissible gastro-enteritis viruses. Vet. Microbiol. 4, 11.

Woods, R.D., Cheville, N.F. and Gallagher J.E., 1980. Lesions in the small intestine of newborn pigs inoculated with porcine, feline, and canine coronaviruses. Am. J. Vet. Res. (in press).

DISCUSSION

H. Miller *(UK)*

Does pseudorabies infect epithelial cells in the upper
or lower respiratory tract?

E. Bohl *(USA)*

It is my understanding that it is the upper respiratory
tract.

H. Miller

Do you get an IgA response?

E. Bohl

We get an IgG response in the mammary gland. We have not
tested the respiratory secretions. I assume there would be an
IgA response there.

K. Petzoldt *(FRG)*

You mentioned antibody response in defence against enteric
diseases. Is there any evidence that cellular immune mechanisms
also play a role. There has been work in humans for example
which shows that following breast feeding tubercle negative
babies become tubercle positive, for a short period of time.

E. Bohl

There are both lymphocytes and macrophages in milk and
there is much interest in what role they play. I know of no
evidence to suggest that they are involved in passive immunity,
however, they probably do contribute and the reason I say this
is that if you have a sow which is immune to TGE, and you take
pigs off that sow for about eight hours, then they become susceptible to TGE. If you want to have good lactogenic immunity,
it is imperative that the pigs keep nursing about every hour and
a half, this is the normal nursing period of pigs. This may go
against the idea of establishment of live cells in the gut which

would give a semi-permanent type of immunity from cells rather than from immunoglobulins, but I can envisage that it would play a considerable role in passive immunity.

J. Soothill   *(UK)*

First a comment: there is evidence from Pitt that the macrophages are of value as a passive protective factor. Now a question - you said that you thought that villus tip infections were transmitted by faeces and protected for by secreted antibody and that crypt infections were transmitted by blood and perhaps protected by serum antibody. What evidence underlies this association which is an intriguing one?

E. Bohl

There is a good deal of evidence that serum antibodies play a very small role in protecting villus enterocytes against virus infection with TGE virus or rotavirus, either passively or actively acquired serum antibodies. There does seem to be protection passively by so-called lactogenic immunity, or local active immunity. Now, the evidence in regard to the crypt enterocyte is probably a little more indirect. We immunise cats against panleucopaenia by parenteral injection. Some people think that feline panleucopaenia virus gets to the crypt enterocytes by way of the blood and not by way of the lumen. Obviously, serum antibodies would be protective if the route to the crypt was by the haematogenous route. This is very important in regard to knowing what type of immunising agent is effective.

P. Brandzaeg   *(Norway)*

I just wondered, with regard to the lack of a respiratory mammary link in pigs, do the pigs have tonsils?

E. Bohl

Yes.

P. Brandzaeg

Are they as well developed as in the human species?

E. Bohl

I would think they are.

A. Ferguson   (UK)

Is there solid evidence that IgA antibody completely prevents rotavirus infection, or does it just alter the course?

E. Bohl

I should have emphasised this more. Most passive immune states do not give complete protection. In fact, it is not to the advantage of the animal to be completely protected. There may be complete protection for the first two weeks of life and then partial protection at 3, 4 or 5 weeks.

A. Ferguson

I completely follow your argument that amelioration of the clinical features is the ultimate objective. But is there evidence that immunity rather than other factors such as motility, acidity and mucous, is involved? Is there proof that active IgA antibody prevents infection by rotavirus? Could it be that antibody has nothing to do with protection against rotavirus?

E. Bohl

Infection occurs in pigs at one, two or three days of age. Maybe there is a very latent infection in the gut which is held in check by antibodies or certain physiological conditions. Then, at 3 or 4 weeks of age, physiological conditions change or the milk antibody level declines, and latent infection develops with excretion - this doesn't answer your question. I don't know if we can say for absolutely sure that it is the IgA that is preventing these infections. I just think it is the most likely explanation at the present time.

<u>T.J. Newby</u> *(UK)*

Thank you very much Professor Bohl. There will be an opportunity to continue this discussion later.

INDUCTION OF AN INTERFERON ACTIVITY IN THE NASAL MUCUS OF CALVES BY ADMINISTRATION OF INACTIVATED IBR VIRUS AND LEVAMISOLE

C. Lejan and J. Asso

INRA, Station de Recherches de Virologie et d'Immunologie, Route de Thiverval, 78850 Thiverval-Grignon, France.

ABSTRACT

When IBRV infects the respiratory tract of calves there is simult-aneously production of interferon which appears in the nasal mucus with the onset of infection and disappears as soon as the infection subsides.

We have inoculated calves with IBRV intranasally (8 days, 1 month, 3 months old) which were non-immune or which had been already immunised with infectious IBRV. The interferon is detected only if the virus grows; it was not detected if the virus did not multiply, i.e. when the animal was immune.

With uv irradiated virus; there is no virus proliferation in the nose of the animal nor interferon in the nasal mucus. But following the simultaneous administration by a general route of an immunostimulant such as levamisole we observed the presence of interferon in the nasal mucus for several days. It is known that levamisole has special affinity as an anthelminthic for the respiratory tract. Other immunostimulants have been used.

INTRODUCTION

The *in vivo* protective role of interferon against viral
infection is clearly established. This protection could be
explained by its activity on virus susceptible cells, but could
be related to its monitoring effect on immune reactions and
activating effect on cells such as macrophages and natural
killer cells. Interferon could be an important factor in animal
defence in the face of infections with multiple aetiology,
such as respiratory disease in calves. The large number of
possible infectious agents explains the predominant part played
in this disease by any defect of spontaneous defences linked to
the aggressive techniques of intensive husbandry.

To induce protection in the calf we have to induce a
local synthesis of interferon which will limit the spread of
viral infection; we can also stimulate cellular defences: the
interferon would be only one of the several lymphokines
released by activated lymphocytes.

Until now the induction of interferon production in
cattle has not been very successful. Chemical inducers such
as poly IC or tylorone are efficient only at high dosage, near
to the toxic dose, and the transient production of interferon
is followed by a non-reactive period.

Conversely the intranasal administration of a non-pathogenic IBR virus affords protection in calves against challenge
with a rhinovirus four days later. To be protective interferon
has to be in nasal mucus before challenge. Potentially contagious vaccine may not be accepted.

We have stimulated nasal interferon production by the use
of uv irradiated IBR virus concurrent with the systemic administration of the immunostimulant, levamisole. Levamisole is a
stimulant of T dependent functions and of monocytes and macrophages particularly in immunodepressed individuals; in addition
it is exacted via the respiratory route.

MATERIALS AND METHODS

Virus

IBR virus grown in MDBK cells and which is no longer pathogenic in calves was used. The virus was inactivated by uv irradiation.

Experimental animals

Holstein Friesian breed calves aged 8 - 15 days with a body weight of 50 kg were used.

Levamisole

The immunostimulant was given by the intramuscular route as a 15% solution (nemisol Specia batch No. 137).

Treatment of the animals

1) Irradiated virus was given by the nasal route: 5 ml into each nostril of a suspension containing 10^7 UFP/ml before inactivation.

2) Levamisole was given by the intramuscular route.

Virus and levamisole were given simultaneously on day 1. The levamisole dose was repeated every forty eight hours. The regime was repeated after one week.

Sampling of nasal mucus

The mucus was collected with a sponge fragment (sterilised, Spontex) introduced into the nostril for 3 to 5 minutes; 5 ml of lactalbumin was added to each sample which was then frozen.

Test for the presence of virus in nasal mucus

1 ml of a 1/50 dilution of the sample was distributed on 8 wells of a MDBK layer microplaque and incubated for 3 days at 37°C.

Detection for IBRV specific antibodies

1 ml of a 1/5 dilution of the sample was heated for
30 min at 56°C then mixed with 100 and 1 000 PFU of IBRV. After
a 12 h incubation at 37°C the residual virus was detected in
MDBK cells 1/10 dilution.

Detection of interferon activity

0.2 ml of the sample was serially diluted 1/3 on MDBK
cells and the cell layer then incubated overnight at 37°C,
washed and challenged with 200 UFP of VSV which destroys the
controls in 36 h at 37°C. The same technique was used after
pH2 treatment of the sample for 24 h at 4°C. A standard bovine
interferon produced on calf kidney primary cells with Newcastle
virus was included in each test as a positive control.

RESULTS

Interferon activity in the nasal mucus (Table 1)

Calves which had been submitted to irradiated virus by
nasal route and levamisole (5 mg/kg by the intramuscular route)
had interferon activity in the nasal mucus, which persisted after
48 h if the levamisole treatment was repeated.

Calves similarly treated with irradiated virus by nasal
route but receiving a lower dose of levamisole (2.5 mg/kg) had
no interferon activity in the mucus.

Calves submitted to irradiated virus by nasal route only
or to levamisole only (at 7.5 mg/kg) had no interferon activity
in the nasal mucus.

Interferon activity was not detected in the serum of any
group of animals.

TABLE 1

INTERFERON ACTIVITY IN NASAL SWABS OF CALVES WITH OR WITHOUT TREATMENT

Group 1										
	day	0	2	4	6	8	10	12	14	16
Treatment		V+L	L	L		V+L	L	L		
Calf 1		0	30	30	30	0	30	90	30	0
2		0	270	90	90	0	90	90	90	0
3		0	30	90	30	0	90	30	90	0
4		0	90	270	90	0	30	90	30	0
5		0	30	30	0	0	270	90	90	0
6		0	90	90	30	0	30	90	30	0

V = inactivated IBR virus given by nasal route

L = intramuscular inoculation of levamisole (5 mg/kg)

Group 2

Calves inoculated according to the same schedule, but with levamisole at a dose of 2.5 mg/kg: NO INTERFERON DETECTED.

Group 3

Calves inoculated only with inactivated IBR virus (no levamisole administration): NO INTERFERON DETECTED.

Group 4

Calves inoculated only with levamisole (5 mg/kg) (no inactivated virus administration): NO INTERFERON DETECTED.

Results are given as the inverse of the mucus dilution which affords complete protection of MDBK cells against 200 PFU of VSV, in given experimental conditions.

Presence of infectious virus in the nasal mucus

No excretion of IBRV was found in the treated animals or in the control calves.

Anti IBRV antibodies

The local inoculation of irradiated virus in the nostril did not induce synthesis of specific neutralising antibodies in the mucosa even in the presence of levamisole.

Challenge inoculation (Table 2)

A challenge with live IBRV was performed on the 3rd day after the treatment of calves, with levamisole and irradiated virus or with inactivated virus alone. The results demonstrated that giving levamisole in association with inactivated virus prevented the growth of infectious IBRV.

TABLE 2

CHALLENGE OF CALVES WITH LIVE IBR VIRUS

Group 1											
6 calves, inoculated on day 1 with inactivated IBR virus (intranasally) and levamisole (5 mg/kg, intramuscular route)					NO VIRUS ISOLATED						
Levamisole (5 mg/kg) IM, on day 2					IN NASAL SWABS DURING 15 DAYS						
Challenge with live IBR virus on day 4					OF OBSERVATION						
Group 2		day post challenge									
6 calves, inoculated on day 1 with inactivated IBR virus (intranasal route)		1	2	3	5	7	8	9	10	11	13	15
Challenge on day 4 with live IBR virus	Calf 1	+	+	+	+	+	−	−	−	−	−	−
	2	+	+	+	+	−	−	−	−	−	−	−
	3	+	+	+	+	+	+	+	+	−	−	−
	4	+	+	+	+	+	+	−	−	−	−	−
	5	+	+	+	+	+	+	+	−	−	−	−
	6	+	+	+	+	+	−	−	−	−	−	−
	+ = virus in nasal swabs − = no virus isolated											

DISCUSSION

The simultaneous administration of levamisole by the intramuscular route and of uv inactivated IBRV by the nasal route induces the presence of interferon in the nasal mucus. The effect is transient but can be maintained by repetition of levamisole administration. One week after the first induction it is possible to produce again the same sequence of events with a new administration of inactivated virus and of levamisole. This stimulation depends strictly on the levamisole dose.

A double signal is necessary for the induction of local interferon activity; initially contact of the mucosa with inactivated virus; and secondly a systemic administration of levamisole. Several hypotheses could be put forward to explain this.

The inactivated IBRV and levamisole act on two different cell types. Whilst the inactivated virus is in direct contact with the mucosal epithelium, the levamisole may stimulate blood monocytes to migrate to the mucosa. Thus interferon could be produced by levamisole stimulated macrophages in the lympho-epithelial area of the mucosa already in contact with viral antigen. Stimulated macrophages could enhance the interferon synthesis by lymphocytes primed with the inactivated virus. The possible importance of monocytes is demonstrated by the short-lived effect of levamisole on interferon synthesis, a repetition of levamisole inoculation being necessary every 48 h to maintain local interferon production.

Levamisole is known to induce maturation of the T lympho-cytes, but the reconstitution of levamisole susceptible T lymphocytes takes 3 weeks. In the calf 5 mg/kg levamisole enhances the lymphocyte response to mitogens for at least 5 days. So we consider that T lymphocytes by themselves are not the principal agent in local interferon synthesis; at the most they could react with levamisole activated monocytes to produce interferon. The levamisole or its degradation products could stimulate the respiratory mucosa cells already in contact with inactivated virus. It is known that levamisole increases cell metabolism.

The determination of the characteristics of locally produced interferon will give some indications on the cells responsible for its synthesis: we have to discriminate between bovine interferon type I produced by epithelial cells and bovine interferon type II, lymphokine produced by activated lymphocytes.

The calves which produced interferon in their respiratory tracts resisted challenge with infectious virus. The treatment has been tested in the field. For practical reasons levamisole was mixed with milk and encouraging results have been obtained.

DISCUSSION

K. Petzoldt   (FRG)

Dr. Asso, you talked about the minimum effective doses of levamisole. Did you look for the minimum effective doses of IBRV?

J. Asso   (France)

I don't think this is very important. We used two dosage levels: 10.7 and 10.5 before irradiation with the same results, but it is important to administer a large volume of virus in the nose of the animal in order to cover as large a part of the mucosa as possible. In the animals which have had the irradiated virus we have never observed growth of the virus. So it seems that after irradiation, the virus is totally inactivated.

J. Hannon   (Ireland)

When you tested the treatment under commercial conditions, did you have any controls?

J. Asso

Controls were on adjacent farms; we also had information from the preceding batch of animals and on the batch of animals at the same period of the previous year.

H. Miller   (UK)

Do you have any observations on viral induced interferon as opposed to immune interferon?

J. Asso

No.

T.J. Newby   (UK)

Have you tried any other antigen apart from IBR virus?

J. Asso

We tried PI3 and also inactivated PI3 but it seems that IBR is a better interferon stimulator than PI3.

H. Bazin   (Belgium)

The normal values are not able to increase the production of interferon.

T. Newby

Thank you Dr. Asso.

KINETICS OF INTESTINAL ANTIBODY DEVELOPMENT IN CALVES AFTER INFECTION WITH BOVINE ROTAVIRUS

R.G. Hess,* P.A. Bachmann,* G. Dirksen,**
and G. Schmid***

Institute of Medical Microbiology, Infectious and
Epidemic Diseases,* the Clinic of Internal Medicine,**
and the Clinic of Obstetrics,*** Veterinary Faculty,
University of Munich, Veterinärstrasse 13, 8000 Munich 22,
Federal Republic of Germany.

ABSTRACT

Antibodies were demonstrated in the small intestine, in faecal material, and in serum from calves which had been infected with different strains of bovine rotavirus at 6 - 9 days of age.

Antibodies were first detected in the jejunum 2 - 12 days post infection. Two to thirteen days later rotavirus antibodies appeared in the faeces. Serum antibodies were detected between 22 and 38 days after oral infection.

Antibodies were demonstrable in the faeces for up to 65 days post infection. Most antibodies found in the small intestine or faeces were shown to be of the IgG1 class as demonstrated by immunoelectrophoresis, significant amounts of IgA were also present.

INTRODUCTION

Neonatal calf diarrhoea is caused by a number of different infectious agents of which rotavirus is one of the most common bovine enteropathogens. Serological and virological evidence from several areas of the world indicates that rotavirus infections are ubiquitous in cattle populations (Bachmann and Hess, 1981).

Viral infection and replication is mainly concentrated in the epithelial cells of the upper part of the small intestinal villi causing desquamation and necrosis of the cells. This is followed by stunting and, sometimes, atrophy of the villi which consequently leads to malabsorption and diarrhoea. Morbidity and mortality rates depend on the age of the infected animal, on the virulence and origin of the virus and on hygienic conditions. Subclinical infections are common, however, and seem to be the cause of most endemic outbreaks of the disease.

As in almost all intestinal infections, serum antibodies do not correlate with protection against infection or reinfection. Protection is usually associated with local immunity, which either develops actively following intestinal infection, or is transferred by passive 'lactogenic' antibodies via colostrum and milk of immune and immunised mothers.

This passive immunity is most important during the neonatal period when the newborn needs time to build up an active immunity. The efficacy and duration of such 'lactogenic' protection differs considerably, however, among the various species. In Figure 1, for example, the occurrence of rotavirus antibodies in colostrum and milk during the first 6 days of lactation of cows is compared to that of sows in which a much slower decrease of rotavirus antibodies is found even over a 2 week period.

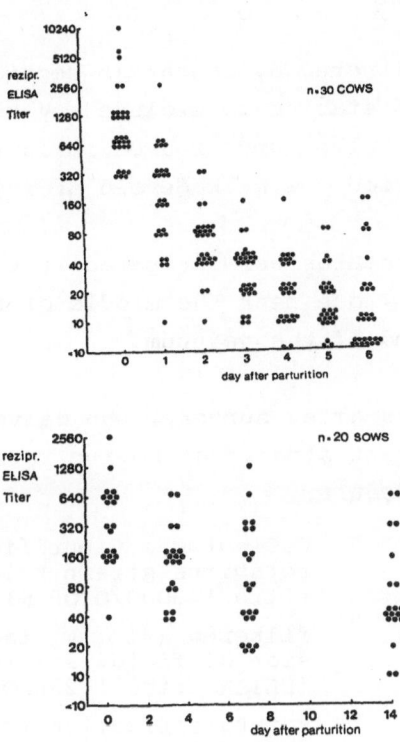

Fig. 1.   ELISA antibody titres in colostral and milk whey during the first
6 days after parturition from 30 cows naturally infected with
rotavirus compared to colostrum and milk titres during the first
14 days after parturition from 20 sows naturally infected with
rotavirus.

With this immunological situation in mind, we investigated
the active production of intestinal antibodies against bovine
rotavirus over a period of about 4 months in colostrum-deprived
newborn calves. One of the aims of the present work, which is
still in progress, is to find an explanation for the various
results obtained following active immunisation of newborn
calves at an age of 3 - 4 days (Acres and Radostis, 1976;
Thurber et al., 1977).

MATERIALS AND METHODS

Six calves delivered by caesarean section were kept in
individual isolation stables to exclude any contact with
infectious agents. Calves were reared colostrum-deprived and
fed reconstituted dried cow milk devoid of rotavirus antibodies.

Two jejunal fistulas were prepared in 4 of the 6 calves
(numbers 4, 5, 6, 8), one near the middle of the jejunum and
the second at the end of the jejunum.

One to two days after surgery, the calves were orally
infected with different strains of bovine rotavirus according
to the following schedule:

Calf No. 4:   CsCl gradient purified bovine
                    rotavirus strain K-2-42 (ELISA
                    titre 1:3000/0.05 ml)

Calf No. 5:   filtered (450 μm) faecal suspen-
                    sion of field isolate (V 1158)
                    (ELISA titre 1:256/0.05 ml)

Calf No. 6:   natural infection from calf No. 5

Calf No. 8:   chloroform-treated faeces suspen-
                    sion of strain K-2-42. (ELISA
                    titre 1:256/0.05 ml)

Each calf received 1 ml of virus suspension which was
diluted in 4 ml of phosphate-buffered saline (PBS).
Reinfection was performed with homologous virus of the same
preparation on days 65, 67 and 50 in calves numbers 4, 6 and
8 respectively. During the first 14 days following infection,
samples were taken daily from the fistulas and faeces. Serum
samples were obtained every third day during the first 4 weeks
after infection and thereafter at weekly intervals.

Jejunal fluids were inactivated at 56°C for 30 minutes,
and pH was regulated to 4.5 within 5 minutes after sampling.
Twenty grammes of faecal material was diluted in 20 ml of
sodium-acetate-buffer, pH 4.5, and treated like jejunal fluids.
Calves numbers 2 and 3 were orally infected only in order to
follow virus shedding. They served as controls.

Determination of rotaviral antibody titres was carried out using a microenzyme-linked immunosorbent assay antibody blocking technique described elsewhere (Bachmann, 1979).

Immunelectrophoresis was carried out according to the technique described by Grabar and Williams (1953) in a flat bed chamber (FBE 3000, Pharmacia) using 1.5% agarose (purified, Serva) and 0.03 m diethylenbarbiturate, 0.065 m acetate buffer pH 8.2. H-chain specific antibovine IgA, IgM, IgGl and IgG2 sera prepared in rabbits were employed (Miles Labs).

RESULTS

Development of intestinal antibodies against bovine rotavirus in jejunal fluid, faeces and serum:

Table 1 shows the results of the demonstration of rotavirus found in the jejunal fluid and/or faeces of six orally infected calves. The control calves numbers 2 and 3 which had been infected on the first day of life excreted virus for 4 - 5 days. The calves with fistulas (numbers 4, 5, 6, 8) which had been infected between days 6 - 9 of life excreted virus for only 2 - 3 days (except calf number 8). The time lapse between infection and excretion of virus was, however, 1 - 2 days longer than in the control calves.

Antibodies against rotavirus always occurred first in the jejunal fluids collected from the fistulas.

In calf number 4 antibodies first appeared in the jejunal fluid at a very low level 12 - 13 days following infection. In the faeces (Figure 2) and in faeces examined 14 days after infection, titres remained at a level of 1 : 10 and 1 : 20 until reinfection on day 65. In the serum, anti-rotavirus activity first began 25 days after infection.

TABLE 1

SHEDDING OF BOVINE ROTAVIRUS BY JEJUNAL FISTULAS AND BY FAECES OF ORALLY INFECTED COLOSTRUM DERIVED NEWBORN CALVES AT DIFFERENT DAYS OF LIFE

Calf-no.	Infection at day	Assay	Sample	Day after infection															
				1	2	3	4	5	6	7	8	9	10	11	12	13	14	15	16
2	1	IEM	faeces	O	***	****	**	O	O	O	O	O	O	O	O				
		ELISA	faeces	O	****	****	**	(*)	O	O	O	O	O	O	O				
3	1	IEM	faeces	O	*	**	***	(*)	O	O	O	O	O	O					
		ELISA	faeces	O	***	***	****	**	*	O	O	O	O	O					
4	9	IEM	faeces	O	O	(*)	**	**	(*)	O	O	O	O	O					
		ELISA	faeces	O	O	*	**	***	O	O	O	O	O	O					
			fist 1	O	O	O	**	*	O	O	O	O	O	O					
			fist 2	O	O	O	**	*	O	O	O	O	O	O					
5	6	IEM	faeces	O	*	***	*	O	O	O	O	O	O	O					
		ELISA	faeces	O	*	**	*	O	O	O	O	O	O	O					
			fist 1	O	O	O	O	O	O	O	O	O	O	O					
			fist 2	O	*	O	O	O	O	O	O	O	O	O					

TABLE 1 (cont.)

Calf-no.	Infection at day	Assay	Sample							Day after infection									
				1	2	3	4	5	6	7	8	9	10	11	12	13	14	15	16
6	by contact (1 or 2)	ELISA	faeces	O	O	***	***	O	O	O	O	O	O	O					
			fist 1	n.t.	n.t.	**	*	O	O	O	O	O	O	O					
			fist 2	n.t.	n.t.	**	*	O	O	O	O	O	O	O					
8	8	ELISA	faeces	O	O	O	O	O	O	*	**	O	O	O	O	***	***	**	O
			fist 1	O	O	*	O	O	O	O	O	O	O	O	O	O	O	O	O
			fist 2	O	O	*	O	O	O	O	O	O	O	O	O	O	O	O	O

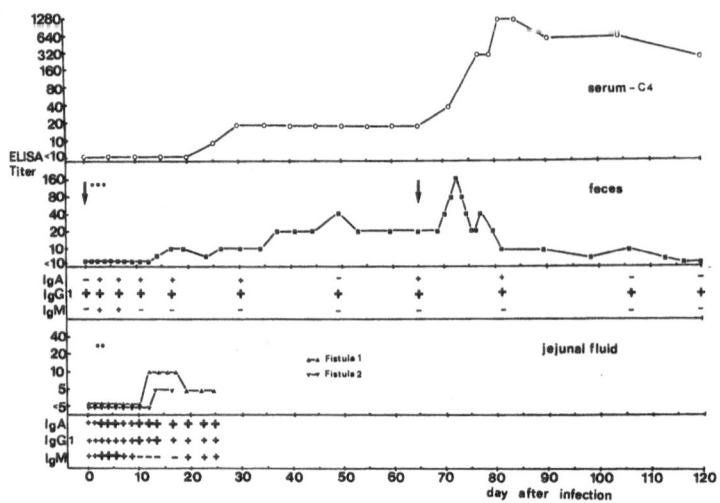

Fig. 2. Comparison of ELISA antibody titres in jejunal fluids, faeces and
serum of calf number 4, which was orally infected with purified
rotavirus on day 9, and class specificity of jejunal and faecal
immunoglobulins.

Seven days after reinfection, (65 days after priming), an
8-fold increase of faecal antibodies occurred. But this
antibody response lasted only 16 days and after that the same
low titres as during the initial phase were detected. One
hundred and seventeen days after infection and 52 days after
oral reinfection, faecal antibodies were no longer demonstrable.
A 64-fold increase in antibody titres was observed in the serum
within 17 days after reinfection, and titres remained unchanged
at this level up to day 117.

Concerning class specificity of antibodies found in the
jejunum, more IgA that IgM or IgGl were observed, whereas in
the faeces, IgGl was the predominant immunoglobulin with IgA
present in smaller amounts.

A very similar antibody profile was found in calf
number 8 (Figure 3) which had been infected with chloroform-
treated faecal material of the same virus strain which had been

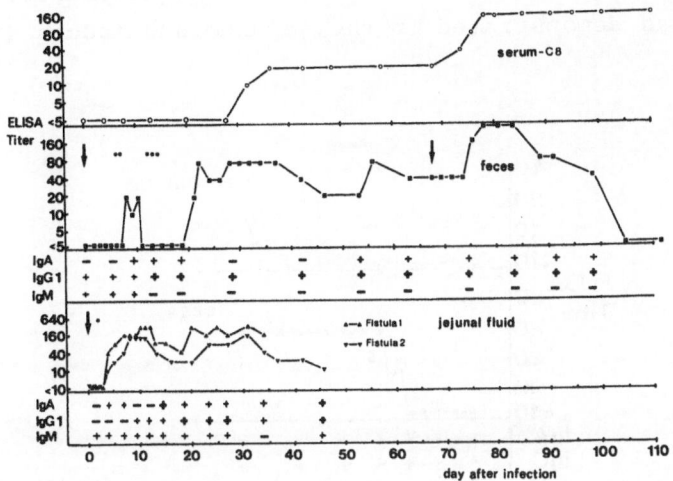

Fig. 3. Comparison of ELISA antibody titres in jejunal fluids, faeces, and serum of calf number 8, which was orally infected with chloroform-treated rotavirus-containing faeces on day 8, and class specificity of jejunal and faecal immunoglobulins.

given to calf number 4. In contrast to calf number 4, rotaviral antibodies appeared much earlier in the jejunum (day 4) and in the faeces (between days 8 and 10). Antibody activity in the faeces disappeared, however, after day 10 and a new virus excretion period began for 3 days. On day 21 following infection, a second antibody response resulting in higher titres in the faeces was observed.

Antibodies were first demonstrated in the serum 32 days after infection.

Reinfection on day 67 led to an 8-fold increase of antibody titres in faeces. This level decreased constantly until anti-rotavirus antibodies could not be detected in the faeces on day 104 after priming and day 37 after boosting. An 8-fold increase of antibody titres was observed in the serum 10 days after infection, while the titres remained unchanged until the end of the experiment.

302

In this calf, more IgA was found in the jejunum early after infection, whereas later (3 - 4 weeks post infection) more IgG1 was demonstrated in the jejunum and faeces (Figure 4).

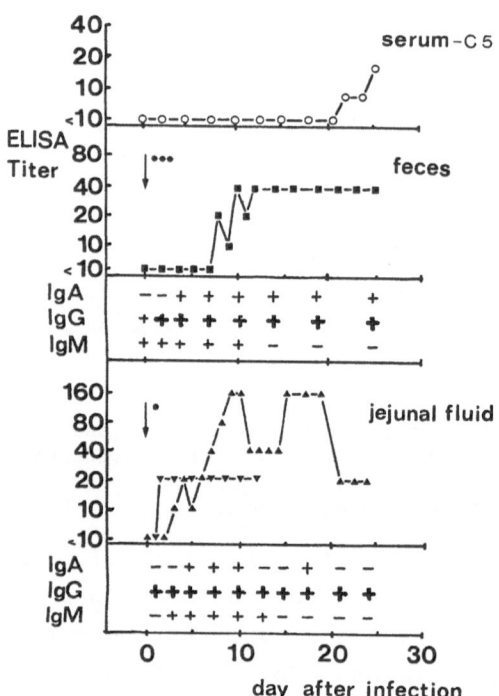

Fig. 4. Comparison of ELISA antibody titres in jejunal fluids, faeces, and serum of calf number 5, which was orally infected with a virulent field strain (V1158) on day 6, and class specificity of jejunal and faecal immunoglobulins.

In calf number 5 a very early anti-rotavirus response in the jejunal fluids was observed (days 2 and 3), and in the faeces (day 8). Serum antibodies first appeared 22 days after infection. In this calf most of the jejunal and faecal immunoglobulins belonged to the IgG1 class.

Calf number 6 which had undergone natural infection was
the only infected and fistulated animal to develop slight
diarrhoea on days 3 and 4 following infection. In the jejunal
fluids, anti-rotavirus antibodies were first seen 5 days after
infection and they increased to very high titres of 1 : 640
on days 10 - 13. Faecal antibodies appeared 18 days after
infection and reached their highest level 10 days later. Twenty
days later they decreased to undetectable levels at which
time reinfection was carried out. Antibodies were first
demonstrated in the serum 38 days after infection.

Following reinfection on day 50, an antibody shedding
profile in the faeces similar to that after the first
infection occurred. Thirty eight days after reinfection and
88 days following the first infection, rotavirus antibody
activity was no longer found in the faeces. Serum titres did
not increase after reinfection in this calf. Immunoglobulins
in the jejunum and faeces of this animal were more closely
associated with IgG and only slightly with IgA in the jejunum.
There were, however, significant amounts of IgA present in the
faeces.

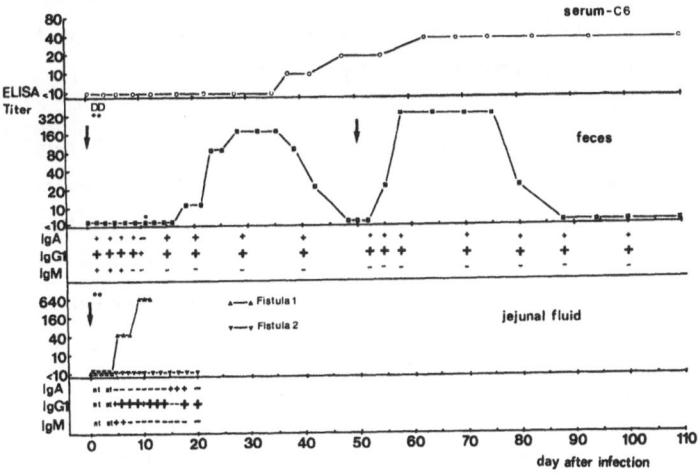

Fig. 5. Comparison of ELISA antibody titres in jejunal fluids, faeces, and
serum of calf number 6, which was infected by contact with calf
number 5 during the first 2 days of life, and class specificity of
jejunal and faecal immunoglobulins.

DISCUSSION

Since rotavirus infections in calves are mainly - if not solely - located in the enterocytes of the villi of the small intestine, the results presented provoke a number of questions.

A wide range of variation has been observed with respect to the time of appearance of rotavirus antibodies in jejunal fluids or faeces. It took 2, 4, 5, and 12 days until rotavirus antibodies were demonstrable in the small intestines of calves numbers 5, 8, 6, and 4 respectively, and then 8, 8, 18, and 14 days until they appeared in the faeces. In serum, the anti-bodies first appeared 22, 32, 38, and 25 days after infection in the animals mentioned above.

There is no explanation for this considerable variation. We believe, however, that strain differences, amount of antigens, and - probably most important - the extent of epithelial infection, may account for these variations. These explanations are supported by the response of calf number 5 which had been infected with a virulent field strain and reacted early and strongly with local antibody production. Calf number 6, however, which had been naturally infected through contact with calf number 5 showed only low activity.

Local antibodies appeared very late in calf number 4 which had been infected with highly purified virus. However, in this calf most of the intestinal immunoglobulins demonstrated were of the IgA class, which is in contrast to the results obtained from all other calves. More animals are to be investigated to clarify this question.

The problem regarding the question whether there is a local 'memory response' in gut associated lymphoid tissue cannot be answered by the results obtained. Calves numbers 4 and 8 were reinfected orally at a time when there was still local rota-virus antibody present. However, in both calves a distinct rise in antibody activity in faeces was observed 7 and 10 days respectively after boosting. Serum antibody titres similarly rose after reinfection. In calf number 6, which had been reinfected at a time when rotavirus antibodies were no longer detectable in the faeces, a second phase of antibody development occurred in the faeces beginning 5 days after reinfection. The duration of antibody presence in the faeces following reinfection was, however, short. They were demonstrable for about 130 days in calf number 8, 50 days in calf number 4, and 25 days in calf number 6. It cannot be determined at this time whether these responses were due to an 'immunological memory' or whether they were simply the expression of a second 'new' infection. Examination of the different immunoglobulin classes found in the small intestine and faeces of these calves also gave conflicting results. Only in one calf (number 4) was IgA the most reactive immunoglobulin in intestinal fluids. In the remaining calves (numbers 3, 5, 8) IgG1 predominated in the intestine.

Newby and Bourne (1976) have found that there is a selective transport system of IgG1 from serum to intestine in cattle, as well as from serum to mammary gland as shown by Kemler et al. (1975). But when we compare anti-rotaviral activity in the serum and faeces during the last ten days of the observation period, high titres are found in the serum, but no rotaviral antibodies are found in the faeces. This does not support evidence for such a selective transport mechanism. IgG2 was found in very poor amounts only in 2 fistulas.

Nevertheless, in some cases and under certain conditions, IgA might possibly be induced in high amounts, the pathways of which are not yet understood.

REFERENCES

Acres, S.D. and Radostis, O.M., 1976. The efficacy of a modified live reo-like virus vaccine and an *E. coli* bacterin for prevention of acute undifferentiated neonatal diarrhoea in beef calves. Canad. Vet. J. <u>17</u>, 1977.

Bachmann, P.A., 1977. Rotavirusnachweis in Fäzes: Erfahrungen mit dem Enzyme-linked-Immunosorbentassay (Elisa). Zbl. Vet. Med. B. <u>26</u>, 835.

Bachmann, P.A. and Hess, R.G., 1981. Viruses and Diarrhoea of Animals IV. Comparative Aspects of Pathogenesis and Immunity. In: Virus Infections of the Gastrointestinal Tract. A.S. Kapikian, D.A.J. Tyrrel, eds. Marcel Dekker, New York, in press.

Graber, P. and Williams, C.A., 1953. Méthode permettant l'étude conjuguée des propriétés électrophorétiques et immunochimiques d'un mélange de protéines application au sérum sanguin. Biophys. Biochem. Acta. <u>10</u>, 193-194.

Kemler, R., Mossmann, H., Strohmaier, U., Kickhoefen, B. and Hammer, D.K., 1975. *In vitro* studies on the selective binding of IgG from different species to tissue sections of the bovine mammary gland. Eur. J. Immunol. <u>5</u>, 603.

Newby, T.J. and Bourne, F.J., 1976. The nature of the local immune system of the bovine small intestine. Immunology. <u>31</u>, 475.

Porter, P., Noakes, D.E. and Allen, W.D., 1972. Intestinal secretion of immunoglobulins in the preruminant calf. Immunology. <u>23</u>, 299.

Thurber, E.T., Bass, E.P. and Beckenhauer, W.H., 1977. Field trial evaluation of a Reo-Coronavirus calf diarrhoea vaccine. Canad. J. comp. Med. <u>41</u>, 131.

DISCUSSION

H. Miller   (UK)

When you looked for early IgA antibodies, is there a
possibility that you were not detecting them because they were
complexed with virus?

G. Hess   (FRG)

That is possible. We examined some faecal samples and
some jejunum fluids by electron microscopy but did not find
immune complexes. However, we did not look at all of them.

D. van Zeane   (Netherlands)

Did you actually prove that IgG1 is directed against
rotavirus?

G. Hess

No, I didn't say that. IgG1 was the predominant immunoglobulin found in faeces and in jejunal fluid. We are now
establishing a class specific ELISA assay to determine this.

K. Petzoldt   (FRG)

How did you quantitate the Ig levels? Secondly, you
showed that in most cases where you were able to detect virus
in the faeces, no virus could be detected in the fistula fluid.
What is the reason for this?

G. Hess

To answer the last question first, we think that it is a
concentration effect in faeces. We looked at jejunum fluid
once a day for the first ten days after infection. We did not
concentrate jejunum fluid and therefore it is necessary to have
an extremely sensitive test to detect viral antigen.

With regard to the first question, immunoglobulins were only measured by the appearance of stronger precipitation in immuno electrophoresis.

T.J. Newby   *(UK)*

I suppose it was fairly surprising that you did not find any antibody in faeces of animals with high circulating anti-body. When we looked at this we found that the majority of the IgG1 in serum had originated from the cells in the lamina propria. Maybe your antibody was made at a distal site. I don't know how much of that would actually get into the gut.

W. Leibold   *(FRG)*

Of what importance is it in diseases which are mostly locally situated, to measure the serum type of antibodies?

G. Hess

We think, and Professor Bohl agrees, that serum anti-bodies are no measure for the protection rate of the animals. Protection lasts about 25 or 30 days although serum antibody disappears before this. On the other hand, after reinfection a very high antibody serum level occurs although none appears in faeces or in jejunum fluid. We think that these animals become infected by rotavirus after a further period of time.

W. Leibold

Despite the serum antibodies?

G. Hess

Yes. This is the cause of such sub-clinical infections.

P. Brandtzaeg   *(Norway)*

In this local production of IgG, what is the state of the intestinal mucosa in these experimentally infected animals? Our experience in the human species is that as soon as the epithelial barrier breaks down, the slightest break in the barrier, the local production will be turned on for IgG, and this may even dominate the normal IgA response locally. I wonder how this might influence your data on the local production of IgA and IgG antibodies.

G. Hess

When you look at the epithelial cells of the small intestine of a rotavirus infected calf you would not find the decimation of epithelial cells all over the small intestine. That is our experience. You often find it scattered in small areas. Then you find completely healthy areas.

P. Brandtzaeg

That's more than enough to explain the stimulation of a local IgG response; you don't need a complete decimation. Even a break would change the physiological situation of the local immune system.

G. Hess

That's right.

T.J. Newby

If there are no more questions I will thank the speakers and close this session.

IMMUNE RESPONSE TO SUBUNIT VACCINES AGAINST ENVELOPED VIRUSES

B. Morein*, K. Simons**, M. Horn af Rantzien*
T. Waller* and M. Sharp***

* National Veterinary Institute, Stockholm, Sweden;

** European Molecular Biology Laboratory, Heidelberg,
Federal Republic of Germany;

*** Moredun Institute, Edinburgh, United Kingdom.

ABSTRACT

Antibody can be extracted from different organs, and specific activity against microorganisms can be measured on such material with good accuracy (Waller et al., 1980).

This method has been applied on bovine lungs and trachea to measure the antibody activity against PI-3 virus and was compared to that activity in serum from corresponding animals. In general the antibody titres in extracts from lungs and trachea correlated with that in serum when measured with the HI-test, although the titres were lower.

The immune responses to PI-3 virus in the IgG and IgA classes were assayed with the ELISA technique. It was then found that the PI-3 titre within the IgG class in the lung extracts varied between the different animals in parallel with the titres in serum. On the other hand, the response in the IgA class in the lung extracts varied independently with the serum titres between the animals.

Efficient subunit vaccines can be prepared consisting of the spike proteins of membrane viruses in forms of micelles or with the spike proteins integrated into lipid vesicles, so called virosomes (Morein et al., 1978). From PI-3 virus (Morein et al., submitted) protein micelles were prepared and used as vaccines on pathogen-free lambs. Antibody response as well as protective immunity was induced by such a micelle vaccine containing 15 µg spike protein per dose after two vaccinations, when an oil adjuvant was included at the first vaccination. The antibody response was measured in serum in haemagglutination inhibition (HI) and serum neutralisation (SN) assays. The protective effect was shown by reduced virus excretion and pneumonic lesions in the vaccinated animals compared to non-vaccinated animals.

The immune response of the PI-3 spike protein micelles were tested in BALB/c mice. They were vaccinated twice 3 weeks apart with different doses of protein micelles (0.1 to 10 μg protein). The antibody response in serum was followed with weekly intervals until the end of the experiment 6 weeks after the second vaccination. Antibodies to PI-3 were measured in extracts from lungs and trachea with the HI-test and the ELISA technique. One μg spike protein micelles induced clearcut antibody response in serum and in extracts from lung and trachea. The IgA response in the extracts was low compared to the IgG response.

INTRODUCTION

The effectiveness of viral vaccines depends often on the method used to convert the virus into a vaccine. Whole viruses that have been attenuated or killed may be effective, but especially the killed virus vaccines have undesirable side effects which limit their use (Chanock et al., 1975; Ginsberg, 1975; Salk and Salk, 1977). The components in the virus preparations that give rise to the side effects seem not to be important for the protective immune response in the host organism. The preparation of so-called subunit vaccines which contain only the viral antigens needed for immunogenicity has therefore become a central aim in vaccine development.

For the enveloped viruses the surface glycoproteins seem to be the antigens responsible for induction of protection (Bachmayer et al., 1976; Bolognesi, 1976; Hilleman, 1976). However, subunit vaccines available have generally proved less efficient than whole virus vaccines in stimulating protective immunity. Little is known, however, about the physical state of the glycoproteins in the vaccine preparations used. It seems conceivable that the procedures to isolate the proteins have been too harsh, and that the form in which the proteins have been administered is not optimal (Chanock et al., 1975).

These questions were first studied with subunit vaccines prepared from Semliki Forest virus (a Toga virus) the lethal strains of which cause acute encephalomyelitis in mice (Bradish et al., 1971; Mussgay and Weiland, 1973). The viral glycoproteins were isolated in non-denaturated form using mild non-ionic detergents. The proteins were then injected into mice either in a monomeric form, an octameric form, or in a reconstituted phospholipidbound form. It was found that the protective immune response depended dramatically on the physical state of the proteins, the two latter forms inducing protection against a 10^3 fold higher challenge dose of virus than the monomers.

PREPARATION OF THE VACCINES

The molecular structure of Semliki Forest virus has been studied in detail. The surface glycoproteins are integral membrane proteins forming spike-like projections on the external surface of the virus particle. Each spike is a three chain structure containing three glycopolypeptides E1 (molecular weight 40×10^3), E2 (52×10^3) and E3 (10×10^3) (Garoff et al., 1964). The spikes span the lipid bilayer membrane by hydrophobic carboxy terminal polypeptide segments in E1 and E2. The spikes can be solubilised in lipid-free form using non-ionic detergents such as Triton X-100 (p-tert-octylphenolpolyoxyethylene 9-10). In Triton X-100 the spikes occur as monomers complexed to a micelle of Triton X-100 (4.5S complexes) (Simons et al., 1978). When the detergent is removed in absence of added lipid octameric spike aggregates (29S complexes) are formed (Helenius and Von Bonsdorff, 1976). When detergent is removed in the presence of egglecithin reconstitution occurs and vesicles (virosomes) are obtained which contain spike proteins inserted into egglecithin bilayers in a way similar to the viral membrane (Almeida et al., 1975; Helenius et al., 1977).

VIROSOMES AND 29S COMPLEXES INDUCE A HIGH DEGREE OF PROTECTION

Groups of 10 mice were first vaccinated with 0.05 - 10 µg of the 29S-complexes (a single immunisation with one third s.c. and two thirds i.p.). The mice were challenged 2 weeks later with 50 LD_{50} (10^4 pfu) virus intraperitoneally. It was found that 0.5 µg induced protective immunity in 50% of the mice and that all mice were protected following vaccination with 10 µg. In subsequent vaccinations 10 µg spike protein was used irrespective of vaccine used. Challenge was performed intraperitoneally with 50 to 10^7 pfu.

As shown in Figure 1 most of the mice vaccinated with 29S-complexes or virosomes survived a challenge dose of 10^7 pfu, the largest dose tested. Mice vaccinated with the monomer form (4.5S-complexes) resisted a challenge of only $10^{3.4}$. These doses corresponded to 10^4 and $10^{0.8}$ LD_{50} of non-vaccinated mice respectively. For further details see Morein et al., 1978.

The dependence on T-cells for induction of protective immunity was studied by comparing the response of BALB/c mice with that of BALB/c nude (nu/nu) mice. The mice were vaccinated with virosomes. No difference in survival time or rate was found between non-vaccinated and vaccinated nude mice.

The total antibody response was measured in serum with a solid phase radioimmunoassay (Morein et al., 1978). No antibodies were detected in vaccinated nude mice, which were challenged after two weeks and tested after four weeks, whereas the antibody titres kept rising from the first to the fourth week after immunisation of normal mice (Figure 2). Our results thus suggest that T-cells are required for protective immunity as well as for antibody formation against Semliki Forest virus as earlier shown for other viruses (Vierelizier et al., 1974; Bloom and Rager-Zisman, 1975).

The high protective effect, resistance to more than 10^4 LD_{50}, induced by the 29S and virosome vaccines shows that highly effective subunit vaccines can be prepared when these proteins are assembled into multimer aggregates. Monomeric spike proteins give only a low degree of protection. Earlier studies have shown that solubilisation of Toga viruses with different mild detergents leads to vaccines with low efficacy (Mussgay and Weiland, 1973). From other enveloped viruses stable monomeric forms of spike proteins have been isolated, and they are poor immunogens. The Friend leukaemia virus spike glycoprotein (gp 70) is in contrast to the Semliki Forest virus spike protein a typical peripheral membrane protein which does not need detergent for solubility. It is attached to the viral membrane through another membrane protein (Schäfer and Bolognesi, 1977). This glycoprotein had to be injected with adjuvant in two doses of about 100 µg per mouse to give partial protection against leukaemia (Schäfer and Bolognesi, 1977; Hunsman et al., 1976). A monomer preparation of the influenza virus haemagglutinin can be

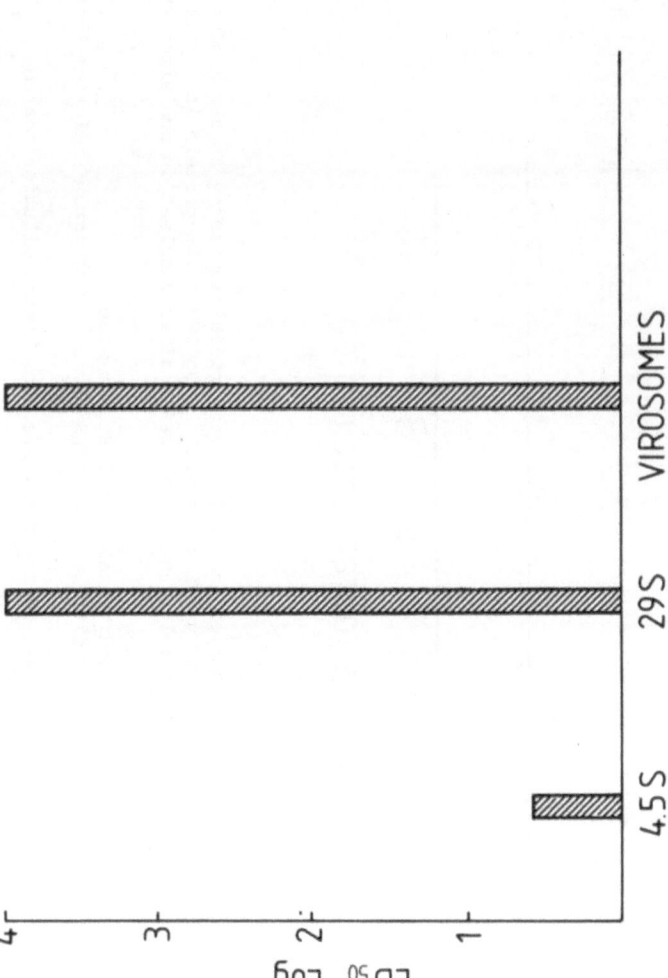

Fig. 1. Vaccination against Semliki Forest virus encephalomyelitis in BALB/c mice: the protective effect induced by different forms of purified spike protein vaccines.

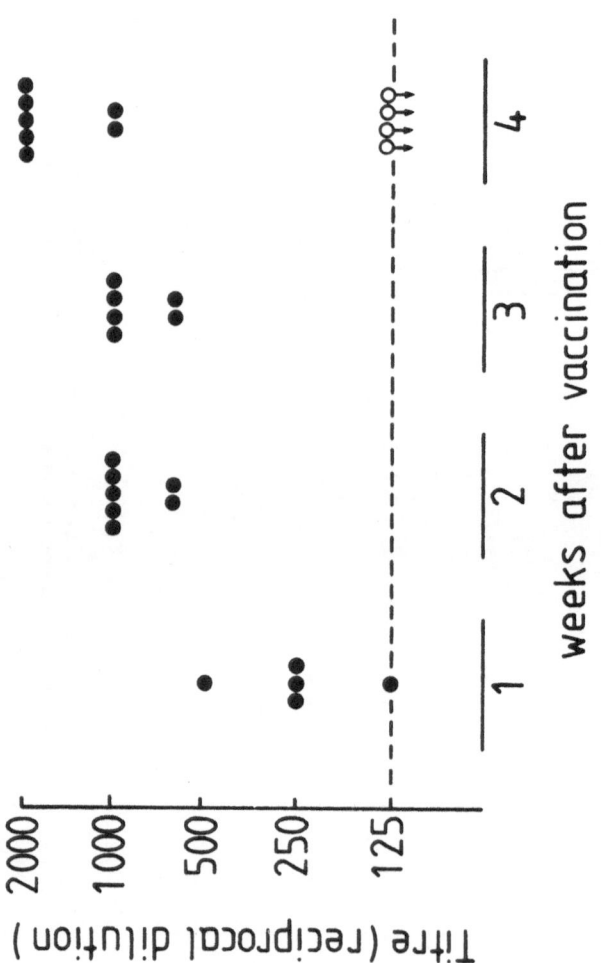

Fig. 2. The antibody responses assayed in a solid phase radioimmunoassay in serum of normal BALB/c, and BALB/c nude (nu/nu) mice following vaccination with 10 μg SFV spike protein in virosomes. The nude mice were challenged with 10^3 pfu virulent virus two weeks after vaccination and after two weeks the sera from survivors were collected.

● indicates titres from individual normal BALB/c mice

o indicates titres from individual nude BALB/c mice. The arrow indicates that the titre was below dilution tested

– indicates threshold level of the test, i.e. the lowest dilution tested.

isolated by cutting off its hydrophobic tail by protease treatment (Brand and Skehel, 1972). This was only weakly immunogenic in hamsters (Jennings et al., 1974) and in man (Tyrrell, 1974).

PARAINFLUENZA 3 VIRUS (PI-3)

PI-3 was selected for the next vaccination experiments since it causes a typical local infection in the respiratory tract in man and many animals. Parainfluenza 3 virus has two species of glycoproteins in the virus envelope, corresponding to the haemagglutinin and the fusion proteins found in other paramyxoviruses (Shibuta et al., 1979).

Protein micelles from PI-3 virus were prepared by the same method as used for SF virus. The virus is solubilised with Triton X-100 and applied to a Beckman SW40 centrifuge tube containing a 20 - 50% sucrose gradient devoid of detergent with a top layer (0.3 ml) of 15% sucrose with 1% Triton X-100 (Figure 3). During centrifugation the non-glycosylated proteins are pelleted. The surface glycoproteins are solubilised by the detergent and delipidated in the Triton X-100-containing layer. When the glycoproteins enter the detergent-free gradient, bound detergent dissociates and the proteins associate to form soluble aggregates with a sedimentation constant of about 30 S. The SDS gel electrophoresis pattern of the resulting protein micelle preparation is shown in Figure 3. Only the two surface glycoproteins are present. The other virus proteins were recovered in the pellet.

We were not able to reconstitute the spike proteins of PI-3 virus with egglecithin using the same conditions that had been successful for SFV. Our aim was to obtain lipid vesicles with a high density of glycoproteins exposed on their surface to mimic the appearance of the virus envelopes in the intact virus particles. For this purpose reconstitution was performed at protein to lipid ratios of 1 : 1. However, most of the proteins did not associate with the lipid but formed aggregates with one another instead. Similar problems have been encountered in

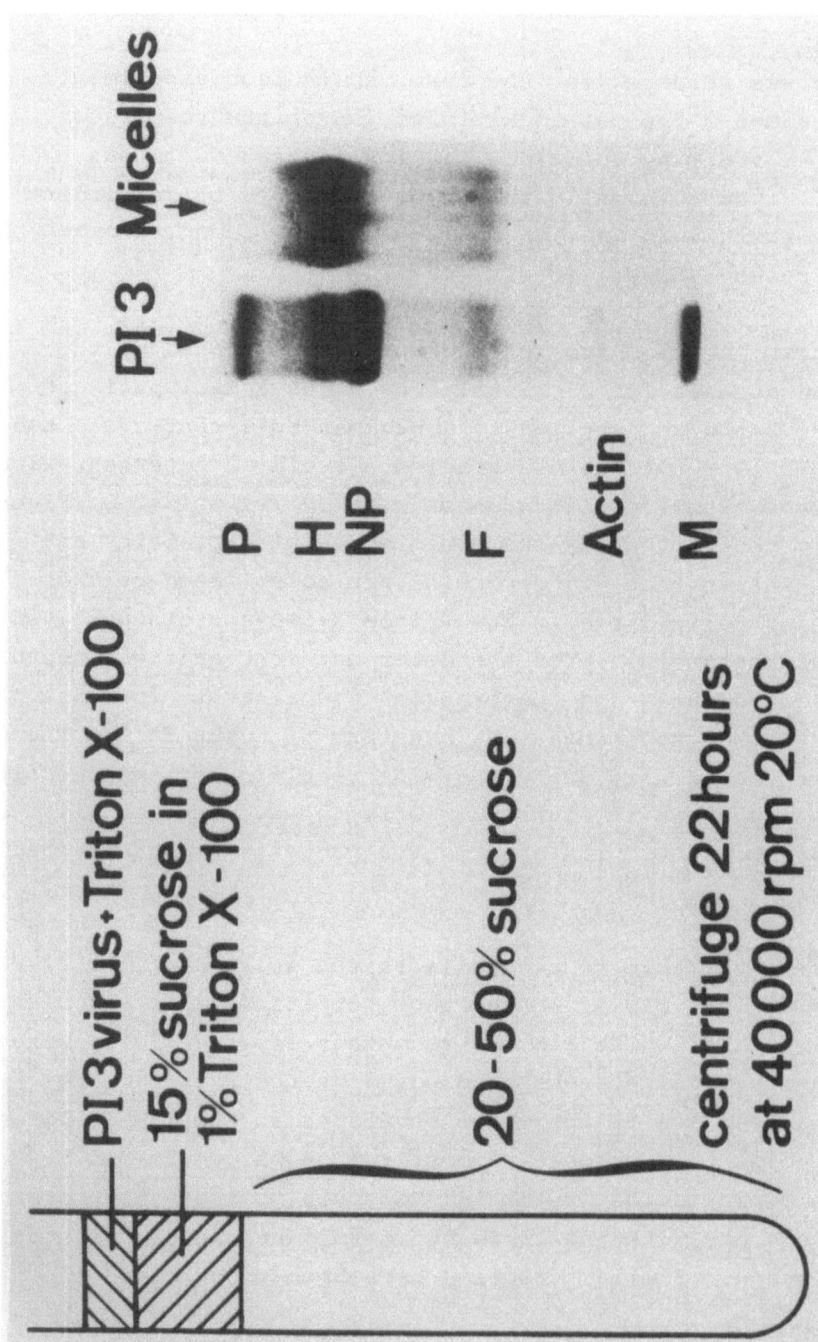

Fig. 3. Sucrose density gradient centrifugation to isolate the protein micelles from PI-3 virus. To the right SDS-gel electrophoresis of the resulting preparation is shown. Two proteins (H and F) are seen in the protein micelles.

reconstitution studies using influenza and Sendai virus glycoproteins (M.J. Gething, M. Waterfield and A. Helenius,
unpublished findings). Only at high lipid-protein ratios did
the PI-3 glycoproteins quantitatively associate with the
egglecithin. Under such conditions egglecithin vesicles are
obtained in which the density of glycoproteins is so low that
the spikes can barely be detected in the electron microscope.
Thus the outcome of the reconstitution seems to be dependent
on the lipid-protein ratio; high ratios favour self-association
of the protein whereas at lower ratios reconstitution is
observed. Another variable which probably also influences the
outcome is the protein concentration. One expects self-association
of proteins to be concentration dependent in the same way as
detergent molecules associate to form micelles above a certain
concentration the so-called critical micellar concentration
(Helenius and Simons, 1975).

To study the efficacy of the PI-3 virus glycoprotein
micelles as vaccines, a test series was started in specific
pathogen-free lambs. Previous studies have shown that formalin-
inactivated whole PI-3 virus when administered twice can protect
the lambs against the disease caused by the virus (Smith, 1975;
Wells et al., 1976). The experimental protocol used for the first
tests is shown in Table 1. The lambs were monitored by checking
virus excretion in nasopharyngeal swabs taken from the lambs after
intranasal and intratracheal challenge with infective PI-3 virus
and examination of pneumonic lesions in the lung at necropsy.
The haemagglutination inhibition activity was tested in serum
samples. The results from the swab tests and necropsy show that
the group of lambs that received the protein micelles together
with adjuvant in the first immunisation seemed to be protected
against the virus infection (Table 2). No significant protection
was seen in the group which received 15 µg of the protein
micelles alone. The haemagglutinin inhibition tests confirm
this interpretation (Table 3).

TABLE 1

VACCINATION OF SPF-LAMBS WITH P-13 VIRUS PROTEIN MICELLES

Group	No. of lambs	Weeks after vaccination*			
		0	3	6	7
A	4	Not vaccinated	Not vaccinated	Inoculate intranasally and intra-tracheally	Kill and necropsy lambs
B	7	15 µg micelles	15 µg micelles		
C	6	15 µg micelles (Adjuvant: Bayol/Falba)	15 µg micelles		

* The vaccines were injected intramuscularly

TABLE 2

RECOVERY OF PI-3 VIRUS FROM NASAL SWABS

Group	Days after inoculation						
	1	2	3	4	5	6	7
A	4/4*	3/4	4/4	4/4	4/4	4/4	4/4
B	7/7	6/7	7/7	7/7	5/7	0/7	0/7
C	1/6	0/6	1/6	1/6	1/6	0/6	0/6

*   No swabs positive
No lambs in the group

TABLE 3

HAEMAGGLUTINATION INHIBITION ACTIVITY AGAINST PI-3 VIRUS*

Group	0	2	3	4	5
A	–	–	10	–	10
B	–	10	10	10	10
C	10	20	40	160	160

               ↑   ↑
              1st   2nd
     vaccination   vaccination

* Reciprocal of serum dilution

The lambs vaccinated with PI-3 micelles without adjuvants did not respond with increased serum titres in contrast to the results obtained in vaccination experiments on mice with SFV micelles. The lack of an antibody response to the PI-3 micelles without adjuvants could be due to too low a dose being used or to species differences of viruses or experimental animals. But even after two injections with 50 µg of the micelles without adjuvants the lambs showed no serological response (Sharp, personal communications). Further experiments were therefore performed in mice, which were vaccinated with protein micelles, and monomers of the PI-3 glycoproteins were also included. The monomers were prepared as described for SFV. The experimental protocol is shown in Table 4. The serological response measured with an enzymelinked immunosorbent assay (ELISA) is shown in Figure 4. Two striking observations can be made.

1. Monomers in complex with detergents give a good antibody response.

2. In mice a clear-cut antibody response is obtained with 10 and 1 µg of the micelle vaccine.

Why the monomers induce a high antibody response in contrast to what was found with a similar preparation of SFV monomers is not clear, but one explanation is that the monomers aggregate soon after injection of the animals. However, the monomers seem to induce a faster antibody response than the micelles and at least part of it is within the IgM class (Figure 4). These results indicate a basic difference between the two types of vaccine. The antibody response was also measured in extracts from lungs and trachea (Waller et al., 1980). Generally the IgG response to PI-3 correlated with the results from serum. The IgA result was very weak, which can be expected after a parenteral immunisation.

The above results indicate that protein micelles can be effective vaccines and monomers in certain cases are not effective. The procedure to prepare the micelles can be used for most membrane proteins. Regarding PI-3 micelles in sheep, an oil adjuvant had to be included to obtain a potent vaccine. It is of interest to study in which physical form different antigens should be presented in vaccines to elicit maximal protective effect and adjuvants of different kinds may be necessary to obtain effective vaccines.

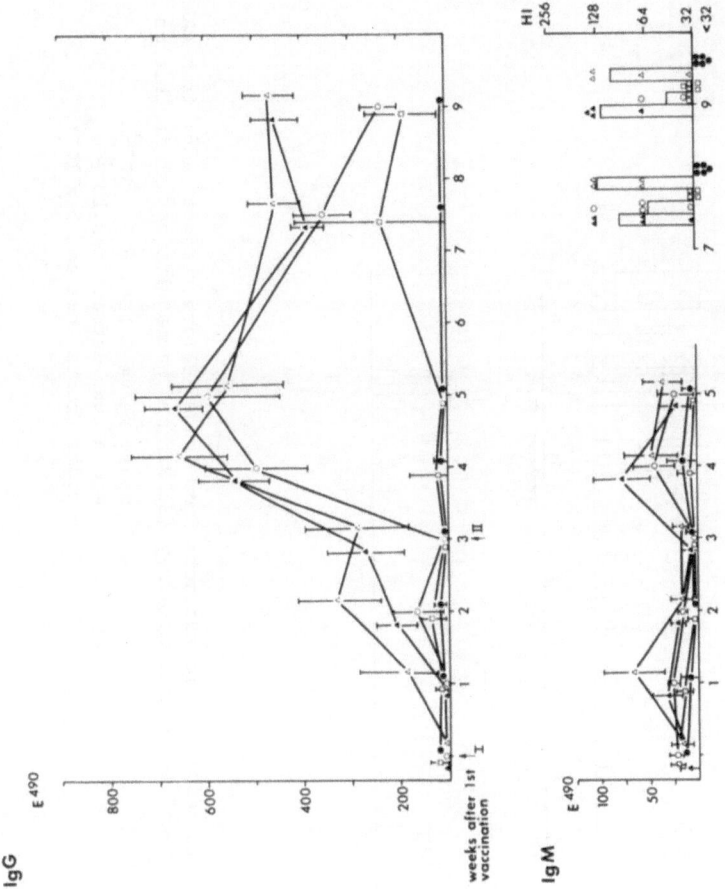

Fig. 4 (A)

324

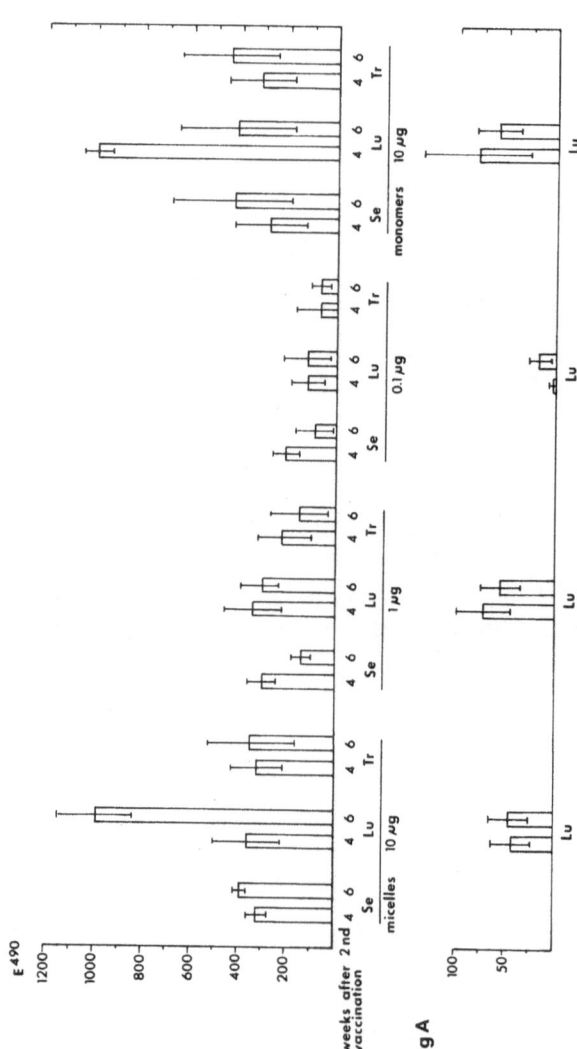

Fig. 4 (B)

Fig. 4   The antibody response in serum (A) and extracts from lungs (B) and trachea* (26) from BALB/c mice
         measured in an enzymelinked immunosorbent assay (ELISA) and haemagglutination inhibition (HI).

         ▲ 10 μg micelles   * mouse serum dilution 5 x 10⁻³
         ○ 1 μg   mouse lung extract 5 x 10⁻²
         ▫ 0.1 μg   mouse trachea extract 5 x 10⁻²
         △ 10 μg monomers
         ● non-vaccinated

REFERENCES

Almeida, J.D., Brand, C.M., Edwards, C.D. and Heath, T.D., 1975. Lancet 2: 899.

Bachmayer, H., Liehl, E. and Schmidt, G., 1976. Preparation and properties of a novel influenza subunit vaccine. Postgrad. Med. J., 52: 360.

Bloom, B.R. and Rager-Zisman, B., 1975. Viral Immunology and Immunopathology (ed. A.L. Notkins) 113. Academic Press, New York.

Bolognesi, D.P., 1976. Potential leukemia subunit vaccines. Cancer Res., 36: 655.

Bradish, C.H., Allner, B. and Maber, H.B., 1971. J. Gen. Virol., 12: 141.

Brand, C.M. and Skehel, H.H., 1972. Nature, New Biology, 238: 145.

Chanock, R.M., Richmann, D.D., Murphy, B.R., Spring, S.B., Schnitzer, T.J. and Richardsson, L.S., 1975. Current approaches to viral immunoprophylaxis. In: Notkins, A.L. (ed), Viral Immunology and Immunopathology. New York: Academic Press, p 291.

Garoff, H., Simons, K. and Renkonen, O., 1964. Virology, 61: 493.

Ginsberg, H.S., 1975. Subunit viral vaccines. In: Notkins, A.L. (ed), Viral Immunology and Immunopathology. New York: Academic Press, p 317.

Helenius, A., Fries, E. and Kartenbeck, J., 1977. J. Cell Bio., 75: 866.

Helenius, A. and Simons, K., 1975. Solubilization of membranes with detergents. Biochim. Biophys. Acta., 415: 29.

Helenius, A. and Von Bonsdorff, C.H., 1976. Biochem. Biophys. Acta., 436: 895.

Hilleman, M.R., 1976. Herpes simplex vaccines. Cancer Res., 36: 857.

Hunsman, G., Moening, V. and Schäfer, W., 1976. Virology, 66: 327.

Jennings, R., Brand, C.M., McLaren, C., Shephard, L. and Potter, C.W., 1974. Med. Microbiol. Immunol., 160: 295.

Morein, B., Helenius, A., Simons, K., Pettersson, R., Kääriäinen, L. and Schirrmacher, V., 1978. Effective subunit vaccines against an enveloped virus. Nature, 276: 715.

Mussgay, M. and Weiland, E., 1973. Intervirology, 1: 529.

Salk, J. and Salk, D., 1977. Control of influenza and poliomyelitis with killed virus vaccines. Science, 195: 834.

Schäfer, W. and Bolognesi, D.P., 1977. Contemp. Top. Immunobiol., 6: 127.

Shibuta, H., Kauda, T., Adachi, A. and Yogo, Y., 1979. Microbiol. Immunol., 23: 617.

Simons, K., Helenius, A. and Caroff, H., 1978. Mol. Biol., 80: 119.

Smith, W.D., 1975. The nasal secretion and serum antibody response of lambs following vaccination and aerosol challenge with parainfluenza 3 virus. Research Veterinary Sci., 19: 56.

Tyrrell, D.A.J., 1974. J. Infect. Dis., 129: 766.

Vierelizier, J.L., Postlethwaite, R., Schild and Allison, A.C., 1974. J. Exp. Med., 140: 1559.

Waller, T., Lyngset, A., Elvander, M. and Morein, B., 1980. Veterinary Immunology and Immunopathology. In press.

Wells, P.W., Sharp, J.M., Burrells, L., Rushton, B. and Smith, W.D., 1976. The assessment in sheep of an inactivated vaccine of parainfluenza 3 virus incorporating double stranded RNA as adjuvant. J. Hyg. Camb., 77: 255.

DISCUSSION

P. Brandtzaeg   *(Norway)*

Would it not be necessary to have some indication of blood contamination?

B. Morein   *(Sweden)*

Yes, I agree. Mice are bled out as is slaughterhouse material.

W. Leibold   *(FRG)*

Can you expand a little on why your virosomes are particularly efficient. What is the mechanism behind it?

B. Morein

At the moment I can't see any difference between the virosomes and the micelles.

W. Leibold

You need the adjuvant, if I understand correctly.

B. Morein

Yes, in sheep, but probably not in mice. Let us consider the reason why the multimer forms are so efficient in mice. To get a T helper cell response, at least in mice, you need the antigen to be presented by a cell carrying the same IA antigen as the immuno-competent cells. If you have a multimer form, this will attach to cells with a factor of 10 for each added binding site.

W. Leibold

Do you think it is only a matter of presentation together with the IA antigens?

B. Morein

That is one of the reasons. It is also known that the
soluble antigen, for instance, will stimulate suppressor cells
and particulate antigens will stimulate helper cells better.
But I don't know if you can say that a micelle is a particulate
antigen because it is kept in solution.

J. Bienenstock *(Canada)*

If you put these virosomes into the animal, where do they
go? Is there any evidence that those virosomes have a peculiar
distribution in the body?

B. Morein

I don't know. I have heard that certain lipids might
have a peculiar distribution to the lungs. No doubt that is
why you are asking. But that is a development area. You could
choose lipid which is known to be excreted in the lung to see
if parenteral injected material can get there. I would like to
do that. In this case the virosomes were not better than the
micelles. We used the virosomes which were Egg lecithin actually. That is supposed to be very neutral with no adjuvant
activity as such. But the adjuvant activity could just be the
physical shape in which the adjuvant is presented. I would say
that the virosomes are not better than the micelles unless you
do something with the lipids in them and include something which
modulates the immune response. In sheep, for example, they need
some sort of modulation of the antibody response in order to get
an immune response and get protection. I don't think it is a
question of the amount of antigens, not in the way that we can
produce them anyway.

J. Bienenstock

Certainly work done about thirty years ago in the lung
suggested that giving material in complete Freund's adjuvant
produced granulomas in the lung of extraordinary degrees and
it is not surprising that you would get a very good IgG antibody
response - but that is a granulomatous, inflammatory, peripheral

type of response which is a very poor way of stimulating IgA
antibody. You get a very poor IgA response but you still may
get good protection and it does not exclude the possibility of
cells, whatever they are, being very important as well as serum
antibody in resistance and recovery in this virus infection.

F.J. Bourne   *(UK)*

This is interesting because it could influence the whole
rationale of vaccination against respiratory disease. In the
gut, for instance, with TGE it is accepted that IgA is protective and that the other immunoglobulins are less significant in
protection. The situation in the lung is less clear but in
purely quantitative terms, the further you go down the respiratory tract, the greater is the predominance of IgG relative to
IgA. But the work of Kenton Morgan in the pig suggested that
this, even so, was locally produced rather than serum derived.

J. Bienenstock

Oh, I think so; if you look at these lungs they are
absolutely full of small to big granulomas in which you find
extraordinary numbers of plasma cells and extraordinary amounts
of antibody that can be extracted.

F.J. Bourne

If there are no further points we will move on to the
next paper.

IMPORTANCE OF LOCAL ANTIBODY IN RESISTANCE TO MYCOPLASMA INFECTIONS OF THE RESPIRATORY TRACT

Geraldine Taylor and C.J. Howard

ARC, Institute for Research on Animal Diseases,
Compton, Berkshire RG16 ONN, UK.

ABSTRACT

A solid-phase micro-radioimmunoassay was used to study the development of class-specific antibodies to Mycoplasma pulmonis in sera and lung washings of mice after inoculation with live or inactivated mycoplasmas by a variety of routes. Attempts were made to correlate these findings with resistance to a subsequent intranasal challenge with M. pulmonis. These investigations indicated that resistance to M. pulmonis in mice correlated with the presence of antibody in lung washings and that antibody of any Ig class may mediate resistance. Similar studies in calves vaccinated with inactivated M. bovis also suggested that antibody in lung washings is important in resistance and that this antibody was predominantly IgG.

Further evidence that antibody of any Ig class in the respiratory tract can mediate resistance to mycoplasma infections was obtained from an examination of the ability of intranasal administration of purified mouse immunoglobulins to protect against infection with M. pulmonis. Thus, IgG1 and IgG2a were most effective in protecting mice against infection with M. pulmonis, IgG2b less so and IgA was least effective of all. The ways in which antibodies may mediate resistance to mycoplasma infections are discussed.

INTRODUCTION

Mycoplasmas colonise the surface of the bronchial mucosa and in this position stimulate a peribronchiolar and perivascular accumulation of lymphocytes. These lymphoid accumulations are accompanied by a bronchial exudate composed of polymorphonuclear leukocytes and macrophages. Although mycoplasma infections are often prolonged, animals do develop resistance to a subsequent infection, even when the initial infection has not been cleared (see Whittlestone, 1976; Taylor et al., 1977). Resistance may not be long lasting since repeated symptomatic and asymptomatic *M. pneumoniae* infections occur in man at intervals of several years (Foy et al., 1970; Foy et al., 1977). However recurrent infections must eventually result in a more durable immunity since the incidence of disease later in life is low (Foy et al., 1970; 1977).

Antibody appears to be important in resistance to mycoplasma infections, since passively transferred convalescent serum can protect animals against respiratory disease.(Masiga et al., 1975; Cassell et al., 1973; Taylor and Taylor-Robinson, 1976). However, attempts to produce effective vaccines have not met with great success despite the ability of these vaccines to induce serum antibodies (see Whittlestone, 1976). Because mycoplasmal diseases begin as a superficial infection of the respiratory tract, local immunity should be of major importance in preventing disease. The importance of antibodies in the respiratory tract and investigations of the most effective means of inducing such antibodies are discussed below.

RESISTANCE INDUCED BY LOCAL AND PARENTERAL IMMUNISATION WITH VIABLE MYCOPLASMAS

A comparison of intranasal (i.n.) and intraperitoneal (i.p.) inoculation of hamsters with live, virulent *M. pneumoniae* organisms, indicated that mycoplasmas inoculated by the i.n. route induced a greater protection against a subsequent i.n.

challenge than did i.p. administration of organisms (Fernald
and Clyde, 1970). These differences were more marked when
animals were inoculated with an attenuated strain of
M. pneumoniae. Similarly, an avirulent strain of *M. pulmonis* only
induced resistance in mice to i.n. challenge with virulent
mycoplasmas, after i.n. inoculation. Mice receiving the
avirulent organisms intravenously (i.v.) were not immune
(Taylor et al., 1977). These findings indicated the importance
of local immunity in the development of resistance to
mycoplasma infections of the respiratory tract. However, there
are examples where immunity following parenteral administration
of live mycoplasmas can be as effective as that following i.n.
immunisation. For example, an attenuated strain of *M. mycoides*
subsp. *mycoides* administered subcutaneously (s.c.) to cattle
(Lloyd and Trethewie, 1970), a virulent strain of *M. pulmonis*
administered i.v. to mice (Taylor et al., 1977) and virulent
M. bovis inoculated i.v. in calves (Howard et al., 1977), all
induced resistance to a subsequent challenge via the respiratory
route with virulent organisms. In fact, i.v. administration of
M. pulmonis to rats not only induced complete protection against
the development of pneumonic lesions but also reduced the
incidence and severity of lesions in the upper respiratory
tract (Cassell and Davis, 1978).

The ability of mycoplasmas to induce resistance to i.n.
challenge following parenteral inoculation may be related to
their ability to persist and replicate for a period, thereby
increasing the antigenic stimulus and the levels of serum
antibody. However, there is not always a correlation between
the levels of serum antibody induced by parenteral inoculation
of live mycoplasmas and resistance to i.n. challenge (Fernald
and Clyde, 1970; Taylor et al., 1977). A more important
factor may be the ability of the mycoplasma to spread to the
respiratory tract and induce a local immune response. Thus,
mycoplasmas can be isolated for several weeks from the lungs
of mice inoculated i.v. with a virulent strain of *M. pulmonis*
and from the lungs of calves inoculated i.v. with *M. bovis* and
such animals are resistant to i.n. or intratracheal (i.t.)

challenge (Taylor et al., 1977; Howard et al., 1977). In contrast, mycoplasmas do not persist in the lungs of mice inoculated i.v. with an avirulent strain of *M. pulmonis* and such animals were not immune.

Another possibility is that after parenteral inoculation, mycoplasmas colonise other mucosal sites, such as the genital tract which is colonised in rates by *M. pulmonis*, and the existence of a common mucosal immune system may provide a protective effect in the respiratory tract (Cassell and Davis, 1978). A similar phenomenon may account for the observation that resistance to pneumonia in hamsters induced by *M. pneumoniae* was stimulated by prior selective infection of the upper respiratory tract with this organism. However, whereas there was a 40 to 60% reduction in the severity of pneumonia in hamsters whose previous infection was confined to the upper respiratory tract, there was an 80 to 100% reduction in animals whose previous infection also involved the lower respiratory tract. Replication of challenge organisms was also significantly suppressed only in the latter group of hamsters (Jemski et al., 1977). It appears, therefore, that it is the immune response in the lower respiratory tract which is most important in resistance to pneumonia induced by mycoplasmas.

ANTIBODY RESPONSES AFTER LOCAL AND PARENTERAL IMMUNISATION WITH VIABLE MYCOPLASMAS

The development of Ig-containing cells in the lungs of hamsters inoculated i.n. with *M. pneumoniae* and of mice inoculated i.n. with *M. pulmonis* follows the sequence IgM, IgG and IgA (Fernald et al., 1972; Cassell et al., 1974). Whereas IgA-containing cells became the predominant cell in the lungs of mice from 3 to 8 weeks following i.n. inoculation with *M. pulmonis*, the number of IgA-containing cells in the lungs of hamsters changed very little after infection with *M. pneumoniae*. Cassell and colleagues (1974) suggested that the lungs and draining lymph nodes were the primary sites of antibody production in mycoplasma infected animals and that antibody diffuses from these sites into serum and respiratory tract secretions. IgM, IgG1, IgG2 and IgA antibodies were all detected in sera and lung washings (LW) from mice inoculated i.n. with *M. pulmonis* although the appearance of IgA was delayed in comparison with the other antibodies (Cassell et al., 1974). Since the presence of antibodies in LW was only assessed qualitatively by Cassell et al., (1974), a quantitative assessment of Ig class-specific antibodies was made using a solid-phase radioimmunoassay. Mice were inoculated either i.n. or i.v. with a virulent strain of *M. pulmonis* and their sera and LW were examined at intervals for antibodies to the mycoplasma (Taylor and Howard, 1980a).

Mice inoculated i.n. with 5×10^3 CFU *M. pulmonis* do not develop pneumonic lesions, although mycoplasmas can be isolated from the lungs for several weeks and such animals are resistant to a subsequent i.n. challenge 35 days after immunisation with a dose of *M. pulmonis* sufficient to induce severe pneumonia in control mice (Taylor et at., 1977). IgG2 and IgM antibodies were first detected in sera from these mice 14 days after inoculation. IgG1 antibody was detected 21 days after inoculation and became the major antibody at the time of challenge. IgA antibody was not detected until 28 days after inoculation. Antibody was first detected in LW 28 days after inoculation and was present in both IgG1 and IgG2 classes. IgA and IgM antibodies appeared 7 days later, but IgG1 and IgG2 predominated. Thus, at the time of challenge, the predominant antibodies in both sera and LW were IgG1 and IgG2, with lower levels of IgA and IgM (Table 1).

Mice inoculated i.v. with 2×10^6 CFU *M. pulmonis* are also resistant to i.n. challenge (Taylor et al., 1977). Such animals rapidly develop antibodies in both sera and LW, although little or no IgA antibody can be detected (Taylor and Howard, 1980a). At the time of i.n. challenge, 35 days after i.v. immunisation, IgG1 and IgG2 antibodies predominate in sera although only IgG2 antibody was detected in LW (Table 2). After i.n. challenge mice developed a secondary antibody response in

LW that involved both IgG1 and IgG2 classes. Thus, IgA does
not appear to be of importance in resistance of mice immunised
by the i.v. route. If it is the availability of antibody in
the respiratory tract which is important in immunity, these
studies suggest that IgG1 and IgG2 antibodies may be involved.
IgA may also contribute to resistance, but only in those mice
immunised by the i.n. route. IgA antibodies are thought to
play some part in resistance to *M. pneumoniae* in man. Thus, only
pre-existing IgA antibody in human nasal secretions correlated
with resistance to respiratory disease induced by this
mycoplasma (Brunner et al., 1973).

TABLE 1

CLASS-SPECIFIC ANTIBODIES IN SERA AND LUNG WASHINGS (LW) OF MICE 35 DAYS
AFTER INTRANASAL INOCULATION WITH 5×10^3 CFU OR INTRAVENOUS INOCULATION
OF 2×10^6 CFU VIABLE *M. pulmonis*

Route of inoculation	Sample	$\log_{10}$ U antibody* at challenge			
		IgG1	IgG2	IgM	IgA
Intranasal	Serum	4.0	3.8	3.0	3.0
	LW	2.5	2.6	1.7	2.0
Intravenous	Serum	3.5	3.9	2.7	1.4
	LW	< 0.7	1.6	< 0.7	<0.7

* Mean Units of antibody for 5 mice per group

RESISTANCE INDUCED BY LOCAL AND PARENTERAL IMMUNISATION WITH
INACTIVATED MYCOPLASMAS

Parenteral administration of inactivated mycoplasmal
vaccines have met with limited success in inducing resistance
to i.n. challenge with live mycoplasmas. Since the route of
administration of live mycoplasmas appeared to be important
in determining resistance to a subsequent i.n. challenge, a
comparison of the ability of local and parenteral administration
of inactivated organisms to induce resistance has been carried
out.

TABLE 2

PROTOCOL FOR VACCINATION OF MICE WITH FORMALIN-INACTIVATED *M. pulmonis*

Vaccine group	Treatment on indicated day			
	0	7	14	21 or 42
Controls	PBS s.c.*	—	PBS i.n.	
s.c. + i.v.	Antigen s.c.+	—	Antigen i.v.	5×10^5 CFU *M. pulmonis* i.n.
s.c. + i.n.	Antigen s.c.	—	Antigen i.n.	
3 x i.n.	Antigen i.n.	Antigen i.n.	Antigen i.n.	

* All subcutaneous (s.c.) inoculations given in Freund's incomplete adjuvant

+ Antigen = suspension of formalin-inactivated *M. pulmonis*; each dose contained 50 µg total protein, administered either s.c., intravenously (i.v.) or intranasally (i.n.) into group of 5 mice

Formalin-inactivated *M. pneumoniae* administered s.c. to hamsters did not significantly reduce the frequency of pneumonia after i.n. challenge with live organisms. In contrast, inactivated organisms inoculated i.n. on three occasions at weekly intervals reduced both the frequency and severity of pneumonia after challenge (Greenberg et al., 1977).

Mice primed with a s.c. inoculation of formalin-inactivated *M. pulmonis* in adjuvant and boosted 14 days later either i.v. or i.n. were resistant to i.n. challenge with live mycoplasmas. However, resistance was significantly greater in mice boosted i.n. than in those boosted i.v. (Taylor et al., 1977). Resistance to i.n. challenge with live *M. pulmonis* was also induced in mice by three i.n. inoculations of inactivated mycoplasmas at weekly intervals (Atobe and Ogata, 1977; Taylor and Howard, 1980$_a$). Resistance to i.t. challenge with live *M. bovis* was only induced in calves primed with inactivated *M. bovis* administered intramuscularly (i.m.) in adjuvant and boosted i.t. and not in those animals boosted i.m. (Howard et al., 1977). The failure to induce resistance either to *M. bovis* infection in calves by i.t. administration of inactivated mycoplasmas (Howard et al., 1980) or to *M. pulmonis* in rats by i.n. inoculation of inactivated organisms (Cassell and Davis, 1978) may have been due to insufficient amounts of antigen administered to the respiratory tract. Immunity has also been induced in animals that have been hyperimmunised by repeated parenteral administration of antigen in adjuvant (Hayatsu, 1978; Howard et al., 1980). However, in general these studies indicate the importance of administration of mycoplasmal antigen to the lungs for the development of resistance to mycoplasma disease.

ANTIBODY RESPONSES AFTER LOCAL AND PARENTERAL IMMUNISATION WITH INACTIVATED MYCOPLASMAS

An examination of the development of antibody in animals vaccinated with inactivated mycoplasmas failed to show a correlation between the levels of complement-fixing antibodies in sera and resistance to i.n. challenge (Greenberg et al., 1977; Taylor et al., 1977; Howard et al., 1977; Atobe and Ogata, 1977). However, there was a correlation between the levels of complement-fixing antibodies (as measured by the single radial haemolysis test) in LW of calves vaccinated with inactivated *M. bovis* and resistance to i.t. challenge (Howard et al., 1980). Thus, calves inoculated by the two regimes that induced immunity, namely i.m. + i.t. or 3 x s.c., developed antibodies in LW at the time of challenge (i.e. 7 days after completion of vaccination). In contrast, antibodies were not consistently demonstrated in LW from calves vaccinated by those procedures that failed to induce immunity, namely i.m. + i.m. and i.t. + i.t. (Howard et al; 1980).

The Ig class-specific antibody response to *M. pulmonis* in sera and LW from mice vaccinated with inactivated mycoplasmas was examined to elucidate the relative importance of the various Ig classes in the development of resistance (Taylor and Howard, 1980a). Mice were vaccinated either s.c. + i.v., s.c. + i.n. or 3 x i.n. with inactivated *M. pulmonis* as shown in Table 2. Such animals were examined 7 and 28 days after completion of vaccination for their susceptibility to i.n. challenge with live *M. pulmonis* and the presence of antibodies in sera and LW. When challenged 7 days after vaccination, all three groups of vaccinated mice were protected against the development of pneumonia and there was a significant reduction in the numbers of mycoplasmas isolated from the lungs when compared with controls (Table 3). *M. pulmonis* was isolated from the lungs of all of 5 mice vaccinated s.c. + i.v. and all of 5 of those vaccinated s.c. + i.n., but from only 1 out of 5 mice vaccinated 3 x i.n. IgG1, IgG2 and IgM antibodies were present in the sera from all vaccinated mice (Table 4). However, there was no clear correlation between the levels of such antibodies and resistance. For example, although resistance was greatest in mice vaccinated 3 x i.n., Ig class-specific antibodies in sera from those animals were either the same or significantly less than those of mice vaccinated by the other two regimes. Only IgG1 antibody was detected in LW from mice

TABLE 3

COMPARISON OF VARIOUS ROUTES OF ADMINISTRATION OF FORMALIN-INACTIVATED *M. pulmonis* ON THE ISOLATION OF
MYCOPLASMAS FROM THE LUNGS OF MICE AFTER INTRANASAL CHALLENGE WITH 5 x 10⁵ CFU *M. pulmonis*

Animals challenged at indicated days after completion of vaccination	Vaccine* group	No. mycoplasmas in lungs+ at indicated days after challenge	
		1	14
7	Controls	ND	6.9 ± 0.1
	s.c. + i.v.	ND	3.4 ± 0.5
	s.c. + i.n.	ND	3.6 ± 0.2
	3 x i.n.	ND	0.8 ± 0.8
28	Controls	5.5 ± 0.1	7.0 ± 0.1
	s.c. + i.v.	4.0 ± 0.2	4.1 ± 0.4
	s.c. + i.n.	2.7 ± 0.6	3.7 ± 1.0
	3 x i.n.	3.1 ± 0.6	3.5 ± 1.0

* See Table 2 for details of vaccination protocol

+ Mean no. mycoplasmas isolated ($\log_{10}$ CFU/ml ± standard error)

vaccinated s.c. + i.v., whereas IgGl, IgG2 and IgA antibodies
were detected in LW from mice vaccinated by the other two
regimes. Only IgGl antibody was detected in LW from mice
vaccinated s.c. + i.v., whereas IgGl, IgG2 and IgA antibodies
were detected in LW from mice vaccinated by the other two
regimes. The greater resistance of mice vaccinated 3 x i.n.
when compared with those animals vaccinated s.c. + i.n. or
s.c. + i.v. appeared to correlate with the significantly
greater levels of IgA antibody in LW from the former group of
mice.

TABLE 4

CLASS-SPECIFIC ANTIBODIES IN SERA AND LUNG WASHINGS (LW) OF MICE 7 DAYS
AFTER VACCINATION WITH INACTIVATED *M. pulmonis*

| Vaccine* group | Sample | Log_{10} U antibody at challenge[+] | | | |
		IgGl	IgG2	IgM	IgA
Controls	Serum	< 1.0	< 1.0	< 1.0	< 1.0
	LW	< 0.3	< 0.3	< 0.3	< 0.3
s.c. + i.v.	Serum	5.0	2.1	3.8	< 1.0
	LW	1.5	< 0.3	< 0.3	< 0.3
s.c. + i.n.	Serum	4.7	3.4	3.1	< 1.0
	LW	1.8	0.3	< 0.3	1.6
3 x i.n.	Serum	4.2	3.5	2.7	< 1.0
	LW	1.4	0.5	< 0.3	2.1

* See Table 2 for details of vaccination protocol

[+] Mean Units of antibody

When challenged 28 days after vaccination, all three
groups of vaccinated mice were still resistant to challenge
with live *M. pulmonis* and this resistance was apparent as early
as 24 h after challenge (Table 3). At this time, there were
approximately 10 fold fewer organisms isolated from the lungs
of mice vaccinated s.c. + i.n. or 3 x i.n. compared with those
vaccinated s.c. + i.v. This increased resistance was not
associated with the levels of serum antibodies, which were
highest in mice vaccinated s.c. + i.v., but rather with the
presence of IgA antibody in LW (Table 5). The only other
antibody present in LW from vaccinated mice at this time was

IgG1, which was present in all three groups of vaccinated animals.

TABLE 5

CLASS-SPECIFIC ANTIBODIES IN SERA AND LUNG WASHINGS (LW) OF MICE 28 DAYS AFTER VACCINATION WITH INACTIVATED *M. pulmonis*

Vaccine* group	Sample	Log_{10} U antibody at challenge +			
		IgG1	IgG2	IgM	IgA
Controls	Serum	< 1.0	<1.0	< 1.0	<1.0
	LW	< 0.3	<0.3	< 0.3	<0.3
s.c. + i.v.	Serum	5.2	2.9	3.2	1.1
	LW	1.9	<0.3	< 0.3	<0.3
s.c. + i.n.	Serum	4.4	1.8	1.8	1.4
	LW	1.6	<0.3	< 0.3	0.5
3 x i.n.	Serum	3.9	1.8	1.4	1.5
	LW	0.8	<0.3	< 0.3	0.8

* See Table 2 for details of vaccination protocol

\+ Mean Units of antibody

The antibody detected in LW from mice vaccinated s.c. + i.n. or 3 x i.n. appears to have originated in the respiratory tract. Thus, 7 days after vaccination IgA antibody was detected only in LW and not in sera (Table 4). Furthermore, there was an accumulation of lymphocytes in the peribronchiolar and perivascular areas of the lungs of these animals 7 days after vaccination. Immunofluorescence studies showed that these cells contained IgG1, IgG2 or IgA (Taylor and Howard, 1980a). In contrast, there was little or no increase in Ig-containing cells in the lungs of mice vaccinated s.c. + i.v., indicating that most of the antibody detected in LW from this group of animals was derived from the serum. Thus, following vaccination with inactivated mycoplasmas, resistance of mice to i.n. challenge with live *M. pulmonis* appears to be related to the presence of IgG1 and IgA antibody in LW. In mice immunised with live organisms resistance may be related to IgG2 as well as IgG1 and IgA in LW.

An examination of the Ig class of antibodies present in LW from calves vaccinated with inactivated *M. bovis* has also been made (Howard et al., 1980). The predominant antibodies in LW from immune calves i.e. those vaccinated i.m. + i.t. or 3 x s.c. were IgGl and IgG2. These antibodies were present only in low levels in LW from non-immune calves, i.e. those vaccinated i.m. + i.m. or i.t. + i.t. It is interesting to note, however, that both i.m. + i.t. and i.t. + i.t. were the only regimes to induce IgA antibody in LW.

These studies suggest that antibody of any Ig class present in the lungs may be capable of mediating resistance. Further support for this suggestion was obtained from an investigation into the abilities of purified mouse immunoglobulins to protect mice against i.n. challenge with *M. pulmonis*.

PASSIVE IMMUNISATION WITH PURIFIED MOUSE IMMUNOGLOBULINS

Convalescent mouse serum obtained from mice inoculated i.n. 6 weeks previously with *M. pulmonis* was fractionated on a Protein A-sepharose column eluted with buffers of differing pH (Taylor and Howard, 1980$_b$). The Ig class-specific anti-bodies to *M. pulmonis* as measured by radioimmunoassay, in the various fractions are shown in Table 6. Although antibodies of two or three Ig classes could be detected in all fractions, one Ig class always predominated and contamination by the other Ig classes was usually minimal. Thus, fractions were enriched for one particular Ig class. The ability of these fractions to protect mice against i.n. challenge with *M. pulmonis* was investigated by incubating the fractions with the mycoplasma at 37°C for 30 min prior to i.n. inoculation into mice. There was no reduction in the numbers of viable mycoplasmas following incubation with the various Ig fractions, so all mice were inoculated with 3.5 x 10^4 CFU *M. pulmonis*. Twenty-four hours after inoculation, mycoplasmas were isolated from the lungs of all 10 out of 10 mice that had been inoculated i.n. with a mixture of *M. pulmonis* and normal mouse serum. In contrast, mycoplasmas were not isolated from any of the 10 mice inoculated with mycoplasmas mixed with whole convalescent

TABLE 6

ISOLATION OF MYCOPLASMAS FROM THE LUNGS 24 HOURS AFTER INTRANASAL (I.N.) INOCULATION OF MICE WITH A SUSPENSION OF *M. pulmonis* MIXED WITH IG FRACTIONS OF CONVALESCENT MOUSE SERUM ELUTED FROM A PROTEIN A-SEPHAROSE COLUMN

pH of fraction	Specific antibody titre					No. mycoplasmas isolated from lungs after incubation of inocula with serum fractions*
	IgG1	IgG2a	IgG2b	IgM	IgA	
8.0	160	< 20	<20	< 20	<u>517</u>	2.3 ±0.79† (8/11)‡
6.0	<u>6,761</u>	32	44	< 20	78	<1.6 (0/10)
4.5	113	<u>955</u>	26	< 20	< 20	<1.6 (0/10)
3.5	132	91	<u>251</u>	< 20	23	1.7 ±0.51 (5/10)
Convalescent serum	32,359	12,589	4,898	288	16,218	1.6 (0/10)
Normal serum	< 20	< 20	<20	< 20	< 20	3.4 ±0.61 (10/10)

* After incubation of equal volumes of *M. pulmonis* at 2×10^6 CFU/ml and various serum fractions for 30 min at 37°C, groups of mice were inoculated i.n. with $3.5. \times 10^4$ CFU of *M. pulmonis*

† Mean of number of mycoplasmas isolated ($\log_{10}$ CFU/ml ± S.D.)

‡ Proportion of mice from which *M. pulmonis* was isolated

serum, or from any of the mice that had received mycoplasmas
and the IgG1 or IgG2a enriched fractions (Table 6). *M. pulmonis*
was isolated from the lungs of 5 out of 10 mice inoculated
i.n. with a mixture of mycoplasmas and the IgG2b fraction and
from 8 out of 11 mice inoculated with mycoplasmas and IgA.
However, the number of mycoplasmas isolated from the latter
two groups of animals was significantly less than that from
control animals receiving normal mouse serum ($p < 0.001$ and
< 0.05 respectively). Although the differences were not great,
the IgG2b fraction appeared to be more protective than the IgA
fraction. Further the number of mycoplasmas isolated from
mice that had been inoculated with *M. pulmonis* mixed with a 1/50
dilution of the IgG1 fraction was not significantly different
from that isolated from control animals. As this dilution of
the IgG1 fraction is equivalent to the levels of IgG1 in the
IgG2b and IgA fractions, it is unlikely that the protective
properties of these fractions was mediated by contaminating
IgG1. These studies confirm the suggestion that antibody of
any Ig class present in the lungs is capable of mediating
resistance to mycoplasma infections.

Antibodies to mycoplasmas may exert their protective
effects by a variety of mechanisms. For example, antibody of
any Ig class could reduce the attachment of mycoplasmas to
bronchial epithelial cells, a process which appears to be
important in the pathogenesis of mycoplasma infections.
Preliminary studies examining the attachment of radioisotope-
labelled *M. pneumoniae* to hamster tracheal organ cultures have
shown that attachment can be blocked by serum antibodies
(Powell, quoted by Fernald, 1979). In addition, antibodies
can inhibit mycoplasma growth, although this property has not
been demonstrated for mouse serum containing antibodies to
M. pulmonis (Cole et al., 1970). IgG antibodies could mediate
resistance by their ability to promote phagocytosis or
complement-mediated lysis of mycoplasmas. Mouse IgG1, IgG2a
and IgG2b antibodies all appear to promote the phagocytosis of
mycoplasmas by lung macrophages and to mediate killing of
mycoplasmas by complement (Table 7), (Taylor and Howard, 1980b).

All these properties of antibodies would result in the increased clearance of mycoplasmas from the respiratory tract.

TABLE 7

BIOLOGICAL PROPERTIES OF PURIFIED Ig CLASS-SPECIFIC ANTIBODIES TO
M. pulmonis

Characteristics	IgG1*	IgG2a	IgG2b	IgA
Metabolism inhibition titre	< 2	< 2	ND	ND
Complement-mediated lysis titre	40	10	2	< 2
% lung macrophages showing phagocytosis of *M. pulmonis*-coated erythrocytes	32	63	6	< 1
% protection against infection†	100	100	50	27

* Convalescent mouse serum eluted from protein A-sepharose column at pH 8.0 = IgA, pH 6.0 = IgG1, pH 4.5 = IgG2a, pH 3.5 = IgG2b

† Passive immunisation with Ig fractions as described in Table 6

CONCLUSIONS

Resistance to mycoplasma infections of the respiratory tract appears to be related to the presence of specific antibody in the lungs. Although local presentation of antigen seems to be the most efficient route for the stimulation of such antibodies, repeated parenteral administration of antigen in adjuvant may stimulate sufficiently high levels of serum antibodies that protective titres may be achieved in the lungs. Resistance can be correlated with the presence of IgG as well as IgA antibody in the lungs suggesting that the Ig class of the protective antibody is not critical.

REFERENCES

Atobe and Ogata, M., 1977. Protective effect of killed *Mycoplasma pulmonis* vaccine against experimental infection in mice. Jap. J. vet. Sci. <u>39</u>, 39.

Biberfeld, G. and Sterner, G., 1971. Antibodies in bronchial secretions following natural infection with *Mycoplasma pneumoniae*. Acta path. microbiol. Scand. Sect. B, <u>79</u>, 599.

Brunner, H., Greenberg, H.B., James, W.D., Horswood, R.L., Couch, R.B. and Chanock, R.M., 1973. Antibody to *Mycoplasma pneumoniae* in nasal secretions and sputa of experimentally infected human volunteers. Infect. Immun. <u>8</u>, 612.

Cassell, H. and Davis, J.K., 1978. Protective effect of vaccination against *Mycoplasma pulmonis* respiratory disease in rats. Infect. Immun. <u>21</u>, 69.

Cassell, G.H., Lindsey, J.R. and Baker, H.J., 1974. Immune response of pathogen-free mice inoculated intranasally with *Mycoplasma pulmonis*. J. Immunol. <u>112</u>, 124.

Cassell, G.H., Lindsey, J.R., Overcash, R.G. and Baker, H.J., 1973. Murine mycoplasma respiratory disease. Ann. N.Y. Acad. Sci. <u>225</u>, 395.

Cole, B.C., Golightly-Rowland, L., Ward, J.R. and Wiley, B.B., 1970. Immunological response of rodents to murine mycoplasmas. Infect. Immun. <u>2</u>, 419.

Fernald, G.W., 1979. Humoral and cellular immune responses to mycoplasmas. In: The Mycoplasmas, volume II, p. 399. Academic Press, New York.

Fernald, G.W. and Clyde, W.A., 1970. Protective effect of vaccines in experimental *Mycoplasma pneumoniae* disease. Infect. Immun. <u>1</u>, 559.

Fernald, G.W., Clyde, W.A. and Bienenstock, J., 1972. Immunoglobulin-containing cells in lungs of hamsters infected with *Mycoplasma pneumoniae*. J. Immunol. <u>108</u>, 1400.

Foy, H.M., Kenny, G.E., McMahan, R., Mansy, A.M. and Grayston, TJ., 1970. *Mycoplasma pneumoniae*. J. Amer. Med. Assoc. <u>214</u>, 1666.

Foy, H.M., Kenny, G.E., Sefi, R., Ochs, H.D. and Allan, I.D., 1977. Second attacks of pneumonia due to *Mycoplasma pneumoniae*. J. infect. Dis. <u>135</u>, 673.

Greenberg, H., Helms, C.M., Grizzard, M.B., James, W.D., Horswood, R.L.
    and Chanock, R.M., 1977. Immunoprophylaxis of experimental
    Mycoplasma pneumoniae disease: Effect of route of administration
    on the immunogenicity and protective effect of inactivated
    M. pneumoniae vaccine. Infect. Immun. 16, 88.

Hayatsu, E., 1978. Acquired immunity to *Mycoplasma pneumoniae* pneumonia
    in hamsters. Microbiol. Immunol. 22, 181.

Holmgren, N., 1974. On the immune response in porcine serum and
    tracheobronchial secretions following experimental infection
    with *Mycoplasma hyopneumoniae*. Zentbl. Vet. Med., Reihe B. 21, 188.

Howard, C.J., Gourlay, R.N. and Taylor, G., 1977. Induction of immunity
    in calves to *Mycoplasma bovis* infection of the respiratory tract.
    Vet. Microbiol. 2, 29.

Howard, C.J., Gourlay, R.N. and Taylor, G., 1980. Immunity to *Mycoplasma
    bovis* infections of the respiratory tract of calves. Res. vet.
    Sci. 28, 242.

Jemski, J.V., Hetsko, C.M., Helms, C.M., Grizzard, M.B., Walker, J.S. and
    Chanock, R.M., 1977. Immunoprophylaxis of *Mycoplasma pneumoniae*
    disease: effect of aerosol particle size and site of deposition
    of *M. pneumoniae* on the pattern of respiratory infection, disease,
    and immunity in hamsters. Infect. Immun. 16, 93.

Lloyd, L.C. and Trethewie, E.R., 1970. Contagious bovine pleuro-pneumonia.
    In: The role of mycoplasmas and L-forms of bacteria in disease,
    ed. J.T. Sharp, p. 172, C.C. Thomas, Springfield, Illinois.

Nasiga, W.N., Roberts, D.H., Kakoma, I. and Rurangirwa, F.R., 1975.
    Passive immunity to contagious bovine pleuropneumonia. Res. vet.
    Sci. 19, 330.

Taylor, G. and Howard, C.J., 1980$_a$. Class-specific antibody responses
    to *Mycoplasma pulmonis* in the serum and lungs of infected and
    vaccinated mice. Infect. Immun. (In press).

Taylor, G. and Howard, C.J., 1980$_b$. Ability of purified mouse
    immunoglobulins to protect against *Mycoplasma pulmonis* infection
    of mice. Manuscript in preparation.

Taylor, G., Howard, C.J. and Gourlay, R.N., 1977. Protective effect of
    vaccines on *Mycoplasma pulmonis*-induced respiratory disease of
    mice. Infect. Immun. 16, 422.

Taylor, G. and Taylor-Robinson, D., 1976. Effects of active and passive
    immunization on *Mycoplasma pulmonis*-induced pneumonia in mice.
    Immunol. <u>30</u>, 611.

Whittlestone, P., 1976. Immunity to mycoplasmas causing respiratory
    diseases in man and animals. Adv. vet. Sci. comp. Med. <u>20</u>, 277

DISCUSSION

F.J. Bourne   *(UK)*

How did you infect your mice intranasally?

G. Taylor   *(UK)*

We anaesthetise them with sodium pentobarbitone; when
they are deeply anaesthetised we inoculate 50 μl intranasally.
You can actually sense that most of it goes down to the lungs
because the mice have difficulty in breathing. I am sure a
lot goes elsewhere but certainly a lot of it gets to the lungs.
It was intratracheal.

K. Petzoldt   *(FRG)*

Did you use anaesthetic with the calves?

G. Taylor

No, we put it straight into the trachea.

J. Soothill   *(UK)*

In other contexts I have heard you discussing the damaging
effect of immunisation with a certain respiratory virus, namely
Channock's work with RSV. Are there any other examples of
disease due to a respiratory virus being made worse by immunisation?

G. Taylor

Not that I am aware of, unless you count measles virus
which is not particularly a respiratory virus. Some of the
early work with inactivated measles vaccines did induce a more
severe measles infection, including pneumonia, in humans.

J. Soothill

What I am saying is that we must remind our colleagues
that in one species immunisation is known to do harm in the
field of respiratory viruses if it is done clumsily.

G. Taylor

Yes. With mycoplasma pneumoniae, there has been one report of an inactivated vaccine administered to some prison volunteers. Two of these volunteers did get a more severe disease than the rest. However, this has never been repeated and there have been quite a number of vaccine trials with inactivated mycoplasma pneumoniae vaccines with no adverse effects.

B. Morein   (Sweden)

In bacterial diseases, it has been reported with *Pasturella haemolytica*, that there has been worse disease after vaccination, in calves. In Canada it was reported that there were more losses countrywide in animals vaccinated against virus diarrhoea than in non-vaccinated animals.

J. Soothill

But were they immunising only the animals which were at greater risk?

B. Morein

As I understand it, a survey was made of all the animals vaccinated with virus diarrhoea in the whole of Canada. All of these had a lower production rate and a higher morbidity rate, etc. This was in relation to attenuated strains.

F.J. Bourne

What would you think was the mechanism operating here?

J. Soothill

In the field of Channock's work on human RSV infection, it is suspected that one is disturbing the balance of IgG response, cell mediated response and local immunity response. If the immunisation produces a potentially damaging sensitisation, you get greater disease. That was also the thought in the field of using inactivated measles virus.

G. Taylor

I think the measles group of viruses are different from all other viruses. The problem is that they have a fusion antigen; if you do not make antibodies to the fusion antigen then you don't protect and, in fact, you may get an imbalance, not perhaps to the type of immune response but the antibodies directed to different antigens. That may be the problem.

J. Soothill

Do you not have such viruses in non-human animals?

G. Taylor

Well, there is PI-3 in mice.

A. Ferguson   (UK)

Just to supplement Professor Soothill's point, there is no doubt at all that immune responses which may be involved in protection may substantially contribute to pneumonia and tissue damage. We see that in the iactrogenic immune deficiencies that we produce clinically.

I would like to ask a question about the induction of immunity to mycoplasma in a natural infection. It is an intra-lumenal parasite or organism. Is the induction phase thought to be a macrophage getting into the alveolus or the trachea, phagocytosing mycoplasma and then coming back in again, or do you actually see mycoplasma penetrating the mucosa over the lymphoid nodules?

G. Taylor

Workers in America have done some studies looking at the distribution of *Mycoplasma pulmonis* in mice at intervals, after inoculation, by fluorescence. Immediately after inoculation the mycoplasmas are distributed throughout the respiratory tract, so there are some attached to the bronchial epithelial walls and some attached to the alveolar walls. They persist there until

the development of antibody; as antibody develops, the mycoplasmas are cleared from the lung parenchyma and you can see
them inside macrophages in the alveolar spaces. They have become localised on the surface of the bronchial epithelium and
they persist there.

A. Ferguson

But how is the antigen presented to the immune system?

G. Taylor

I think it is phagocytosed from the alveolar side.

H. Miller   (UK)

I believe that mycoplasma is extremely mitogenic for T
lymphocytes in mice but we have looked at this in sheep and we
have not been able to demonstrate any mitogenesis of mycoplasma
on sheep lymphocytes. This was *Mycoplasma ovis*.

G. Taylor

Mycoplasmas do vary; *Mycoplasma pulmonis* is interesting
because it is mitogenic and they may have contributed to the
protection that we got. But there are a number of other mycoplasmas which are not mitogenic.

F.J. Bourne

Did you not show at one time that pathogenic mycoplasma
in thymectomised mice led to no lesion at all?

G. Taylor

Yes, that's right; we thymectomised some mice and although
the numbers of organisms in the lungs was greater and the mycoplasmas spread from the lungs to non respiratory sites, there
were no lung lesions at all.

K.L. Morgan (UK)

Does the interaction between the epithelium and the mycoplasma take place with the dead organism as well?

G. Taylor

     I don't think so. You can do various treatments to see what inhibits the attachment; I think heating the mycoplasmas is one of the things that stops attachment.

K. Dalsgaard   (Denmark)

     Was there any reason, other than tradition, to choose formaldehyde for the inactivation?

G. Taylor

     No, it was just the first thing that we tried and it worked.

K. Dalsgaard

     I would have thought that in a rather complex protein structure such as the mycoplasma, formaldehyde might be rather harmful.

G. Taylor

     Yes, in retrospect I think it might have been better to use something else.

K. Dalsgaard

     It could be dissolved in some organic medium or detergent and then reconstituted without nucleic acid, perhaps.

G. Taylor

     Yes, these were whole washed organisms that we used.

F.J. Bourne   (UK)

     We heard this morning from John Bienenstock of success using inactivated vaccines with PI-3 and with mycoplasma. In general, would this tie up with clinical success rates in humans?

354

J. Bienenstock   *(Canada)*

No - if you consider measles, it is still true that regardless of whether it is respiratory or elsewhere, the question of whether it is live is rather important. Dr. Taylor showed quite clearly that there was a fairly short memory, at least with the killed intratracheal immunisations in mice. Obviously, that would have very significant implications as far as immunisation is concerned. I don't think you showed memory in the calf.

G. Taylor

No, in fact, the calves have only been challenged one week after vaccination. We may only need one or two other injections to keep them immune because the time period for which we are trying to protect calves against respiratory diseases is relatively short. So that may not be such a problem if we can boost them regularly.

J. Bienenstock

I was a bit surprised; I am familiar with the disparities between the various species in mycoplasma - we studied mycoplasma in the hamster some time ago. There, at least, IgM is a very significant component and certainly, in man, the major antibody appears to be IgM although there is some controversy in the literature. You are showing almost no IgM whatsoever. Is that surprising?

G. Taylor

That was true in these mice; if you look at mice that had been infected then there is quite a persistent IgM response following an infection. But in mice inoculated with inactivated organisms there is not very much IgM response. Also, the G1 and G2 ratios are different between mice vaccinated by inactivated organisms and those infected with live organisms. There is more G1 in the mice vaccinated with inactivated organisms where the predominant immunoglobulin is G2.

J. Bienenstock

So the response to the immunisation protocol is different from the normal natural series of events?

G. Taylor

Yes.

J. Bienenstock

What about the numbers of T cells? Certainly, in the hamster, the numbers of non-immunoglobulin containing cells in the infiltrates are almost hundreds to one greater than the numbers of antibody producing cells. We always assumed they were T cells although it was never proven.

G. Taylor

Most of the cells seemed to be accounted for in the classes IgG1, IgG2 or IgA. As you know, there is a rapid accumulation of cells in the lungs of hamsters after challenge which are mainly immunoglobulin negative. When we challenged these mice we looked 24 hours, 3 days and 1 week after challenge to see if we could see a similar accelerated response. There was a very slight one but nothing like as great as that in hamsters.

F.J. Bourne

How far away are you from conducting field trials with these vaccines in the calf.

G. Taylor

We have been instructed to go straight into attempting to get a combined vaccine. Just recently we have combined two mycoplasmas and two viruses, RSV and PI-3, and *Mycoplasma dispar* and *Mycoplasma bovis*, and mixed them together and put them into just a small trial, just to see if they interfere with the antibody response. They don't so we are going to try to get a test certificate.

F.J. Bourne

    Will this be a double subcutaneous?

G. Taylor

    In fact, we are going to give three subcutaneous inoculations with adjuvant because it is much easier to do that in the field than to do intratracheal.

H. Williams Smith   *(UK)*

    What is the importance in this country of mycoplasma infection in calves?

G. Taylor

    All calves have mycoplasmas in the respiratory tract - *Mycoplasma dispar* or the ureaplasmas. Recently *Mycoplasma bovis* has been introduced into this country and when that occurs it seems to be of major importance in those outbreaks. The role of *dispar* and the ureaplasmas is less clear and probably interact with the viruses in a combined, mixed infection.

H. Williams Smith

    Would a vaccine be practical in this country?

G. Taylor

    It would be for *Mycoplasma dispar* and *Mycoplasma bovis* but the ureaplasmas are a little different because there are several serotypes of ureaplasmas and work has not yet started on what cross-protection there is between the different serotypes. There is not one serotype which is particularly associated with disease.

H. Williams Smith

    These are pure infections we are talking about, are they?

G. Taylor

    No, they are mixed infections.

H. Williams Smith

And this is where all the problems start, I presume?

G. Taylor

Yes. One of the approaches we had was that perhaps
respiratory disease was initiated by the virus and that the
mycoplasmas and the bacteria appeared as secondaries causing
the disease. We thought that if we could break the chain by
vaccinating against the viruses we may be able to protect
against pneumonia. But as we have got some mycoplasma vaccines
as well, that work, we thought we would put those in as well.

H. Williams Smith

If you just had the mycoplasma vaccines, would the other
things go away?

G. Taylor

We don't know. That would be something to try.

F.J. Bourne

There is fairly convincing evidence, is there not, from
Compton, that PI-3 plays no part in the epidemiology of calf
pneumonia.

G. Taylor

Well, we had an inactivated PI-3 vaccine that experimentally provided complete protection against PI-3 challenge. It
was tried on a local farm and although PI-3 went to that farm -
it was isolated from the farm during the period of observation.
Although the infection rate in the vaccinated calves was less
than that in the non-vaccinated calves there was no significant
difference in the incidence of disease between the vaccinated
and non-vaccinated calves. From that we deduced that in that
year, at that time, at that farm, PI-3 did not contribute to
that outbreak. But that is not to say that in other areas, at

other times, PI-3 may not contribute. At Compton we feel at the moment that RSV is probably more important.

J. Soothill

Earlier on, Dr. Asso ascribed much of the respiratory virus trouble to crowding of calves together. Is there any evidence from non-human animals that separation from the mother contributes to respiratory infection, particularly virus infection, as opposed to the gastro-intestinal infection we were talking about before? Have you accumulated evidence that mothers feeding the child provide protection against respiratory virus and mycoplasma infections?

G. Taylor

I don't know of any evidence; somebody else may be able to answer that better. All I can say is that you do see outbreaks in calves that have maternal antibodies and you quite often see that especially when RSV is associated with those outbreaks. I believe there is some evidence that the incidence is less in calves that have received colostrum.

F.J. Bourne

Yes, there is evidence that calves with high colostrum antibody levels do suffer less from respiratory disease. It is also true to say that if you don't house calves you get less respiratory disease.

J. Soothill

But how about continued suckling?

F.J. Bourne

Well, if you continually suckle you don't usually house the animals. There are some suckler systems where calves are housed during the period in which they are suckled. Personally I don't know of any outbreak of disease in such a unit because there are not many units in this area. What is the situation

in Ireland? Perhaps Professor Hannon might be able to throw
some light on this.

J. Hannon   (Ireland)

I can't comment on that; I don't think the numbers are
large enough to make a valid observation.

H. Williams Smith

Surely single suckler systems are usually out of doors?

F.J. Bourne

Systems have been developed now where they are housed in
kennel systems, so they are part in, part out.

H. Williams Smith

I think the point Professor Soothill was making was that
when calves are crowded together they have come from many
different farms. I think crowding is a major factor.

F.J. Bourne

Yes, in epidemiological terms there is no question about
it, the intermixing of calves is a very serious component in
the development of disease.

K. Petzoldt

I would like to ask another question for general discussion. Professor Bohl talked about the so-called mammary gut link.
I wonder if there is also a mammary lung link.

E. Bohl   (USA)

This is very interesting. I have been trying to find
out if anybody has any evidence that IgA antibodies that would
come from milk would protect against respiratory tract infections. It looks as though passive immunity against respiratory
infections may be associated with IgG class of antibodies,
mainly because there is considerable diffusion of serum IgG

antibodies in the lower respiratory tract which would provide passive immunity. We tried this one experiment which I mentioned where we infected pregnant swine with pseudorabies virus to see if we could detect any IgA type of link between the respiratory tract and the mammary gland and we could not do that.

K. Petzoldt

The reason I asked the question was that in 1975 I believe Tomassi reported that cell traffic between gut and lung tissue is comparable to that between gut and mammary gland.

J. Bienenstock

Well, actually that is my work! There is some evidence. I would accept Professor Bohl's comments insofar as pseudorabies is concerned. However, I do not accept them as a generalisation because he only has information on one specific thing. Paul Montgomery has evidence in the rabbit, if he takes DNP linked pneumococcal cell walls and puts those into the lung of a rabbit, he can obtain IgA specific anti DNP pneumococci in the mammary gland, in the lactating rabbit at a time at which he is unable to see or detect those antibodies in the serum by an extremely sensitive ELISA and/or radio immunoassay technique. That is the work; that is the evidence. In addition there is other evidence. Lars Hanson has some evidence for a urinary tract potential mammary link. There is also the evidence which we have reported that there are cells within the bronchial lymph nodes which will traffic in relatively small numbers; they do traffic to the breast and other mucosal sites. The question is whether there is any significance to all this. I believe it is significant but only as a priming event. Cells originating in the lung are disseminated to other sites and unless the antigen is met again, at other sites, it is of no use since the numbers of cells are insufficient. However, on secondary immunisation there is an amplification system which could seed the rest of the body. So, my feeling is that there is a common mucosal system for Iga. It is primarily related to gut and the other mucosal sites. At least for the lung there is a

mechanism for seeding these other sites. It is of major significance only as a priming event.

E. Bohl

Do you think the migration is IgA type cells or IgG?

J. Bienenstock

In the mouse, there is a population of IgG cells in the
mesenteric node that has a tendency to go back to the gut, and
in the reverse sense there is also a tendency for a population
from the lung to go back to lung. We do not know if these
cells are in the mucosa or in the peripheral lung parenchyma.

G. Mayrhofer (UK)

I think the argument that John Bienenstock is putting
forward relates to the migration of cells which, in most studies,
have been at a stage of differentiation with large dividing
plasma viruses. The migration of those cells is probably an
end stage in differentiation. It is dangerous to think of them
conveying memory. The memory probably resides in small lymphocytes which may have completely different migratory properties.

J. Hall (UK)

I would just like to make the point that in the rat, at
any rate, (and this is probably something which may not happen
in ordinary infections because there are more peripheral
defences) if you instil a bacterial suspension through the
diaphragm so that it is picked up by the lymphatics and conveyed to the mediastinal lymph nodes, you get a systemic IgA
response which is quite as big as anything you can get by
stimulating the gut. This does make the point that in the rat,
at any rate, the lymph nodes are capable of generating a very
vigorous IgA response.

F.J. Bourne

Yes, but this may be a feature of the rat where IgA predominates in the gut. It may be different for other species.

J. Hall

Sure, but call it secretory immunoglobulin for want of a better term; it would probably embrace IgG1 in cattle.

F.J. Bourne

We must close this session now and thank all the speakers.

THE MAMMARY GLAND IMMUNE RESPONSE AND ITS RELATIONSHIP TO INTESTINAL ANTIGENIC EXPOSURE

Barbro Carlsson, José R. Cruz*, Lotta Mellander
and Lars Å. Hanson

Department of Clinical Immunology and Department of
Pediatrics, University of Goteborg, Goteborg, Sweden.
*Institute of Nutrition of Central America and
Panama (INCAP), Guatemala City, Guatemala.

ABSTRACT

Human milk contains antibodies of the secretory IgA (SIgA) type
directed against a variety of enterobacteria, viruses and food proteins.
The appearance of these milk antibodies with specificity against antigens
of intestinal origin is difficult to explain, unless there is a close link
between the immune response in the mammary gland and intestinal exposure.
There is some evidence which suggests that antigens in the intestine may
stimulate lymphoid cells from the Peyer's patches which are committed to
IgA synthesis to home to various exocrine glands, including the mammary
gland. As a consequence of the enteromammaric link, the breast-fed baby is
supplied with SIgA milk antibodies against micro-organisms which are common
in the environment. These antibodies have the capacity to prevent bacterial
attachment to mucous membranes which is the initial step in most infections.
Determination of milk antibodies also provides epidemiological information
concerning intestinal pathogens and can be used to reflect mucosal immunity
in response to various vaccinations.

INTRODUCTION

Human milk is rich in factors with anti-infectious properties. There are specific ones like B-lymphocytes, mainly producing secretory IgA (SIgA) antibodies, T-lymphocytes and phagocytes including macrophages (Smith and Goldman, 1968; Diaz-Jouanen and Williams, 1974; Hanson and Brandtzaeg, 1980). Unspecific components like iron-binding lactoferrin, lysozyme, complement factors, bifidus factor and B-12 binding protein work in co-operation with the specific immune factors to protect the mucosa (Hanson and Winberg, 1972; Goldman and Smith, 1973; Hanson et al., 1978).

As long ago as in 1892, Ehrlich (1892) demonstrated that mice suckling from immunised mothers were resistant to challenge with toxic substances by antibodies in the milk. The antibody activity in milk has later been shown mainly to belong to the SIgA type which also dominates other secretions bathing various mucosal surfaces. Obviously, this composite molecule is well-fitted to function in variable milieux since it is more resistant to extreme pH changes and proteolytic enzymes than serum antibodies, including IgA (Tomasi and Bienenstock, 1968). These antibodies seem to pass through the gastro-intestinal tract of the breast-fed baby with retained antibody activity (Gindrat et al., 1972; Haneberg, 1974).

THE LOCAL ANTIBODY RESPONSE IN THE MAMMARY GLAND

There are indications that the mammary gland is the site of a local immune response. The fact that the dominating immunoglobulin is SIgA indicates that the mammary gland belongs to a unique SIgA system common to other mucous membranes and important for local immune defence. SIgA antibodies are produced by specialised plasma cells found in close connection with submucosal glands, like in the respiratory or gastro-intestinal tract. Similar cells can also be found in the mammary, lacrimal and salivary glands. The dimeric IgA with its J-chain, is produced by the plasma cells and the secretory component SC

coming from the epithelial cells is added to the dimer during
the passage through these cells to the glandular secretion
(Brandtzaeg, 1976). The consistent finding of a higher ratio for
IgA antibodies to different *E.coli* antibodies in milk versus serum
with a mean of 10.5 and a much lower ratio for IgG (mean 0.3)
and IgM (mean 0.9) speaks for a local response (Mellander et al.,
1980).

IMMUNE RESPONSE IN THE MAMMARY GLAND FOLLOWING INTESTINAL
EXPOSURE

Experimental studies in rabbits (Montgomery et al., 1974)
and swine (Bohl and Saif, 1975) have suggested that intestinal
exposure may be the initiator of milk antibodies. Intestinal
colonisation of women in late pregnancy with a non-pathogenic
E.coli strain was also followed within a few days by the
appearance in milk of leucocytes forming plaques against the
colonising strain (Goldblum et al., 1975). A probable explanation
for this link between the intestine and the mammary gland involves
a selective transport of committed precursors of IgA producing
cells which home to the mammary gland via the lymph and the
blood from a central site of antigenic stimulation, e.g. the
Peyer's patches. This concept was first indicated by Craig and
Cebra (1971) which showed that lymphocytes from the Peyer's
patches could repopulate the intestinal mucosa of irradiated
animals with IgA producing cells normally dominating these
tissues. It was also shown in rabbits that when a single Peyer's
patch was stimulated with bacterial antigen, IgA antibodies were
produced in other parts of the intestine (Robertson and Cebra,
1975). Precursors to IgA producing cells leave the Peyer's
patches after antigenic exposure and home specifically to the
intestinal mucosa via the mesenteric lymph glands, ductus
thoracicus and the blood (Pierce and Gowans, 1975).

During pregnancy and beginning of lactation an increase in
the number of plasma cells intra-epithelially was demonstrated
(Weisz-Carrington et al., 1977). The development of the
glandular epithelium also paralleled the proliferation of IgA

producing cells found in close connection to the mammary gland
cells. After weaning or interruption of suckling for more than
ten days, a drastic decrease in epithelial cells and also IgA
producing cells was noted. There are also indications that the
homing is dependent on the hormonal situation, since it was
possible to direct IgA producing cells to the mammary gland in
virgin animals by giving them progesterone, oestrogen and
prolactin (Weisz-Carrington et al., 1978).

ANTIBODIES TO MICROBIAL ANTIGENS

As a consequence of the homing mechanism, it is obvious
that exposure of the intestinal mucosa will result in a transfer
of secretory IgA response also to distant glands like the
mammary gland. Early colostrum contains as much as 20 g/l of
SIgA and the levels decrease to about 0.25 - 0.50 g/l in the
mature milk. This rapid fall is compensated by a simultaneous
increase of the milk volume, so that the child's daily intake is
fairly constant through the lactation period (Mellander et al.,
1980). This substantial amount of antibodies is provided by
privileged as well as underprivileged mothers. Comparison
between milk samples from different groups of mothers in Ethiopia,
Guatemala and Sweden showed very similar levels of milk antibodies (Cruz et al., 1980). Severely undernourished mothers
under heavy stress may, however, produce extremely small milk
volumes which means that the total output of SIgA/day becomes
limited although the concentration is the same as in milk of
privileged mothers (Carlsson et al., 1976).

The milk SIgA antibodies are directed against a variety
of *Enterobacteria*, for instance against a number of O and K
antigens of *E.coli*. Such antigens are important virulence
factors of *E.coli*, where especially the K1 antigen is found on
80% of the strains causing neonatal sepsis meningitis (Robbins
et al., 1974). This disease seems to be more common in infants
who have obtained significantly less breast milk than matched
controls (Winberg and Wessner, 1971). Pakistani mothers who are
exposed to 'enteropathogenic' *E.coli*, EPEC, also have higher milk

antibody levels to O antigens from these strains than unexposed
Swedish mothers (Ahlstedt et al., 1977). This might explain
why diarrhoea caused by EPEC is relatively seldom registered in
breast-fed babies in developing countries despite a frequent
exposure (Mata and Urrutia, 1971).

Milk antibodies have also been demonstrated against O
antigens from various *Salmonella* and *Shigella* strains as well as
against enterotoxins from *V.cholerae* and *E.coli* (Holmgren et al.,
1976; Cruz et al., 1980). These antibodies may help to protect
the breast-fed baby since it has been shown that diarrhoeal
disease increases in frequency after weaning in developing
countries (Mata and Urrutia, 1971).

The milk also contains antibodies against viruses such
as rota-virus and polio-virus (Simhon and Mata, 1977; Yolken
et al., 1978). Furthermore, antibodies against parasites like
Entamoeba histolytica and *Giardia lamblia* (Hult et al., personal
communication) have been demonstrated in milk.

SIgA antibodies in milk against various microbial antigens
are probably present because they represent a repeated exposure
of the intestinal mucosa which should result in a continuous
production of antibodies. Otherwise, it would be difficult to
understand how the SIgA response, which is reported to be short-
lived, can be present against such an array of antigens.

ANTIBODIES TO FOOD PROTEINS

As a result of the gut-mammary link, dietary antigens
could also be expected to give rise to a milk antibody response.
We have been able to demonstrate antibodies against various
food proteins like cows' milk proteins, soy protein and protein
from black beans. Significantly lower levels of SIgA milk antibodies to cows' milk proteins were found in groups of mothers
from Guatemala, where cows' milk is not included in the diet,
than in urban elite mothers with a regular cows' milk intake
(Carlsson et al., 1979). Further studies are needed to define

whether these antibodies play an antiallergic role. It has
been suggested that elimination of potential allergens lowers
the frequency of allergic reaction (Matthew et al., 1977). Breast
feeding the baby means that possible allergens are eliminated
and the antibodies in milk might help to protect against allergens
when they are introduced to the child (Hanson et al., 1977).

VACCINATION CAN IMPROVE THE MILK CONTENT OF SIgA ANTIBODIES

The possibility to improve mucosal defence by stimulation
of secretory IgA antibodies has been extensively studied.
Secretory IgA antibodies against *V.cholerae* and its enterotoxin
have clearly been shown to provide protection in mice (Lange
and Holmgren, 1978). Parenteral cholera vaccination induced a
significant titre increase of milk and saliva antibodies as well
as serum antibodies in earlier non-vaccinated women living in
endemic areas. Swedish women showed no similar increase in
their milk antibody levels after parenteral vaccination and
boosting. This indicates that an existing local response can
be boosted by a parenteral vaccination, but a primary SIgA
reponse cannot be induced (Svennerholm et al., 1980). The same
increase in milk SIgA levels was seen after parenteral polio-
vaccination of women in Pakistan. Surprisingly the milk
antibodies decreased if a booster was given perorally with live
poliovaccine (Svennerholm et al., 1980). This decrease was
especially evident if a cholera vaccination was performed
simultaneously. The interpretation of this is not evident, but
it might be related to immunological unresponsiveness which has
been shown to occur in animals after peroral antigen exposure.
T suppressor lymphocytes specific for IgA antibody formation
might be the mediators (Richman et al., 1978). Another
explanation could be that a consumption of virus antibodies at
a local level can take place.

Further experimental as well as clinical studies of doses,
timing and types of vaccine are evidently needed to confirm
these observations. Anyhow, these studies indicate that it is
possible to modulate the local antibody response in the

mammary gland. This means that vaccination of lactating women does not only protect the mother, but via her milk SIgA antibodies, the baby will also be provided with mucosal immunity. Such milk antibodies could presumably provide the infant with protection against infections and might be especially important in many developing countries where the risk of infection is high. It also seems possible to use milk SIgA for studying epidemiology of intestinal pathogens.

ACKNOWLEDGMENT

These studies were supported by grants from the Swedish Medical Research Council (Nos 215 and 3382), SAREC and the Ellen, Walter and Lennart Hesselman Foundation for Scientific Research.

L. Hanson was an International Fogarty Scholar-in-Residence at the Fogarty International Centre, National Institutes of Health from August 1979 through September 1980.

REFERENCES

Ahlstedt, S., Carlsson, B., Fällström, S.P., Holmgren, J., Lidin-Janson, G.,
    Lindblad, B.S., Jodal, U., Kaijser, B., Sohl Akerlund, Å. and
    Wadsworth, C., 1977. Serum and secretory IgA antibodies induced by
    enterobacteria and food proteins. In: Ciba Foundation Symposium,
    46: Immunology and the gut, Excerpta Medica, Elsevier, Amsterdam,
    p. 115.

Bohl, E.H. and Saif, L.J., 1975. Passive immunity in transmissible gastro-
    enteritis of swine: Immunoglobulin characteristics of antibodies in
    milk after inoculating virus by different routes. Infect. Immun.,
    11: 23.

Brandtzaeg, P., 1976. Complex formation between secretory component and
    human immunoglobulins related to their content of J-chain. Scand.
    J. Immunol., 5: 411.

Carlsson, B., Ahlstedt, S., Hanson, L.Å., Lidin-Janson, G., Lindblad, B.S.
    and Sultana, R., 1976. *Escherichia coli* O antibody content in milk
    from a very low socio-economic group of a developing country. Acta
    Paediatr. Scand., 65: 417.

Carlsson, B., Cruz, J.R., Garcia, B., Hanson, L.Å. and Urrutia, J.J., 1979.
    Immune factors in human milk. In: Nutrition and metabolism of the
    fetus and infant. H.K.A. Visser (Ed.), Nijhoff Publ. Hague, p. 263.

Craig, S.W. and Cebra, J.J., 1971. Peyer's patches: an enriched source of
    precursors for IgA-producing immunocytes in the rabbit. J. Exp. Med.,
    134: 188.

Cruz, J.R., Carlsson, B., Garcia, B., Holme, D.T., Svennerholm, A.-M.,
    Urrutia, J.J. and Hanson, L.Å., 1980. Studies of human milk. IV.
    Antibodies to *Escherichia coli* enterotoxin and to *Salmonella* and
    Shigella somatic antigens. Submitted to Infect. Immun.

Diaz-Jouanen, E. and Williams, Jr. R.C., 1974. T and B lymphocytes in the
    rabbit. Clin. Immunol. Immunopath., 3: 248.

Ehrlich, P ., 1892. Über immunität durch vererbung und saugung. Zeitsch.
    für Hygiene und Infektions-Krankheiten, 12: 183.

Gindrat, J.-J., Gothefors, L., Hanson, L.Å. and Winberg, J., 1972.
    Antibodies in human milk against *E.coli* of the serogroups most
    commonly found in neonatal infections. Acta Paediatr. Scand., 61: 587.

Goldblum, R.M., Ahlstedt, S., Carlsson, B., Hanson, L.Å., Jodal, U.,
    Lidin-Janson, G. and Sohl Åkerlund, Å., 1975. Antibody-forming cells
    in human colostrum after oral immunization. Nature, 257: 797.

Goldman, A.S. and Smith, C.W., 1973. Host resistance factors in human milk.
    J. Pediatr., 82: 1082.

Haneberg, B., 1974. Immunoglobulins in feces from infants fed human or bovine
    milk. Scand. J. Immunol., 3: 191.

Hanson, L.Å., Ahlstedt, S., Carlsson, B. and Fällström, S.P., 1977.
    Secretory IgA antibodies to cow's milk and their possible effect in
    mixed feeding. Int. Arch. Allergy Appl. Immunol., 54: 457.

Hanson, L.Å., Ahlstedt, S., Carlsson, B., Fällström, S.P., Kaijser, B.,
    Lindblad, B.S., Sohl Åkerlund, A. and Svanborg Edén, C., 1978. New
    knowledge in human milk immunology. Acta Paediatr. Scand., 67: 577.

Hanson, L.Å. and Brandtzaeg, P., 1980. Mucosal defence systems. In:
    E.R. Stiehm and V.A. Fulginiti (Eds.), Immunologic disorders in
    infants and children. W.B. Saunders, Philadelphia, 2nd ed., p. 137.

Hanson, L.Å. and Winberg, J., 1972. Breast milk and defence against
    infection in the newborn. Arch. Dis. Childh., 47: 845.

Holmgren, J., Hanson, L.Å., Carlsson, B., Lindblad, B.S. and Rahimtoola, J.,
    1976. Neutralizing antibodies against *E.coli* and *V.cholerae*
    enterotoxins in human milk from a developing country. Scand. J.
    Immunol., 5: 867.

Lange, S. and Holmgren, J., 1978. Protective antitoxic cholera immunity in
    mice: Influence of route and number of immunizations and mode of
    action of protective antibodies. Acta Path. Microbiol. Scand. Sect. C.,
    86: 145.

Mata, L.J. and Urrutia, J.J., 1971. The uniqueness of human milk, Host
    resistance to infection. Am. J. Clin. Nutr., 24: 976.

Matthew, D.J., Norman, A.P., Taylor, B., Turner, M.W. and Soothill, J.F.,
    1977. Prevention of eczema. Lancet, 1: 321.

Mellander, L., Carlsson, B., Dahlgren, U. and Hanson, L.Å., 1980. Humoral
    and cellular immunities transmitted by breastmilk. Colloquia at
    The Medical Society of London, Sept. 1979, (in press).

Montgomery, P.C., Rosner, B.R. and Cohn, J., 1974. The secretory antibody
    response. Anti-DNP antibodies induced by dinitrophenylated type III
    pneumococcus. Immun. Commun., 3: 143.

Pierce, N.F. and Gowans, J.L., 1975. Cellular kinetics of the intestinal immune response to cholera toxoid in rats. J. Exp. Med., 142: 1550.

Richman, L.K., Chiller, J.M., Brown, W.R., Hanson, D.G. and Nelson, M.V., 1978. Enterically induced immunologic tolerance. I. Induction of suppressor T lymphocytes by intragastric administration of soluble proteins. J. Immunol., 121: 2429.

Robertson, S.M. and Cebra, J.J., 1975. A model for local immunity. Ric. Clin. Lab., 6: (Suppl. 3) 105.

Robbins, J.B., McCracken, G.H., Gotschlich, E.C., Ørskov, F., Ørskov, I. and Hanson, L.Å., 1974. *Escherichia coli* K1 capsular polysaccharide associated with neonatal meningitis. N. Engl. J. Med., 290: 1216.

Simhon, A. and Mata, L.J., 1978. Anti-rotavirus antibody in human colostrum. Lancet, 1: 39.

Smith, C.W. and Goldman, A.S., 1968. The cells of human colostrum. I. *In vitro* studies of morphology and functions. Pediatr. Res., 2: 103.

Svennerholm, A.-M., Hanson, L.Å., Holmgren, J., Lindblad, B.S., Khan, Shaukat, R., Nilsson, A., Quereshi, F. and Svennerholm, B., 1980. Parenteral cholera vaccination may increase and oral polio vaccination decrease mucosal immunity. Differences in secretory IgA antibody response in enterally exposed and unexposed individuals. Infect. Immun., (in press).

Tomasi, T.B. and Bienenstock, J., 1968. Secretory immunoglobulins. Adv. Immunol., 9: 29.

Weisz-Carrington, P., Roux, M.E. and Lamm, M.E., 1977. Plasma cells and epithelial immunoglobulins in the mouse gland during pregnancy and lactation. J. Immunol., 119: 1306.

Weisz-Carrington, P., Roux, M.E., McWilliams, M., Phillips-Quagliata, J.M. and Lamm, M.E., 1978. Hormonal induction of the secretory immune system in the mammary gland. Proc. Natl. Acas. Sci. USA., 75: 2928.

Winberg, J. and Wessner, G., 1971. Does breast milk protect against septicemia in the newborn? Lancet, 1: 1091.

DISCUSSION

H. Miller   *(UK)*

Is it possible that the breast is acting in the same
manner as the liver, in rats for example, just simply collecting
IgA that is secreted from the gut? Secondly, do you think that
prolactin has any effect on your immunisation schedules on
lactating mothers?

B. Carlsson   *(Sweden)*

In answer to the first question, I think it is possible
that the same mechanism applies to the breast as to the liver.
We have no proof of it but it might be so. With regard to the
second question, I cannot say at the moment. We suspected this
so we want to repeat the immunisations at different stages,
before and after lactation.

F.J. Bourne   *(UK)*

Dr. Miller, did you ask your first question because you
thought it possible that the IgA in secretions is, in fact,
derived from serum?

H. Miller

Yes, I am asking that question. Just because you have
low levels in serum it does not mean to say that it is not
cleared from the mammary gland or the liver in the same manner.

J. Bienenstock   *(Canada)*

This is right because there is evidence in the mouse
which has been published to indicate that polymeric IgA does
have a selective transport advantage into mouse milk. Whether
that applies to some of the animals we have talked about, or
to the human, is another question. But there seems to be fairly
good evidence in the mouse.

T.J. Newby   (UK)

Ninety percent of the IgA in pig milk derives from the mammary gland.

F.J. Bourne

Taking the argument a stage further, namely that the breast might remove IgA immune complexes from serum, is there any possibility that these might be transferred to the offspring and thereby have an immunogenic effect on the offspring?

J. Bienenstock

There is evidence for that too. I alluded to that yesterday. There are a whole series of papers in fact which suggest that, in fact, you can tolerise the offspring by passively giving immune complexes which are selectively secreted into the milk. Incidentally, nobody has looked to see whether those are IgA immune complexes. In such animals the tolerance occurs before closure but, seemingly, not after closure. There is an accelerated antigen transport and also tolerisation of the offspring seems fairly clear cut, in the rodent systems at any rate.

J. Soothill   (UK)

On that point, administration of antigen with IgA increases the antibody response to the antigen and does not reduce it - this is shown in the data from two people at least, Chris Stokes and a group from America. This is in adult mice. Is there any evidence that it is different in young ones?

P. Brandtzaeg   (Norway)

Coming back to humans and the transfer of serum derived immunoglobulins to glandular sites, there is evidence in man, in patients with myeloma, IgA where you have dimers, and also in Waldenstroms macroglobulinaemia where you have pentameric IgM in high concentrations, these two immunoglobulins will be selectively transferred into the salivary glands, compared with

IgG. In patients with IgG myeloma there will normally be a leakage to the saliva. This probably also applies to human mammary glands but it must not be forgotten that in humans there is very little spill-over of dimeric IgA from the gut into the thoracic duct lymph and into blood. This is in contrast to what is seen in dogs, rats and mice. So I don't think that in the normal situation there is much transfer of IgA from serum into normal human milk.

H. Williams Smith   (UK)

I would like to ask a question about the antibodies Dr. Carlsson found in human milk. I can certainly see the point of having antibodies to entero-pathogens because I can see that they can cope with entero-pathogens in the alimentary tract. However, I cannot see the point of having K-1 antibodies there, which are presumably agglutinating antibodies, because the K-1 strains are invasive. I don't see that they could have any protective effect and I would imagine that K-1 antibodies are there 'just for the ride' - that they happen to be made in human beings and get into the milk. But I can't see how they can function against an invasive type of infection.

B. Carlsson

They could probably function by agglutinating bacteria and hindering them from invading. Actually, they are anti-bodies to K antigens of polysaccharide type. It does not hinder the child from being colonised by those strains but we think they hinder invasion.

J.P. Vaerman   (Belgium)

This may be a trivial question but how do low buffer capacity, high lactose, low protein and low phosphate, con-tribute to non-specific immunity?

B. Carlsson

Maybe they select for other strains of bacteria which are not so prone to be pathogenic.

H. Bazin   *(Belgium)*

Another trivial question: what is the bifidus factor?

B. Carlsson

I don't want to comment on that; I didn't mention it, it was just on the slide.

J. Clamp   *(UK)*

It is an oligosaccharide containing glucosamine, present in human milk. It is synthesised in the breast.

E. Bohl   *(USA)*

It contributes to the propagation of lacto bacillus bifidus in the gut of nursing infants.

Well, if there are no other questions, thank you very much Dr. Carlsson.

THE IMMUNE RESPONSE FOLLOWING ORAL VACCINATION
WITH *E. coli*

T.J. Newby, C.R. Stokes, P.A. Evans and F.J. Bourne
Department of Animal Husbandry, University of Bristol,
Langford House, Langford, Bristol BS18 7DU, UK.

ABSTRACT

The gut responds to colonisation by E. coli with a vigorous immune response principally involving the IgA class of immunoglobulin, which can be shown to protect against subsequent experimental challenge. In lactating sows there is a response also in the secretions of the mammary gland which is more prolonged than that in the intestine.

In contrast to the response to living bacteria, that provoked by inactivated E. coli fed to pigs is less marked and IgA is not consistently involved. Very large numbers of bacteria fed to mice do, however, provoke a local IgA antibody response.

Feeding bacterial antigen also specifically alters the immune responsiveness of the animal to subsequent re-immunisation. In both mice and pigs, feeding the somatic antigen specifically increases the response to subsequent parenteral immunisation. This effect can be transferred by a serum factor of similar molecular size to IgA. In contrast, feeding the pilus antigen K88 to mice reduced their ability to respond to this antigen and this can be transferred by cells but not by serum.

Escherichia coli in the gut of the young pig produces a non-invasive infection that is characterised by profuse diarrhoea and rapid death. Attempts to produce a vaccine for use in the young animal have not yet proved satisfactory and the nature of the local immune response induced by feeding bacteria remains unclear. We have investigated this response in the pig and the mouse.

In studies using larger pigs we have investigated the relationship between colonisation of the gut and the induction of an immune response. Seven groups of four pigs weighing 40 - 50 kg were infected daily for 5 days with doses of *E. coli* varying from 2×10^8 to 2×10^{11}. The infecting strain was nalidixic acid resistant and could be readily identified on agar plates containing this substrate. Faecal swabs were examined daily in all animals for the presence of the vaccinating strain. Two days after the end of dosing all the pigs were killed and antibody to the O antigen was assayed by haemagglutination as previously described (Evans et al., 1980). The results are shown in Figure 1. Two points of interest emerged from this experiment; firstly, only daily doses of 2×10^{10} or 2×10^{11} viable bacteria were large enough to cause multiplication of the organism within the tract so that it was detectable in faecal swabs, and secondly, antibody could only be found in animals showing such evidence of multiplication. From these results it appears that some degree of colonisation is required to provoke a vigorous IgA antibody response in the intestine.

In order to study the duration of the immune response following colonisation of the intestinal tract with *E. coli*, use was made of the link between the immune systems of the gut and the mammary gland; this link has now been established by several investigators who have shown that infection of the intestinal tract with living enteric organisms results in the appearance of specific antibodies in milk (Bohl et al., 1972; Goldblum et al., 1975). Lactating sows were fed 2×10^{11} bacteria per day, a dose which led to the appearance of the

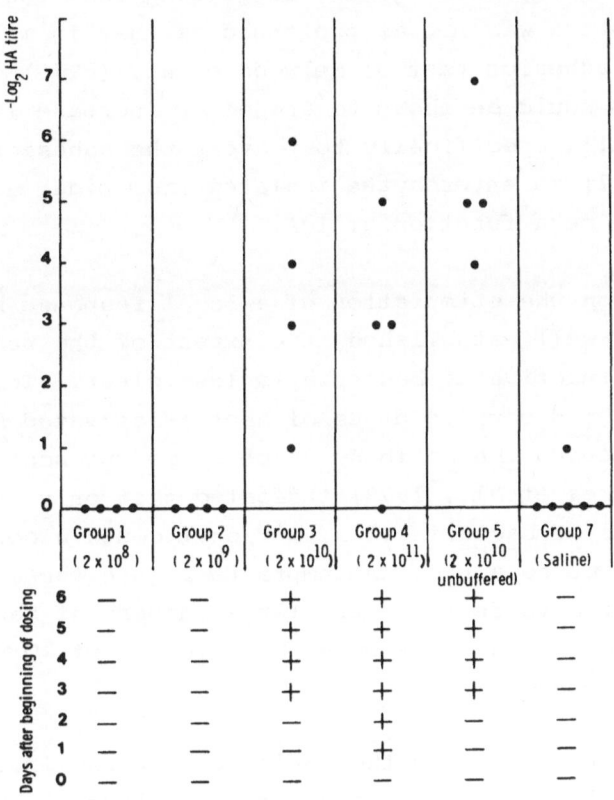

Haemagglutinating (HA) IgA anti-O8 antibody in the intestinal secretions of pigs after oral immunisation with live Escherichia coli, and excretion of organisms during the period of immunisation.

+ indicates presence of inoculum E. coli strain in faeces.

Fig. 1.   Animals were immunised daily for 5 days and intestinal secretions were collected after slaughter on day 7.

organisms in the faeces, and the antibody response was measured in milk.   The results (Evans et al., 1980) confirmed the previous experiment in demonstrating a significant increase in IgA antibody against the infecting organism within seven days

of the start of dosing. The response lasted until the end of
lactation, i.e. at least for 30 days after the start of dosing,
irrespective of whether the organism was fed throughout the
experiment or just for the first four days, but intestinal
antibody, measured at the end of lactation, was only present
in the continually dosed group, suggesting that the response
in the intestine was not as prolonged as that in milk. Using
the *in vitro* adhesion test of Selwood et al. (1975) this
immunisation could be shown to induce an increase in the
ability of milk specifically to prevent the adhesion of K88
bearing *E. coli* to enterocytes isolated from pigs, and this
was shown to be a function of IgA.

Although the stimulation of a local response by live
organisms is well established, the extent of the response
produced by inactivated bacteria is less clear. To investigate
this we have fed varying doses of heat inactivated *E. coli* to
mice and measured the antibody response in gut secretions. The
results (Stokes et al., 1979) indicated that only by feeding
large numbers of bacteria (1×10^{10}/day) could a consistent
IgA response be obtained. Attempts to relate these results
to the pig involve feeding very large numbers of bacteria, since
the pig is larger than the mouse by a factor of 10^3 and eats
10^2 times as much.

In order to compare the antibody response induced by dead
E. coli directly with that stimulated with live organisms,
lactating sows were fed 1×10^{12} heat inactivated *E. coli* for
twenty days. The results (Evans et al., 1980) indicate that the
anti-O response is less marked than that achieved by live
organisms and that IgA was not consistently involved in the
response. Similar results were obtained in young pigs in which
a detectable antibody response could be seen only in those fed
1×10^{11} or 1×10^{12} organisms, and the response was
significantly smaller than that seen in infected animals.

These studies indicate that live bacteria, when they can multiply within the intestine are capable of inducing a vigorous local immune response which persists after the stimulating organism is no longer detectable. In contrast, the response to dead organisms requires very large numbers of bacteria and is smaller than that produced by live. This interpretation of our results is consistent with experiences of the protective capacity of oral vaccination regimes. Sows fed live *E. coli* before parturition produce milk antibody which is highly effective in protecting their litters against experimental challenge (Kohler et al., 1975) and young pigs recovered from *E. coli* enteritis are immune to subsequent re-exposure. In Table 1 are shown the results of an experiment in which 16 pigs were challenged with 1×10^{10} live *E. coli* of the Abbotstown strain. Half the pigs had recovered from an earlier infection with this organism while half had not previously experienced the organism. The results indicate that prior exposure to the organism resulted in a high degree of protection against experimental challenge while the control group were fully susceptible. Four additional animals in each group were killed without challenge and antibody against the infecting organism was detectable in all recovered animals but none of the controls.

TABLE 1

EFFECT OF ORAL CHALLENGE OF THREE-WEEK-OLD PIGS WITH 1×10^{10} *E. coli*

Group	No. infected	No. survivors
Recovered from infection	8	6
Control group	8	0

In contrast, reports of the protection afforded by inactivated oral vaccines indicated that at best only partial protection from experimental challenge can be achieved (Porter et al., 1975).

In addition to the stimulation of local antibody, it is recognised that oral immunisation can result in altered specific

immune responsiveness. The best documented observation is that
of oral tolerance in which the capacity of the animal to respond
to subsequent immunisation is reduced by prior oral immunisation
with T dependent antigens (André et al., 1975; Swarbrick et al.,
1979). Recently it has been reported that feeding the T cell
independent antigen *E. coli* lipopolysaccharide (LPS) resulted in
an increased responsiveness to re-immunisation (Chidlow and
Porter, 1978). We have examined this in relation to the development of oral tolerance by feeding CBA mice with a bacteria
containing both LPS and the K88 antigen, which is a protein and
presumably T cell dependent. The results shown in Figure 2
indicate that tolerance to the protein antigen can coexist in the
same animal with an increased responsiveness to LPS (Stokes et al.,
1979).

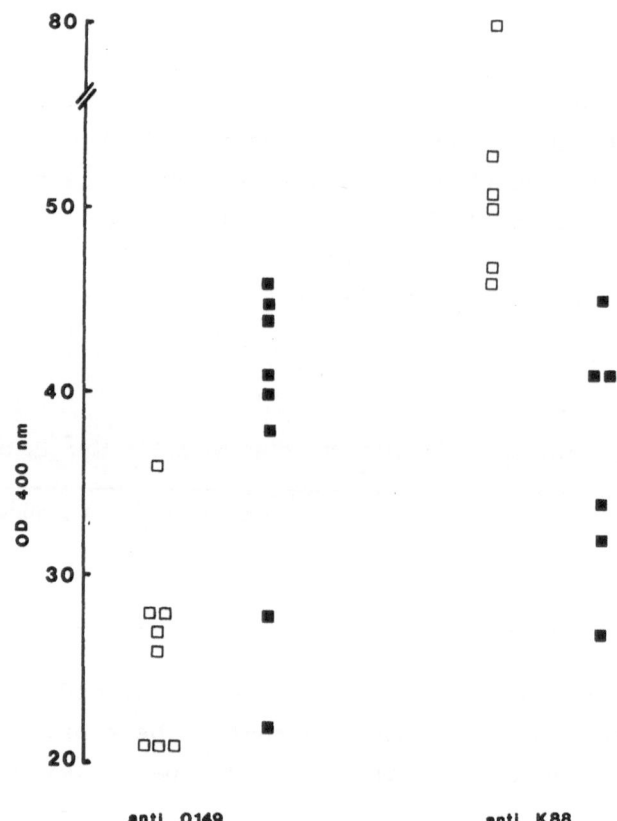

Fig. 2.   The serum antibody response to parenteral immunisation with K88 and
          O149 bearing *E. coli* in normal mice (open squares) and mice previously
          fed 1 x 10^{10} *E. coli* for ten days (closed squares). Antibody was
          assayed by ELISA using an anti mouse immunoglobulin antiserum three
          weeks after immunisation.

Experiments to elucidate the mechanisms underlying these differing responses have indicated that the increased response to LPS can be transferred by a serum factor of similar size to IgA, while spleen cells have no effect. In contrast, the tolerance to K88 can be transferred with spleen cells.

It appears, therefore, that there are at least two mechanisms by which oral immunisation can alter a responsiveness of the immune system to specific antigens: oral tolerance mediated by T cells (Ngan and Kind, 1978) causes a reduction in the response to re-immunisation, while a factor in serum produced as a result of oral immunisation specifically increases the responsiveness of the immune system. It is tempting to assign this latter role to IgA for a number of reasons. Firstly, it can be transferred by a serum factor eluting from gel filtration columns with IgA; secondly, animals showing such increased responsiveness also show an IgA response to endotoxin in intestinal secretions (Stokes et al., 1979); and thirdly, IgA has already been shown to have an enhancing effect upon the immune response (Stokes et al., 1980). Since one would expect vigorous IgA responses to occur to the antigens of pathogenic bacteria this would reduce the possibility of tolerance to enteric bacterial antigens, and explains why feeding endotoxin primes the immune response since this response, in not requiring T cell help, will not be affected by a T cell mediated tolerance.

Acknowledgements

This work was supported by grants from the Leverhulme Trust and the Agricultural Research Council.

REFERENCES

André, C., Heremans, J-F., Vaerman, J-P. and Combiaso, C.L., 1975. A
    mechanism for the induction of immunological tolerance by antigen
    feeding: antigen-antibody complexes. J. exp. Med. 142, 1509.

Bohl, E.H., Gupta, R.K.P., Olquin, F.M.W. and Saif, L.J., 1972. Antibody
    responses in serum, colostrum and milk of swine after infection or
    vaccination with transmissible gastro enteritis virus. Infect.
    Immunity. 6, 289.

Chidlow, J. and Porter, P., 1978. The role of oral immunisation in stimulat-
    ing Escherichia coli antibody of the IgM class in porcine colostrum.
    Res. Vet. Sci. 24, 254.

Evans, P.A., Newby, T.J., Stokes, C.R., Patel, D. and Bourne, F.J., 1980.
    Antibody response of the lactating sow to oral immunisation with
    Escherichia coli. Scand. J. Immunol. 11, 419.

Goldblum, R.H., Ahlstedt, S., Carlsson, B., Hanson, L.A., Jodal, U.,
    Lidin-Janson, G. and Sohl-Akerlund, A., 1975. Antibody forming cells
    in human colostrum after oral immunisation. Nature. 257, 797.

Kohler, E.M., Cross, R.F. and Bohl, E.H., 1975. Protection against neonatal
    enteric colibacillosis in pigs suckling orally vaccinated sows. Am. J.
    Vet. Res. 36, 757.

Ngan, J. and Kind, L.S., 1978. Suppressor T. cells for IgE and IgG in
    Peyer's Patches of mice made tolerant by the oral administration of
    ovalbumin. J. Immunol. 120, 861.

Porter, P., Kenworthy, R. and Allen, W.D., 1974. Effects of oral immunisation
    with E. coli antigens on post weaning enteric infection in the young
    pig. Vet. Rec. 95, 99.

Selwood, R., Gibbons, R.A., Jones, G.W. and Rutter, J.M., 1975. Adhesion of
    enteropathogenic Escherichia coli to pig intestinal brush borders: the
    existence of two pig phenotypes. J. Med. Microbiol. 8, 405.

Stokes, C.R., Newby, T.J., Huntley, J.H., Patel, D. and Bourne, F.J., 1979.
    The immune response of mice to bacterial antigens given by mouth.
    Immunology. 38, 497.

Stokes, C.R., Swarbrick, E.T. and Soothill, J.F., 1980. Immune elimination
    and enhanced antibody responses: functions of circulating IgA.
    Immunology. 40, 455.

Swarbrick, E.T., Stokes, C.R. and Soothill, J.F., 1979. Absorption of
    antigens after oral immunisation and simultaneous induction of specific
    systemic tolerance. Gut. 20, 121.

DISCUSSION

J. Hall   *(UK)*

You seem to have a very satisfactory way of feeding the dead organisms although I realise it is not a procedure which has any place in animal husbandry but if you put the organisms directly into the intestine, does this give a better response?

T.J. Newby   *(UK)*

I am sure it does. The stomach represents an enormous barrier but, as you say, it is hardly a practical possibility.

J. Hall

Do you think it is just the numbers game, the difference between the live and the dead vaccine, or is there an added factor on top of that?

T.J. Newby

The critical feature is that if you give live in sufficient numbers they colonise; then you have a much greater response.

H. Williams Smith   *(UK)*

The question is, where do they colonise? In the mouse I would imagine they colonise in the large intestine, and I would think probably in your pigs too. It is large intestinal immunisation. When you are examining their faeces at intervals afterwards, I would suggest that was because they colonise in the large intestine.

T.J. Newby

Yes, certainly that may be so.

H. Miller   *(UK)*

Regarding the very large doses of bacteria that you were giving to the mice, where you were getting a small response, could that be simply that you had so much endotoxin in the system that you were damaging the lymphoid system?

T.J. Newby

There was a suggestion that the animals fed this large amount were ill.

H. Bazin   *(Belgium)*

What was the molecular weight of your endotoxin?

T.J. Newby

Over a million.

H. Bazin

And how can you verify that you have IgM and IgA anti-bodies? Are you sure it is not just endotoxin? It is a very high molecular weight.

T.J. Newby

Yes, it may not be complexes; it may just be antibody.

H. Bazin

But then you will have IgA antibody with your IgM every time.

T.J. Newby

I can only say that the factor transferred elutes along with IgA and IgM.

K.L. Morgan   *(UK)*

Does anybody know if there is a strain of *E. coli* which is pathogenic for the mouse and which has the same epithelial relationship?

H. Williams Smith

The answer to that is that nobody has found it, if there is one.

P.J. Kilshaw   (UK)

May I clarify a small point. The tolerance of the K antigen, does it or does it not affect the IgA response?

T.J. Newby

I don't know; we are just dealing with serum antibody responses.

J. Seifert   (FRG)

Is it right that you did not find any IgG increase after the immunisation in mice?

T.J. Newby

That's right. There may have been an increase in individual animals but over the groups there was no increase.

J. Seifert

We immunised human beings with *E. coli* and we found an increase of IgG. Perhaps it is specific for mice.

H. Bazin

Can you colonise your experimental laboratory rodents with your *E. coli*?

T.J. Newby

No. I understand from the bacteriologists that there is not a suitable model.

W. Leibold   (FRG)

What is the genetic influence on your results? Are they true for all mice or only certain strains?

T.J. Newby

     Possibly only for certain strains. The work was all done in CBA and A strain mice.

E. Bohl

     Thank you Dr. Newby.

THE ROLE OF MUCUS SECRETIONS IN THE PROTECTION OF THE GASTROINTESTINAL MUCOSA

J.R. Clamp

Department of Medicine, University of Bristol,
Bristol BS8 1TD, UK.

The surfaces of all mucous membranes are protected by a layer of mucus. The protective value of this secretion lies not only in its characteristic physicochemical properties but also in the presence of certain specific constituents. It is a complex secretion, receiving contributions from many types of cell (Jones and Reid, 1978) in addition to material arising by transudation from plasma. Gastrointestinal mucus presents particular problems in this respect when attempts are made to define its nature and role because it is always admixed with copious secretions from sources other than the mucus-producing cell. These secretions, in particular sites, contain powerful proteolytic enzymes and glycosidases which are known to act upon mucus. Any material that survives into the colon is rapidly digested by the large numbers of bacteria that are present in that organ so that faeces contain little or no mucus in the healthy state. The gastrointestinal mucus layer is not likely to be radically different from that in other sites however. In that case, when first secreted, it is a complex secretion containing components arising by transudation (plasma proteins), from cell breakdown (DNA and lipids) or by active secretion (lysozyme, lactoferrin, secretory IgA and glycoprotein). A typical mucus secretion contains about 1% salt, 1% protein and between 1% and 3% glycoprotein (Creeth, 1978).

Mucus glycoprotein is the constituent that determines the physicochemical properties of the mucus layer. It is a large molecule with a molecular weight varying from 2×10^6 in gastric mucus (Allen et al., 1976) to 15×10^6 in colonic mucus (Marshall and Allen, 1978). Although 60 - 80% of the molecule consists of carbohydrate, this is present in relatively small oligosaccharide units. These range in size from disaccharide units to units

containing more than 20 monosaccharide residues, with an
average size of 8 - 10 residues (Clamp, 1978). The glycoprotein
therefore consists of a polypeptide chain with an oligosaccharide
unit attached to every third or fourth amino acid. The carbohydrate surrounds and partially shields the polypeptide chain
from, for example, proteolytic attack. This is an essential
property in the gastro-intestinal tract. However, the polypeptide chains are devoid of carbohydrate at widely spaced intervals ('naked' peptide regions). This is to allow neighbouring
chains to come close enough together to be joined by disulphide
bonds. These cross-linkages are an essential feature of mucus
gel structure. The naked peptide regions and the disulphide
linkages are the most vulnerable regions of the mucus to degradation, whether by proteolytic enzymes or agents that cleave
disulphide bonds.

The linkage of carbohydrate to protein is through N-
acetylgalactosamine to the hydroxyamino acids, serine and
threonine (O-glycosidic linkage). This explains the unusual
amino acid composition of mucus glycoproteins in which serine,
threonine and proline account for over half of the total amino
acids. The oligosaccharide units contain a variety of monosaccharide residues, including L-fucose, D-galactose, N-acetyl-
D-glucosamine, N-acetyl-D-galactosamine and sialic acid. Acidity
would be conferred upon the oligosaccharide units, not only by
sialic acid but also by the presence of sulphated monosaccharide
residues. The number of acid groups and the ratio of sialic
acid to sulphate varies at various levels of the gastrointestinal tract. In general, the acidic nature of mucus increases from the stomach to the colon (Reid et al., 1980).

There are a number of ways in which mucus secretions
protect mucous membranes from attack by micro-organisms.

Obviously physical entrapment and immobilisation can occur
in a similar fashion to that seen with intestinal parasites (see
Miller et al., in this publication). This may well be the most
important method by which the lungs are protected. Indeed those

respiratory diseases in which there is a disturbance of mucociliary clearance, are characterised by repeated infections
even though the immunological defence mechanisms are unimpaired.
Apart from physically trapping any micro-organism and thereby
preventing it from reaching and infecting the mucosal cells,
mucus may contain spurious attachment sites for pathogenic
bacteria (Lindley, 1980). Thus the relationship of mucosal
cells to goblet cell orifices or to the openings of ducts from
mucus-producing submucosal glands is obviously of considerable
importance. This relationship can be demonstrated very easily
for toad mucous membrane, because the tissue can be dehydrated
in the distended state. Electron micrographs show clearly the
epithelial cell boundaries radiating out from a goblet cell
orifice (Figure 1a). Every epithelial cell appears to be in
contact with a mucus-producing cell so that a 'mucus domain'
consists of about 4 to 5 epithelial cells surrounding a central
goblet cell orifice. The pattern is more difficult to demonstrate for human mucous membrane but appears to be similar in
colon (Figure 1b).

The protective role of mucus is augmented by the addition
of specific proteins, namely lysozyme, lactoferrin and secretory
IgA. These proteins do not arise by transudation from plasma,
but are actively secreted into mucus and all appear to play a
protective role against microbial attack. Lysozyme, for example,
interacts with sialic acid residues (Creeth et al., 1979) thus
remaining associated with the mucus layer where it acts against
muramic acid-containing bacterial cell walls. Iron is an
essential requirement for many micro-organisms and lactoferrin
is believed to act by complexing with any iron that is present
in secretions and thereby denying it to the organism (Emery,
1980).

The relationship of secretory IgA to mucus glycoproteins
is of particular interest to this symposium. To understand
this relationship it is necessary to compare the glycoprotein
nature of IgA with that of mucus. Immunoglobulins belong to
the class of proteins known as 'plasma-type' because all the

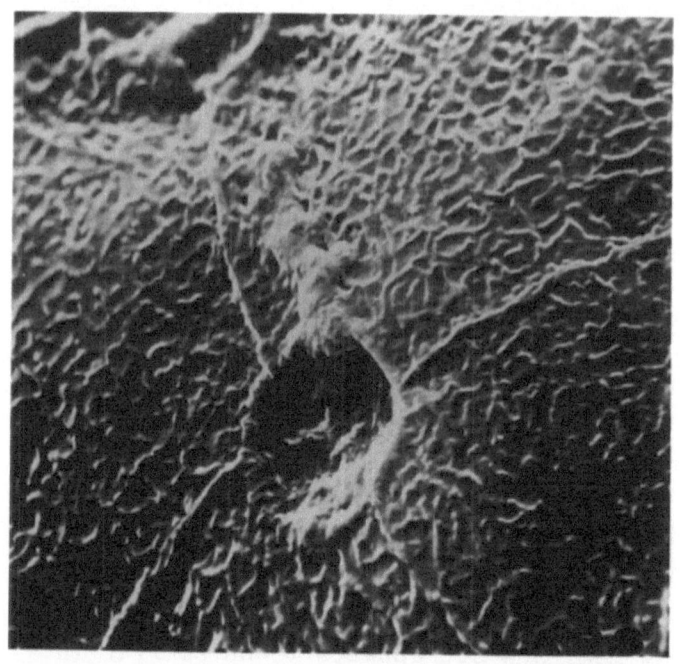

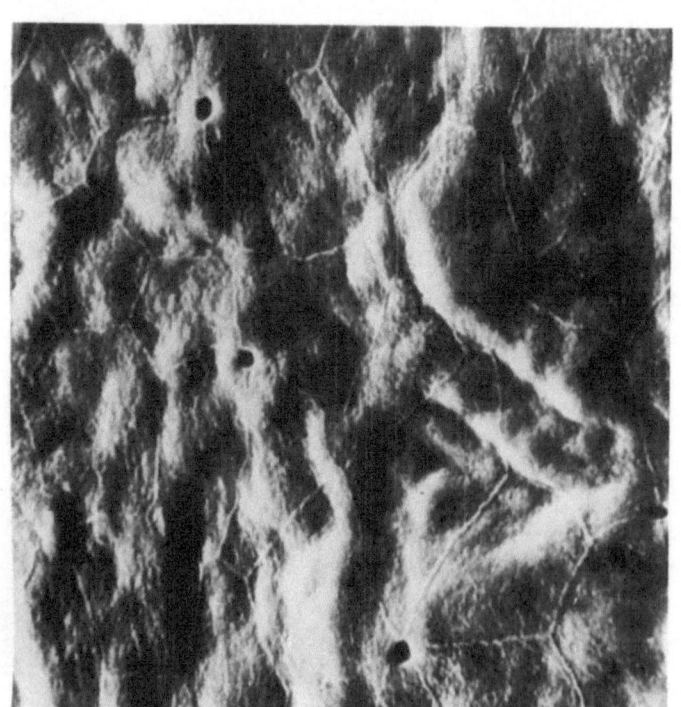

Fig. 1 (a) A scanning electron micrograph of toad
mucous membrane fixed in the distended,
dehydrated state. The orifices of
several goblet cells can be seen with
epithelial cell bounds radiating from
each orifice.

Fig. 1 (b) A similar picture of human colonic
epithelium.

By courtesy of Dr. R. Teague, Department of Medicine, University of Bristol

plasma globulins are similar as far as their glycoprotein characteristics are concerned (Reid and Clamp, 1978). The similarities and differences between immunoglobulins as typical 'plasma-type' glycoproteins and mucus glycoproteins are shown in Table 1.

TABLE 1

COMPARISON OF THE PROPERTIES OF IMMUNOGLOBULINS AS 'PLASMA-TYPE' GLYCO-PROTEINS AND MUCUS GLYCOPROTEINS

	Immunoglobulins	Mucus glycoproteins
Molecular weight	$1.5 \times 10^5 - 1.0 \times 10^6$	$2 \times 10^6 - 15 \times 10^6$
Amino acid content	Amino acid spectrum of a typical protein	High levels of serine, threonine and proline. Low levels of aromatic and S-containing amino acids
Carbohydrate content	Less than 20%	More than 50%
Linkage:		
N-Acetylgalactosamine to serine and/or threonine (O-glycosidic)	Not present in most immunoglobulin classes (exceptions IgAl and possibly IgD)	Main, if not sole, type of linkage
N-Acetylglucosamine to asparagine (N-glycosidic)	Main type of linkage	Possibly present as a minor type of linkage
Monosaccharides:		
Fucose	Present	Present
Mannose	Present	Possibly present as a minor constituent
Galactose	Present	Present
N-Acetylglucosamine	Present	Present
N-Acetylgalactosamine	Absent from all classes except IgAl and IgD	Present
Sialic acid	Present	Present

IgA, of course, exists as two major subclasses, IgA1 and
IgA2 (Grey et al., 1968). IgA1 is unusual among plasma-type
glycoproteins in possessing O-glycosidically-linked oligosaccharide units (Dawson and Clamp, 1967). Indeed the stretch
in the putative hinge region, which is rich in proline and
hydroxyamino acids and which possesses up to 5 such oligosaccharide units, has been called the 'mucus-like' stretch.
The fact that one of the major subclasses of IgA which is involved in the protection of mucous membranes should possess a
'mucus-like' stretch is of considerable theoretical interest.
The O-glycosidically linked oligosaccharide units have been
studied in monomeric plasma IgA1 and are relatively simple.
They are disaccharide units consisting of galactose β-linked to
the 3 position of N-acetylgalactosamine. When IgA1 enters
mucus secretions, however, the oligosaccharide units are larger
and more complex, containing in addition fucose, N-acetyl-
glucosamine and extra residues of galactose (J.R. Clamp and
F.J. Bourne, unpublished findings). It is not known at present
whether the additional monosaccharide residues are added in the
plasma cells synthesising dimeric IgA1 Alternatively, if the
carbohydrate content of dimeric IgA1 is similar to that of
monomeric IgA1 this would imply that the immunoglobulin molecule is processed during passage through some second cell, since
it is unlikely that monosaccharides would be added extra-
cellularly.

The fact that IgA1 possesses a 'mucus-like' stretch
implies that the molecule interacts in some way with either the
mucus gel or with the underlying mucosal cell. This interaction
could be covalent, for example by the formation of disulphide
bonds, although this is not very probable. Much more likely is
that any interaction is mediated by non-covalent forces. Thus
the 'mucus-like' stretch could reversibly hydrogen bond to
similar groups on the gel or at the cell surface. An alternative
possibility is that the mucus gel phase exhibits the phenomenon
of phase separation (Albertsson, 1977). Macromolecules that are
dissimilar to mucus glycoprotein would be excluded and would
remain in the overlying aqueous phase. IgA1 on the other hand,

because of its 'mucus-like' stretch would either enter the
mucus phase or would be orientated at the interface (Edward,
1978). In either case IgA1 would be associated with the mucus
layer whereas IgA2 in which there is a deletion of the 'mucus-
like' stretch, would be associated with the overlying aqueous
phase.

So far I have discussed chemical aspects of mucus and
the nature of the glycoprotein forming the mucus gel, together
with the ways in which immunoglobulins, in particular IgA, may
interact with that gel.

A further intriguing aspect of the influence of immunological mechanisms upon mucus is the effect that antigen (Lake
et al., 1979) and immune complexes (Walker et al., 1977) have
upon the release of mucus. If antigen, in orally-stimulated
rats, or immune complexes in normal rats, are introduced into
the small intestine there is a marked increase in mucus
released from goblet cells. Presumably this helps clear the
antigen complexes from the mucosal surface and may be important
in discouraging infection by pathogenic organisms.

REFERENCES

Albertsson, P.A., 1977. Separation of Particles and Macromolecules by
Phase Partition. Endeavour, 1, No. 2., 69-74.

Allen, A., Pain, R.H. and Robson, T.R., 1976. Model for the Structure of
the Gastric Mucous Gel. Nature, 264, 88-89.

Clamp, J.R., 1978. Chemical Aspects of Mucus. General Considerations.
Brit. Med. Bull., 34, No. 1., 25-27.

Creeth, J.M., 1978. Constituents of Mucus and their Separation. Brit.
Med. Bull., 34, No. 1., 17-24.

Creeth, J.M., Bridge, J.L. and Horton, J.R., 1979. An Interaction between
Lysozyme and Mucus Glycoproteins. Implications for Density-Gradient
Separations. Biochem. J., 181, 717-724.

Dawson, G. and Clamp, J.R., 1967. The Presence of Two Types of Carbohydrate-
Amino Acid Linkage in the same Glycoprotein. Biochem. Biophys. Res.
Commun., 26, 349-352.

Edwards, P.A.W., 1978. Is Mucus a Selective Barrier to Macromolecules?
Brit. Med. Bull., 34, No. 1., 55-56.

Emery, T., 1980. Iron Deprivation as a Biological Defence Mechanism.
Nature, 287, 776-777.

Grey, H.M., Abel, C.A. and Yount, W.J., 1968. A Subclass of Human γA
Globulins (γA2) which Lacks the Disulphide Bonds Linking Heavy and
Light Chains. J. Exper. Med., 128, 1223-1236.

Jones, R. and Reid, L., 1978. Secretory Cells and their Glycoproteins in
Health and Disease. Brit. Med. Bull., 34, No. 1., 9-16.

Lake, A.M., Bloch, K.J., Neutra, M.R. and Walker, W.A., 1979. Intestinal
Goblet Cell Mucus Release. II *In vivo* Stimulation by Antigen in
the Immunized Rat. J. Immunol. 122, 834-837.

Lindley, M., 1980. Adhesion of Pathogenic Microorganisms. Nature, 286,
556-557.

Marshall, T. and Allen, A., 1978. The Isolation and Characterization of the
High-Molecular-Weight Glycoprotein from Pig Colonic Mucus. Biochem.
J., 173, 569-578.

Reid, L. and Clamp, J.R., 1978. The Biochemical and Histochemical
Nomenclature of Mucus. Brit. Med. Bull., 34, No. 1., 5-8.

Reid, P.E., Culling, C.F.A., Dunn, W.L., Ramey, C.W., Magil, A.B. and
    Clay, M.G., 1980. Differences between the O-Acetylated Sialic Acids
    of the Epithelial Mucins of Human Colonic Tumors and Normal Controls:
    A Correlative Chemical and Histochemical Study. J. Histochem.
    Cytochem., 28, 217-222.

Walker, W.A., Wu, M. and Bloch, K.J., 1977. Stimulation by Immune Complexes
    of Mucus Release from Goblet Cells of the Rat Small Intestine.
    Science, 197, 370-372.

DISCUSSION

J. Hall   *(UK)*

The structure you gave of IgA would seem to indicate that it would have some free galactose residues projecting from it.   Would that be correct?

J. Clamp   *(UK)*

Yes, that is true.   There are a number of plasma glyco-proteins which are not cleared by the hepatic mechanisms so it is only semi-specific.   Transferin is another one which is not cleared by this mechanism but ceruloplasmin is and a number of other alpha-1 acid glycoproteins are also cleared by this mech-anism.   So, having a galactose exposed is not sufficient to be cleared by the hepatocyte.

Work has been done which shows that if you alter the galactose with galactose oxidase, or you put the sialic acid back on, it is not cleared.   It is very interesting to look back at some of the early literature because some of the pit-uitary hormones are also cleared by this mechanism and people found that the activity dropped very rapidly in plasma within half an hour.   All kinds of theories were formulated about hormone action on this basis but it was just that they had lost the sialic acid and then when they injected it, it was cleared by the liver.

P. Brandtzaeg   *(Norway)*

Did I understand you correctly when you postulated that perhaps the secretory IgA has to go through the golgi region of the epithelial cell to obtain its hinge region carbohydrate?

J. Clamp

That would be the simplest explanation, yes.

P. Brandtzaeg

But that is not on, the possibility does not exist.

J. Clamp

Well then you must have two populations of plasma cells, one building up the typical unit which is seen in myeloma IgA which just has galactose galactosimine, and then the unit which is present in secretory IgA which has extra fucose, glucosamine and galactose.

P. Brandtzaeg

Yes, it should be easy to analyse. Are the myeloma proteins which you have analysed dimers?

J. Clamp

Most of these were 7-S IgAs. If anyone has got some material which is a dimer and which is non-secretory, we would be delighted to analyse it.

P. Brandtzaeg

I have lots of it.

J. Clamp

Do you? Well, I would be very pleased to analyse it.

J.P. Vaerman   (Belgium)

IgA2 does not seem to have this peculiarity yet the proportion of IgA2 is increased in secretions. How would you reconcile this?

J. Clamp

One could say that you have a double protection, with the IgA1 sitting at the interface and the IgA2 out in the secretions, excluded from the mucous layer. That is a possibility, at any rate.

J. Bienenstock   (Canada)

There has been a suggestion made that secretory IgA is

bound covalently in with mucus, at least in some situations, particularly colostral IgA. Have you any more information in this area?

J. Clamp

We collaborate with Mike Creeth who is a physical chemist in the laboratory adjoining ours. He works with sputum, admittedly from chronic bronchitics and asthmatics, and he has made an observation which he has never published, that after gradient density ultracentrifugation most of the protein is lost. But then if he treats it more vigorously he gets out almost pure IgA. So it looks as if, like lysozyme there might well be a complex between mucus and IgA. He does not know which class it is. I think it is non-covalent linkage.

W. Leibold (FRG)

Just to bring me up do date, how many immunoglobulin classes in the pig have carbohydrate residues in the hinge region? Secondly, do you have any idea whether this carbohydrate in the hinge region has any function as soon as the monomer complexes with an antigen? Does it contribute somehow to the immune complex action after complexing?

J. Clamp

No, I think people have taken off carbohydrate and found that it does not affect the complexing with antigen. Feinstein has shown that one of the oligosaccharide units in IgM is sitting over the complement fixation site. It is a large, bulky unit, of course, being carbohydrate. He postulates that when the legs are pulled down to fix, say, to a bacterial surface, it pulls the carbohydrate away and exposes the complement fixation site. Carbohydrate became attached to protein very early in evolution. You find carbohydrate attached to protein in micro-organisms, in snails and in worms. I believe it has evolved to perform a number of functions; I don't think there is any one function of carbohydrate and it might well be that people working in this field who are looking for one function will never find it.

W. Leibold

Yes, but I am particularly concerned about the carbohydrate residues in the hinge region. In the C-2, C-3 and C-4
domain, it is all right. But how many of the immunoglobulin
classes do have carbohydrate residues, particularly in the
hinge region?

J. Clamp

I was hoping no one would ask that question because IgD,
in fact, is very similar to IgA and carbohydrate is linked in
the hinge region; IgE is very similar to IgM in its carbohydrate.
It was shown some years ago with the rabbit that IgG also has
carbohydrate in the hinge region. I don't know whether anyone
has ever shown that it interferes with antigen complexing at all.

Well, I think perhaps now we should move on to the next
talk.

MUCUS SECRETION IN THE GUT, ITS RELATIONSHIP TO THE IMMUNE RESPONSE IN NIPPOSTRONGYLUS-INFECTED RATS*

H.R.P. Miller, J.F. Huntley and A. McL. Dawson

Moredun Institute, 408 Gilmerton Road, Edinburgh EH17 7JH, UK.

ABSTRACT

The role of mucus in the immune expulsion of Nippostrongylus brasiliensis from the small intestine of the rat was examined. A glycoprotein isolated from intestinal secretions by Sepharose 4B chromatography was characterised by incorporation of (^{35}S) - Na_2SO_4 and D-$(1-^{14}C)$-glucosamine, immuno-diffusion, polyacrylamide gel electrophoresis, and by its immuno-histochemical localisation in goblet cells. These results suggested that the glycoprotein was very similar to a soluble rat intestinal mucin characterised by Forstner et al., 1973. The rate of incorporation of D-$(1-^{14}C)$ glucosamine into acid- precipitable material in intestinal secretions was significantly increased in rats harbouring a primary N. brasiliensis infection. The proportion of this radioactivity which was incorporated into soluble mucin was also increased, to reach a peak 13 days after infection when the worms were being expelled. A new model of infection was also developed, whereby expulsion of immature adult worms occurred within 4 hours of intraduodenal challenge. Macroscopic and microscopic examination of the intestine indicated that mucus may serve both as a barrier to and a trapping agent of N. brasiliensis in immune rats. This is in agreement with similar observations made by Lee and Ogilvie, 1980, for Trichinella spiralis infection in the rat.

*   Part of this work was done while H.R.P. Miller was a member of the Department of Immunology, John Curtin School, Canberra, Australia.

INTRODUCTION

The mechanism by which nematodes are expelled from the gastrointestinal tract is not well understood. Experiments in laboratory animals have established that the immune system initiates the events which lead to parasite expulsion (Ogilvie and Love, 1974; Wakelin, 1978) and there is ample evidence that many species eventually become resistant to gastro-intestinal helminthiasis (Wakelin, 1978). However, in both laboratory and domestic animals worm expulsion appears to be a non-specific process triggered by a specific antigenic challenge (Dineen et al., 1977; Wakelin, 1978).

Worm expulsion is a complex process wherein low molecular weight inflammatory mediators, immunoglobulins, mucus and increased peristalsis may all play a part (Askenase, 1980). Depending on the predilection site of the parasite several or all of these mechanisms could be involved. Those parasites which penetrate the gut wall may be more susceptible to rapidly diffusing inflammatory mediators and inflammatory cells whereas those which dwell in the gut lumen might be affected by changes in the quantity and/or quality of the mucous barrier and to increased peristalsis.

Correlations between age, increased numbers of intestinal goblet cells, and resistance to parasite infection were reported by Ackert and Edgar (1939) in chickens. Similarly, resistance to intestinal parasites in domestic animals (Dobson, 1967) and laboratory rodents (Wells, 1963; Miller and Nawa, 1979) has been related to increased numbers of mucosal goblet cells. Recent data indicate that goblet cell differentiation in parasitised rats is influenced by specific immunological events (Miller and Nawa, 1979).

Intestinal mucus from chickens has been reported to inhibit *in vitro* growth of *Ascaridia galli* (Frick and Ackert, 1948) and more recent experiments by Lee and Ogilvie (1980) suggest that mucus acts as both a barrier to larval challenge and as medium for trapping infective larvae, a process which is aided by specific and non-specific serum-derived factors.

The immune expulsion of *Nippostrongylus brasiliensis* from the intestines of both rats and mice is associated with an increased proportion of goblet cells overlying the intestinal villi (Miller and Nawa, 1979; Uber et al., 1980) but it is not known if there is any change in the rate of synthesis of goblet cell mucin. Consequently, the present work was designed to examine the synthesis of this glycoprotein during primary infection. Since, in certain hosts, nematode parasites can be expelled within hours of challenge (Askenase, 1980), a new model of rapid expulsion of *N. brasiliensis* was developed. The role of mucus in this system was then examined.

MATERIALS AND METHODS

Animals

Female (PVG/cxDA/F$_1$ rats were used for D-(1-14C) glucosamine incorporation studies. Female and male outbred Wistar rats 200 - 300 g weight were used for intraduodenal challenge studies. All rats were fed and watered *ad libitum* .

Parasitological techniques

The methods for culturing *N. brasiliensis* larvae, infection with third stage larvae (l$_3$), and recovering and counting adult worms were those described previously (Nawa and Miller, 1978).

Fourth stage larvae and immature adult worms were recovered from donor rats 4 days after infection with 6 000 l$_3$, they were washed and were distributed in 1 ml volumes of 0.15 M saline for subsequent transfer (Nawa and Miller, 1978) into recipient rats which had been starved 24 - 36 h before challenge.

At intervals after challenge, the rats were bled out under ether anaesthesia and the small intestine was dissected out and

stored at -20°C. To count the worms, the intestines were
divided into 10 equal lengths (Wells, 1962) which were opened
longitudinally. In some experiments intestines were examined
immediately after killing the rats. The worms were counted
with a stereomicroscope at a magnification of x 8.

Incorporation of D-(1-^{14}C)-glucosamine

Female (PVG/cxDA/F$_1$ rats were lightly anaesthetised and
injected intravenously with 2 µCi of D-(1-^{14}C)-glucosamine
hydrochloride (Radiochemical Centre, Amersham 59 mCi/m mol)
(Forstner, 1970). Groups of 4 rats were anaesthetised 1, 2, 4
and 6 hours later and were bled out by section of the carotid
artery. The small intestine was dissected away from the
mesentery, wiped free of blood with damp cotton wool and
divided into two equal lengths, each of which was washed through
with 10 ml of 0.15 M saline and 10 ml of air. The two segments were then gently drawn through damp cotton wool to squeeze
out any remaining adherent mucus. The samples from each half
were pooled, homogenised at 4°C in a teflon-glass homogeniser,
and centrifuged at 36 000 g for 30 minutes to remove insoluble
material. The volume of the supernatant was measured and
replicate 4 ml samples precipitated with 0.4 ml of a mixture
of 100% trichloroacetic acid (TCA) and 10% phosphotungstic acid
(PTA) (Forstner, 1972). After standing in the cold overnight
the samples were centrifuged at 4 000 g for 15 min. The
pellets, washed twice in ice cold 10% TCA/1% PTA, were
collected by centrifugation and finally dissolved in 200 µl of
1N sodium hydroxide. The samples were placed in combustion
cones and allowed to dry before they were oxidised in a model
306 Packard Tri-Carb sample oxidiser.

Acid-precipitated pellets from pooled samples of intestinal
washes from normal and infected rats were resuspended in 10
volumes of chloroform-methanol (1:1, v/v) and recovered by
centrifugation. After 2 further washes in chloroform-methanol,
the solvent was evaporated and the radioactivity in the lipid
fraction measured. Approximately 10% of the radioactivity was
recovered in this fraction from all samples examined.

Incorporation of radioactivity into intestinal washings of infected rats was measured 4 h after intravenous injection of 2 μCi (1-^{14}C) glucosamine on days 8, 11, 13 and 15 after challenge with 4 000 l_3.

Incorporation of (^{35}S)-Na$_2$SO$_4$

The method described by Lake et al. (1980) was used. In brief, Wistar rats were fasted for 36 h and were injected intravenously with 30 μCi of (^{35}S)-Na$_2$SO$_4$ (Radiochemical Centre, Amersham). Five hours later the rats were anaesthetised, bled out, and the intestines removed as described in the previous section. The method for recovering intestinal washings was similar to that described previously except that each segment was washed with 5 ml of 0.1 M sodium phosphate buffer pH 7.0 and 10 ml of air. The intestinal washings were homogenised at 4°C and, after centrifugation, the supernatant was dialysed against 3 x 2l of 0.1 M phosphate buffer pH 7.0 at 4°C.

Column chromatography

Two millilitre samples of intestinal washings from each group of 4 glucosamine-injected rats were pooled, concentrated to 2.5 ml by pressure dialysis, and applied to a 1.6 x 70 cm column (Pharmacia, UK) packed with Sepharose 4B. The column was equilibrated with 0.05 M tris/0.15 M NaCl pH 7.4 and the void volume was determined with blue dextran 2 000 (Pharmacia, UK). Ascending chromatography was used and 9 - 10 ml fractions were collected and precipitated with 1 ml 100% TCA/10% PTA. The precipitates were washed once in 2 ml 10% TCA/1% PTA and dissolved in 200 μl 1N NaOH before being applied to combustion cones.

After combustion in the sample oxidiser the radioactivity of ^{14}C-labelled fractions was measured in a liquid scintillation spectrometer. The recovery or radioactivity was regularly measured with a radioactive standard (Spec-Check, Packard) and was 98-100%. An internal standard (Spec-Check) counted with each sample showed that the samples were unquenched and the counting efficiency was high.

Two millilitre samples of dialysed intestinal washings from recipients of ^{35}S were applied to a 2.6 x 40 cm sepharose 4B column (Pharmacia UK) and chromatographed in 0.1 M Na_2HPO_4, pH 7.0. Five to 6 ml fractions were collected and 1 ml from each was mixed with 10 ml of Aquasol 2 (New England Nuclear, Southampton) and radioactivity was measured in a liquid scintillation spectrometer.

Analysis of protein and hexoses

The levels of protein were measured by the method of Lowry et al., 1951, using bovine serum albumin (Armour, Fraction V) as a standard. Neutral hexoses were measured by the method of Dubois et al., 1956, with galactose as a standard.

Preparation of antiserum

Concentrated gut washings from normal rats were applied to a Sepharose 4B column and the first peak (Fraction I) eluting in the void volume was collected, dialysed against distilled water, and lyophilised (Forstner et al., 1973a). This process was repeated several times.

Rabbits were injected intramuscularly with 1 mg of Fraction I from normal rats emulsified in 1 ml of complete Freund's adjuvant. One milligramme booster doses in 1 ml of incomplete Freund's adjuvant were administered at intervals of two weeks and the rabbits were bled 6 weeks after the first injection and at weekly intervals thereafter. The sera were absorbed twice against normal and *Nippostrongylus*-immune sera insolubilised on Sepharose 4B.

Polyacrylamide disc gel electrophoresis

The methods described by Forstner et al. (1973b) were followed and samples of Fraction I (50 - 200 μg) together with bromphenol blue were run for 2 - 3 h on 4% acrylamide gels in 0.15 M Tris-borate buffer pH 8.6. Some samples were treated with 1% sodium dodecyl sulphate before application. The gels were washed overnight in 7.5% acetic acid and then stained with

periodic acid-schiff (PAS) for carbohydrates or with Coomassie
blue for proteins.

Tissue fixation

For morphological and histochemical studies of goblet
cells, freshly prepared phosphate-buffered 4% paraformaldehyde
(pH 7.4) was injected intraluminally (0.1 - 0.2 ml/cm of gut)
into ligated segments of jejunum which were then immediately
placed in the same fixative held at 0°C. Some tissues were
fixed in the same manner with Baker's formalin and, to study
worm localisation in tissue sections, small segments of
unopened intestine were placed in ice cold Carnoy's fixative.

Segments of intestine (1 - 2 cm) were placed in embedding
medium (Tissue-Tek II, Miles Laboratories) in aluminium foil
boats and immersed in isopentane cooled with liquid nitrogen.
The snap frozen segments were trimmed to give longitudinal
sections of the intestine vertical to the mucosa. Four micron
thick sections were cut in a cryostat and allowed to dry before
they were fixed in paraformaldehyde vapour (80°C) (Lee and
Ogilvie, 1980) Baker's formalin, or Carnoy's fixative.

Adult worms were recovered at various stages after
infection and were embedded in 7% agar before being placed in
paraformaldehyde or Carnoy's fixative. All tissues fixed in
formalin or Carnoy's fluid were dehydrated and embedded in
paraffin wax. Frozen and paraffin sections were stained
either with haematoxylin and eosin or with Alcian blue (pH 2.5)
- PAS.

Histochemical localisation of goblet cell mucin

Endogenous peroxidase activity was removed from tissue
sections with periodic acid and sodium borohydride (Heyderman
and Neville, 1977) and the sections were treated for 15 min
with 0.1% trypsin in phosphate buffer at 37°C then washed in
0.15 M NaCl/0.05 M Tris-HCl buffer pH 7.4. Various dilutions
(1/4 - 1/256) of rabbit anti-Fraction I antiserum in Tris-HCl

buffer were placed on the sections which were left in a moist
atmosphere for 1.5 h. After washing in buffer, the sections
were treated with a 1/40 dilution of sheep F(ab')$_2$ anti-
rabbit Fab labelled with peroxidase by the method of Nakane and
Kawaoi (1974). The sections were washed once more and stained
with diaminobenzidine (Graham and Karnovsky, 1966). For
control purposes sections were either incubated with normal
rabbit serum taken from the rabbit prior to immunisation with
Fraction I antigen or with immune serum which had previously
been absorbed with Fraction I antigen (200 µl of 1/32 dilution
of antiserum against 50 - 100 µl of Fraction I antigen at
5 mg/ml).

Goblet cell mucins were also detected with a wheat germ
agglutinin (WGA) - alkaline phosphatase conjugate. The latter
was prepared by the 1 step glutaraldehyde technique of
Avrameas (1969) and was used at a concentration of 1 mg/ml.
Slides were incubated for 2 h with the conjugate, washed, and
alkaline phosphatase activity revealed by staining with
naphthol AS MX phosphate and Fast Red RT salt for 30 min
(Burstone, 1962). For control purposes, sections were stained
without prior incubation with conjugate or after incubation
with conjugate in the presence of 1M N-acetyl-D-glucosamine
(Sigma, UK).

RESULTS

Identification of soluble rat mucin

The elution of radioactivity after Sepharose 4B
chromatography of intestinal washings from a normal rat injected
with (^{35}S)-Na$_2$SO$_4$ is shown in Figure 1, together with the
elution profiles of protein and neutral hexoses. A distinct
peak of radioactivity (Fraction 1) eluted in the void volume of
the column and contained both neutral hexose and protein
(Figure 1). A similar peak of acid-precipitable radioactivity
was detected in the void volume (Figure 2) after fractionation
of intestinal washings from rats injected with (1-^{14}C)

410

glucosamine. There was, in addition, a second peak of
apparently lower molecular weight but of greater radioactivity
(Figure 2).

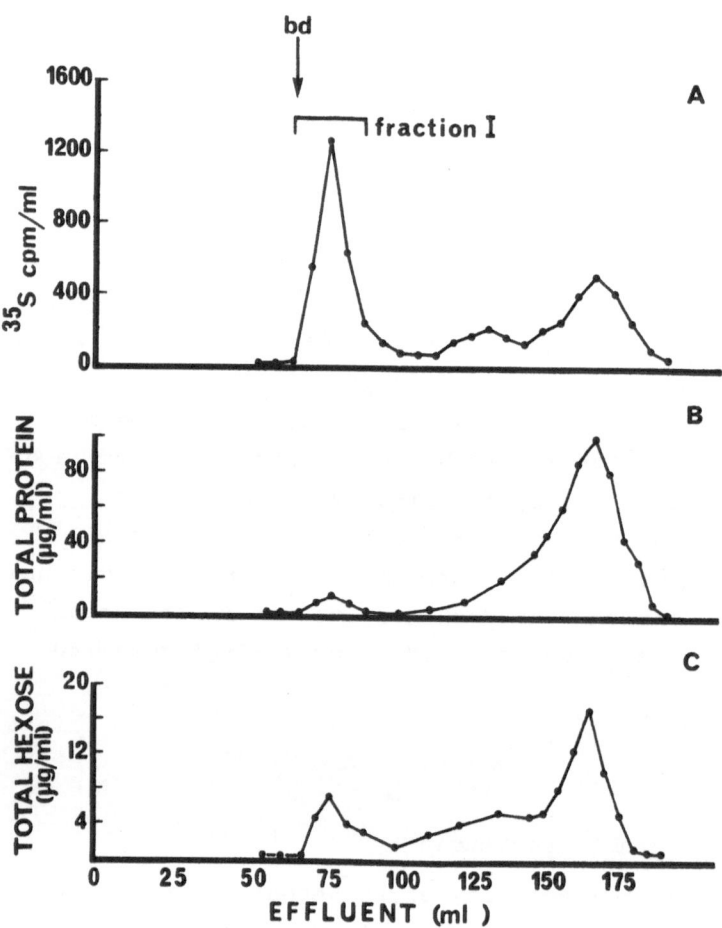

Fig. 1. Elution of ^{35}S-radioactivity from a 2.6 x 40 cm Sepharose 4B
column (panel A) after application of washings from a normal
rat injected 5 hours previously with (^{35}S)-Na$_2$SO$_4$. Also shown
are the protein (panel B) and hexose (panel C) content of each
fraction. The first peak (Fraction I) eluted in the void volume
which was determined by Blue Dextran 2 000 (bd).

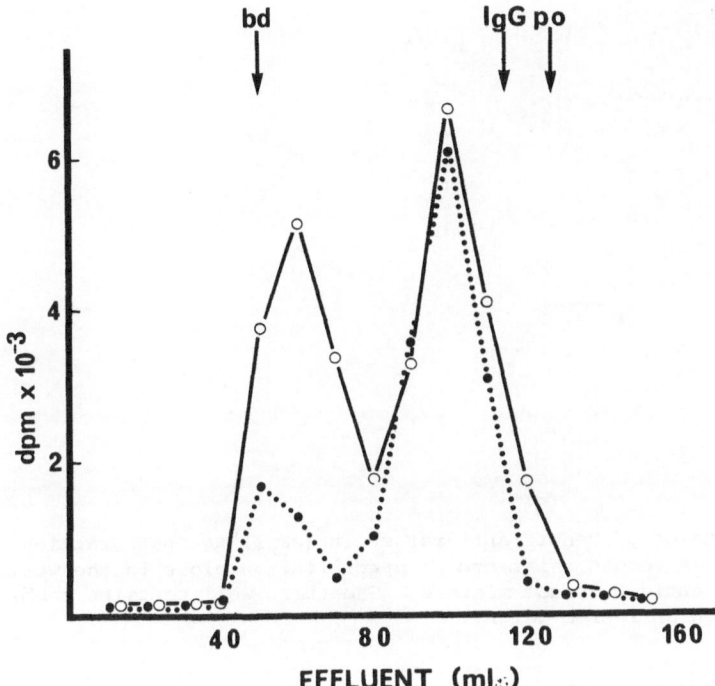

Fig. 2. Elution of acid-precipitable ^{14}C-radioactivity from a 1.6 x 70 cm Sepharose 4B column, after application of 2.5 ml of pooled, concentrated normal (● .... ●) or day 13 post infection (O ———————— O) gut washings. The void volume was determined with Blue Dextran 2 000 and the elution of ovine IgG and horse-radish peroxidase (po) is also shown.

Immunodiffusion of rabbit antisera raised against Fraction I from normal rats gave a major precipitin line and a second very weak arc of precipitation closer to the well containing antigen (Figure 3). These two precipitin lines were also present when the antiserum was tested against Fraction I isolated from *Nippostrongylus*-infected rats. However, immunodiffusion of the antiserum against concentrated gut washings from normal and infected rats revealed only one major line of precipitation.

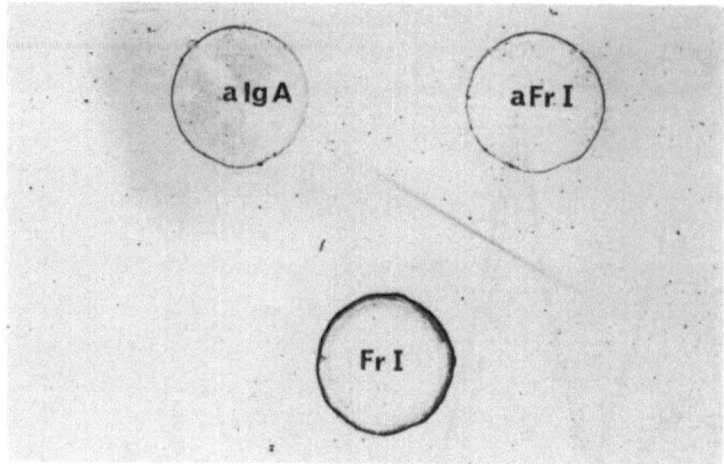

Fig. 3. Immunodiffusion of rabbit anti-rat mucin (aFrI) against Fraction I
(5 mg/ml). A second faint arc of precipitation close to the well
containing antigen is not visible. The third well contains rabbit
anti-rat IgA antiserum (aIgA).

Polyacrylamide gel electrophoresis of Fraction I from
normal rats revealed, after PAS staining, a major band at the
origin of the gel and second band which had migrated 2 - 3 mm
into the gel (Figure 4). After staining with Coomassie blue a
protein band was visible at the origin of the gel only
(Figure 4). Fraction I isolated from infected rats 8 or 13
days after challenge revealed identical patterns of staining
(Figure 4) except that an additional protein band was detected
1 - 2 cm from the origin of the gel (Figure 4).

Immunoperoxidase staining of sections from normal and
Nippostrongylus-infected gut (Figure 5) demonstrated that the
rabbit antiserum raised against Fraction I, stained goblet
cells and associated mucus exclusively. No staining was
observed when normal rabbit serum was substituted for immune
serum, and the intensity of the staining was markedly reduced
although not completely abolished after immune serum had been
pre-incubated with Fraction I.

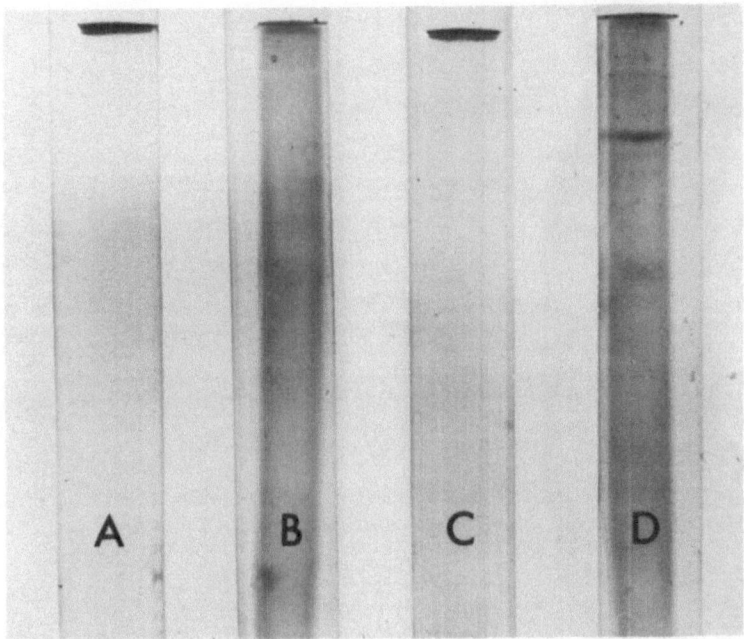

Fig. 4.   Polyacrylamide disc gel electrophoresis of Fraction I from
          Sepharose 4B chromatography.   100 μ g samples purified from
          normal gut washings (A and B) and from day 13 post infection
          washings (C and D) were applied to 4% acrylamide gels in 0.15 M
          Tris-borate buffer pH 8.6.   Gels A and C were stained with
          periodic acid-Schiff for carbohydrates and samples B and D were
          stained with Coomassie blue for protein.

The present results are in good agreement with the more
detailed findings of Forstner and associates (Forstner et al.,
1973a; Forstner et al., 1973b).   These workers have demonstrated that the high molegular weight glycoprotein excluded
by sepharose 4B consists exclusively of rat mucin, consequently
Fraction I described in the present paper will be referred to
as soluble mucin.

414

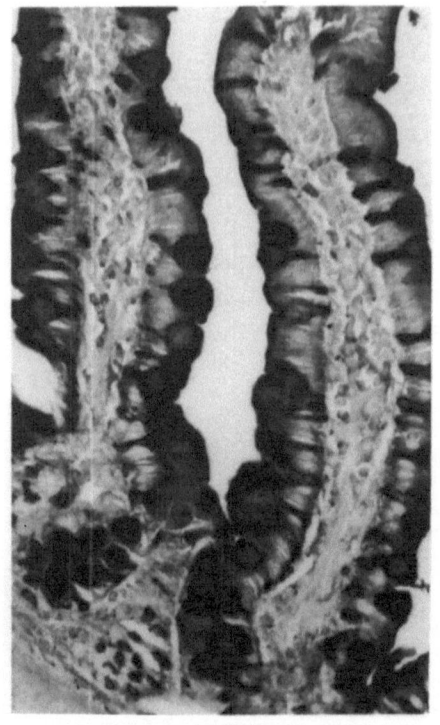

Fig. 5. Immunoperoxidase staining of parasitised (day 13 p.i.) intestine
to reveal the tissue specificity of the rabbit antiserum raised
against Fraction I. Note that specific staining is confined to
the goblet cells and to the epithelial surface x 250.

Turnover of soluble mucin in normal and parasitised rats

Intestinal secretions were harvested from groups of 4
normal rats, 1, 2, 4 and 6 h after injection of isotope by
washing as previously described. The radioactivity incorporated
into acid-precipitable glycoprotein is shown in Figure 6 and,
after sepharose 4B fractionation of pooled samples, the
proportion of the radioactivity present in soluble mucin was
maximal 2 - 4 h after injection (Figure 6). For this reason,
a four hour period after injection of isotope was chosen for
recovering intestinal secretions from *Nippostrongylus*-infected
rats.

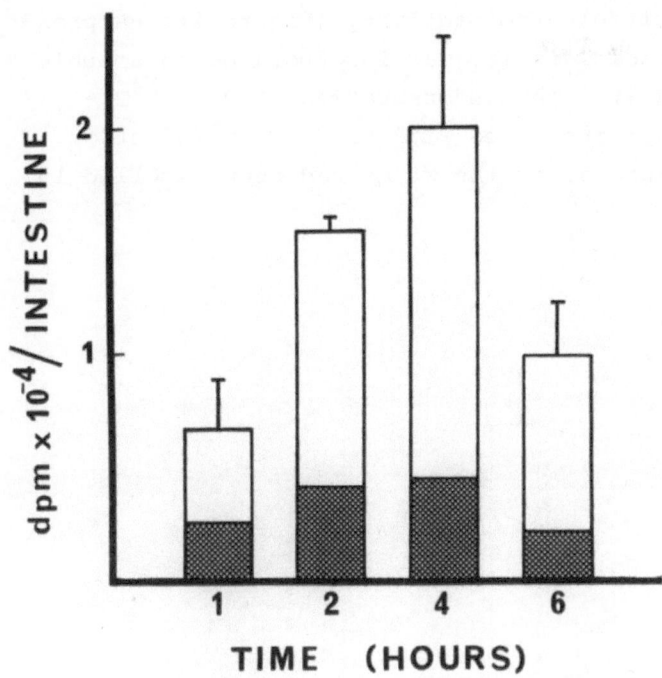

Fig. 6. Incorporation of $(1-^{14}C)$-glucosamine into acid-precipitable gut washings from normal rats (open histogram) is shown together with the proportion of the radioactivity in the sepharose 4B - excluded Fraction I (shaded areas) at intervals after intravenous injection of isotope.

Days 8, 11, 13 and 15 post-infection (p.i.) with *Nippostrongylus brasiliensis* were considered suitable for recovery of intestinal secretions since they coincide with the peak of egg laying activity (day 8) and loss of fecundity by the worms (day 11), with expulsion of the parasite (day 13), and post-expulsion recovery (day 15) in $(PVG/c \times DA)F_1$ rats (Nawa and Miller, 1978).

When compared with normal rats (Figure 7) there was a significant increase in the incorporation of radioactivity into acid-precipitable gut washings recovered from infected rats 8 (P < 0.05), 11 (P < 0.01), 13 (P < 0.005), and 15 (P < 0.01) days p.i. (Figure 7). Sepharose 4B chromatography of pooled

416

samples from normal and from infected rats revealed 2 major
peaks of acid-precipitable radioactivity (Figure 2). Approximately 20% of the radioactivity was incorporated in soluble
mucin (Figures 2 and 7). The incorporation of D-(1-^{14}C)-
glucosamine into mucin increased with time after infection
(Figure 7) but declined after the worms had been expelled 15
days p.i.

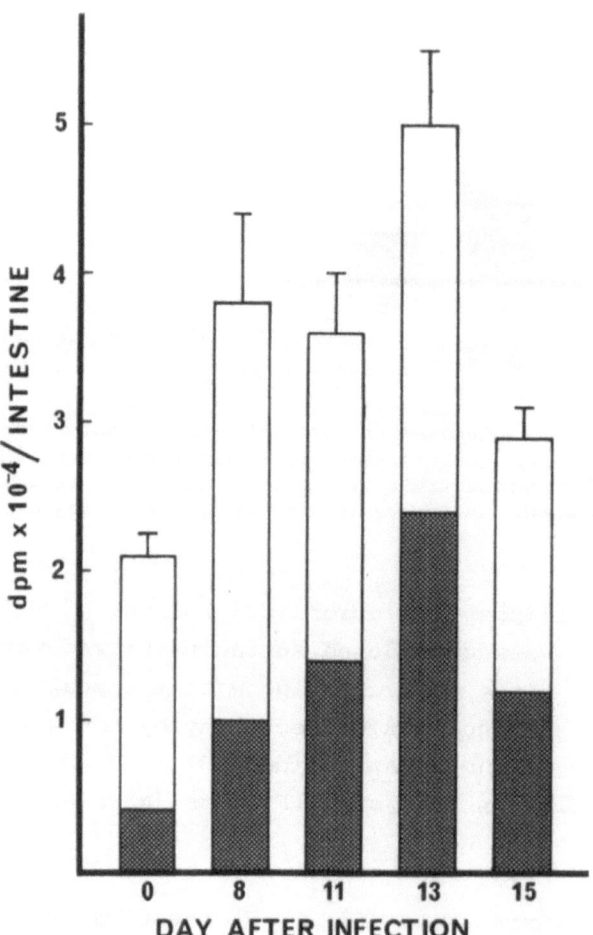

Fig. 7.   Incorporation of (1-^{14}C)-glucosamine into acid-precipitable gut
washings from normal rats and from rats on various days post-
infection with *N. brasiliensis* (open histograms). The proportion
of acid-precipitable radioactivity in soluble mucin (Fraction I) is
represented by the shaded areas.

These results demonstrate that there is a significant increase in the incorporation of D-(1-^{14}C)-glucosamine into intestinal secretions of parasitised rats. Furthermore, it would appear that the maximum incorporation of radioactivity into soluble mucin occurs thirteen days post infection.

Distribution of soluble mucin in the worms

Paraffin sections of parasitised rat intestine, stained with Alcian blue-PAS contained some cross sections of the parasites. The worms were frequently enveloped in mucin and the gut of the parasite itself sometimes contained mucin-like materials. Periodic acid and trypsin treated sections of worms were, therefore, stained to reveal soluble mucins by the immuno-peroxidase technique. The appropriate controls (see earlier) were included (Figure 8). Specific immunoperoxidase staining of the gut was present 30 - 50% of the worms recovered 8 days p.i. (Figure 9) but on days 11 and 13 less than 10% of the worms contained detectable mucin and the staining was much weaker.

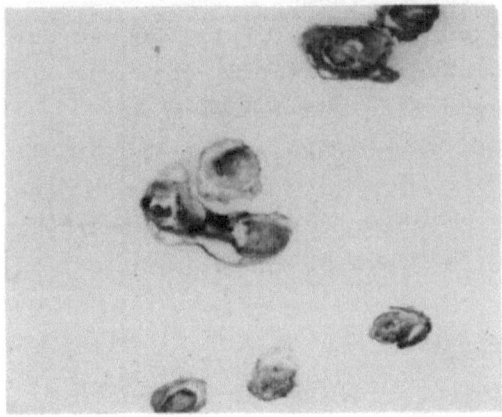

Fig. 8. Cross-sections of 8 day old adult *N. brasiliensis* worms stained with normal rabbit serum and sheep F(ab^1)$_2$ anti-rabbit Fab conjugated to peroxidase. Note absence of specific staining after incubation with substrate x 250.

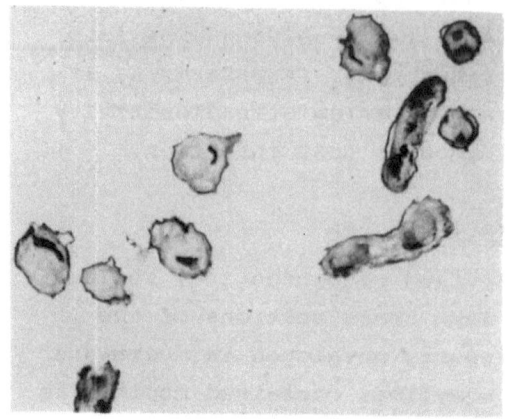

Fig. 9. Specific immunoperoxidase labelling of the gut lumens of 8 day
old worms stained with rabbit anti-rat mucin (Fraction I) and
with peroxidase-labelled sheep $(F(ab')_2$ anti rabbit Fab x 250.

Formalin and Carnoy fixed sections of normal rat intestine,
when stained with WGA-alkaline phosphatase, revealed strong
staining of goblet cell mucin. This is in agreement with
published findings (Etzler, 1979). When Carnoy-fixed sections
of worms were stained with same lectin conjugate there was
strong labelling of the parasite gut (Figure 10) in the pattern
described for immuno-peroxidase. When the lectin-conjugate
was mixed with 1M N-Acetyl-D glucosamine the staining was
abolished.

These findings suggest that soluble mucin is ingested by
parasites early during the first few days of infection.

Rapid worm expulsion from immune rats

Immature adult worms and fourth stage larvae recovered 4
days after infection were injected intraduodenally into naive
and immune recipient rats. Preliminary experiments established
that 17 - 18 days after primary subcutaneous challenge with
4 000 - 6 000 l_3 more than 80% of a secondary challenge given
intraduodenally was expelled from the small intestine within
4 hours. The results of 3 such experiments are shown in
Table 1.

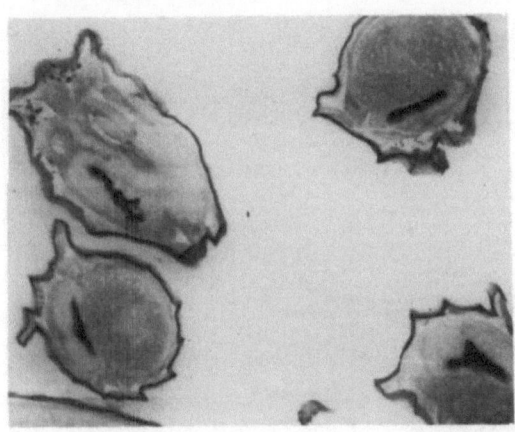

Fig. 10.   Staining of 8 day old worms with wheat germ agglutinin
conjugated to alkaline phosphatase. There is labelling of
the gut lumens in some of the parasites x 400.

The injected worms remained established in the anterior
third of the small intestine throughout the course of the
experiment in normal control rats (Figure 11). The worms
were located in the same region thirty minutes after challenge
in immune rats but, after 2 hours, they had moved into the
posterior half of the intestine and, after a further 2 hours,
less than 10% of the injected dose remained (Figure 11).

Examination of intestines of rats which had not previously
been infected revealed, at all stages after challenge, that the
worms were in close contact with the mucosa and most had some
portion of their bodies embedded between the spatulate villi.
This was readily observed in sections of the parasitised regions
of the gut where there were numerous cross sections of worms
lying between the villi (Figure 12). There were, however, some
parasites apparently lying free in the lumen of the jejunum
(Table 1).

420

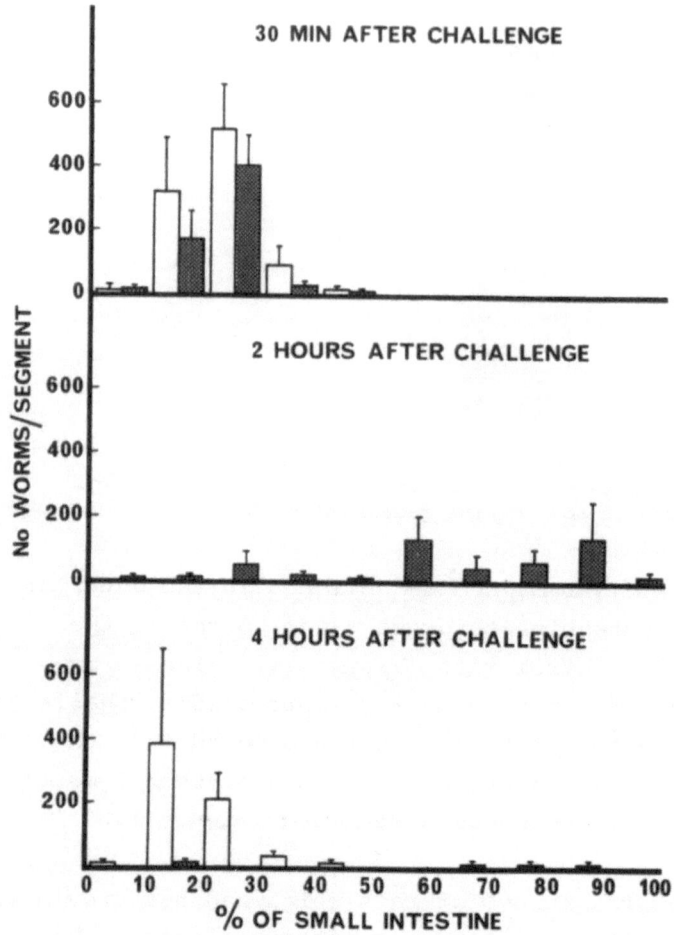

Fig. 11. Distribution of the parasites in normal (open histogram) and immune gut (shaded histogram) 30 minutes, 2 hours and 4 hours after intraduodenal challenge with 1 000 day 4 worms.

TABLE 1

EXPULSION OF *N. brasiliensis* FROM IMMUNE RATS; GOBLET CELL CHANGES AND LOCALISATION OF THE PARASITE

Group (n)	Challenge dose	Worm burden ± SE	Goblet cell discharge	Worm Localisation		
				Mucosa[a]	Lumen[b] (free)	Lumen[c] (in mucus)
Control (5)	500	418 ± 62	±	+++	++	±
Immune (5)	500	55 ± 16	±	+	+	+++
Control (6)	1 000	746 ± 44	+[d]	+++	++	±
Immune (6)	1 000	36 ± 26	+	+	+	+++
Control (4)	2 000	> 1 600	+[d]	+++	++	±
Immune (4)	2 000	113 ± 58	+++	+	+	+++

(a) Attached to mucosa

(b) Free in gut lumen

(c) Entrapped in mucus

(d) Goblet cell discharge localised in vicinity of parasites

Stereo-microspic examination of immune gut revealed the parasites bathed in fluid and lying free in the lumen 30 minutes after challenge. Very few of the worms had penetrated between the villi. This was confirmed in frozen, Carnoy- (Figure 13) and formalin-fixed sections where parasite profiles were predominantly located in the intestinal lumen. Two and 4 hours after challenge the worms were enveloped in globules and strands of viscous mucus (Figure 14) in the lumen of the posterior jejunum and ileum (Table 1).

The different localisation of parasites in normal and immune rats was further emphasised in an experiment in which the intestines were removed and divided in half 2 hours after challenge with 2 000 worms. Each half was washed through with 5 ml phosphate buffer (Lake et al., 1980) and 10 ml air and then drawn through damp cotton wool held lightly between fore-finger and thumb to dislodge adherent mucus. Relatively few worms were recovered from normal rats, the bulk of the population remained attached to the jejunal mucosa. By contrast, the majority of worms in immune rats were recovered in the washings, and were enveloped in strings and globules of mucus which was not readily solubilised in buffer. Very few worms remained attached to the mucosa (Table 1).

These findings demonstrate that immune rats will, when challenged intraduodenally with *N. brasiliensis*, expel the worms very rapidly. The latter are apparently unable to attach to the mucosa and become enveloped in mucus.

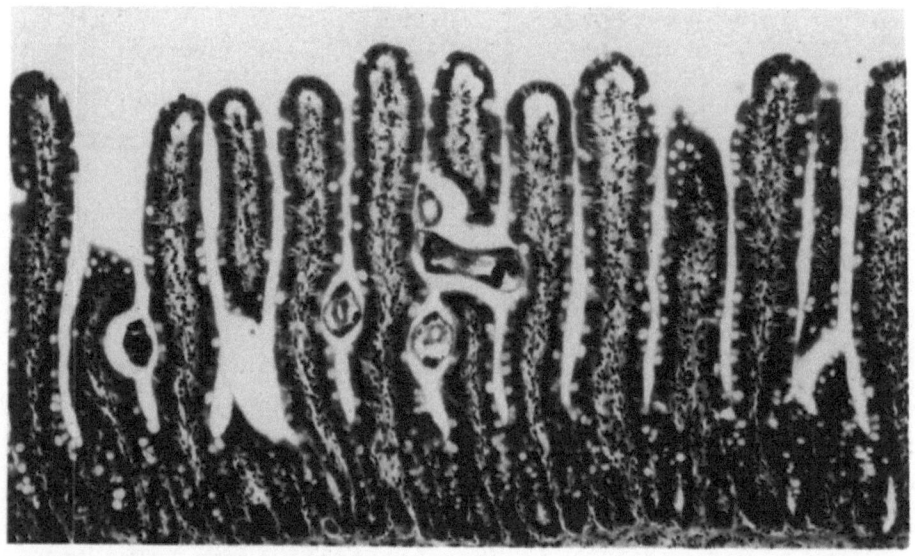

Fig. 12. Carnoy-fixed section of normal intestine 30 minutes after challenge with 2 000 worms. Note that parasites lie in the intervillous spaces x 120.

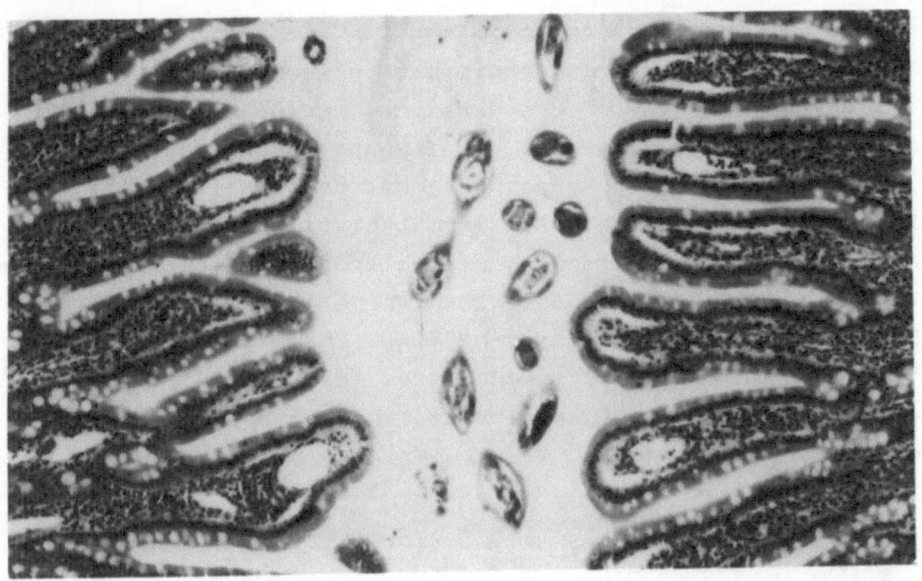

Fig. 13. Section of immune gut 30 minutes after challenge with 2 000
worms. The parasites are confined to the lumen of the jejunum.
x 120.

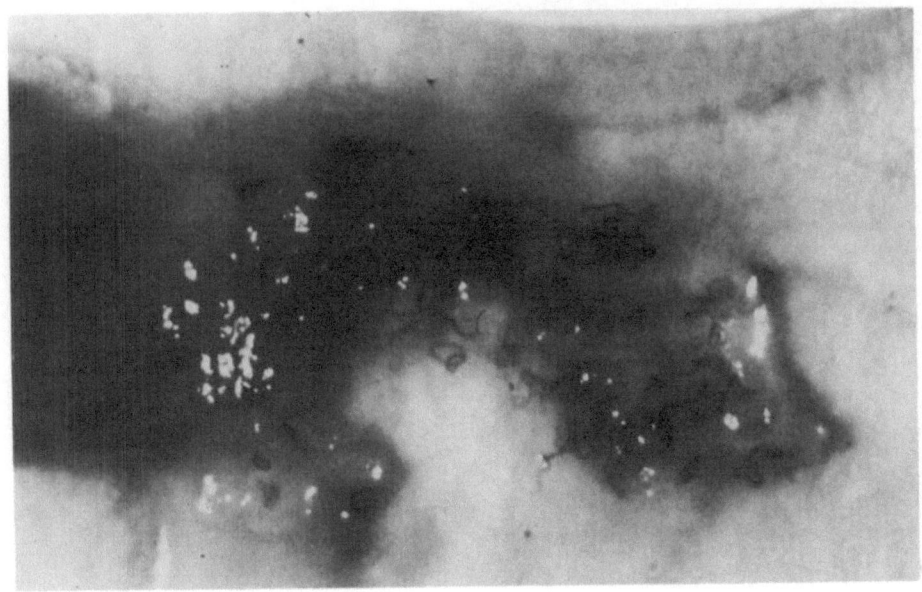

Fig. 14. Envelopment of worms in intestinal mucus 2 hours after challenge
of an immune rat x 5.

Morphology of goblet cells during rapid worm expulsion

Goblet cells in normal recipients of worms were unaltered except in the vicinity of the parasites where there was localised discharge (Table 1). In immune rats given a dose of 500 worms, goblet cell changes were not obvious (Table 1). Following infection with 1 000 worms the villous goblet cells were depleted 4 hours after challenge and, in immune recipients of 2 000 parasites there was extensive goblet cell discharge within 30 minutes at all sites examined, both in snap frozen sections and in formalin-fixed tissues (Figure 15, Table 1). Oedema of the villus also occurred with this challenge dose (Figure 15).

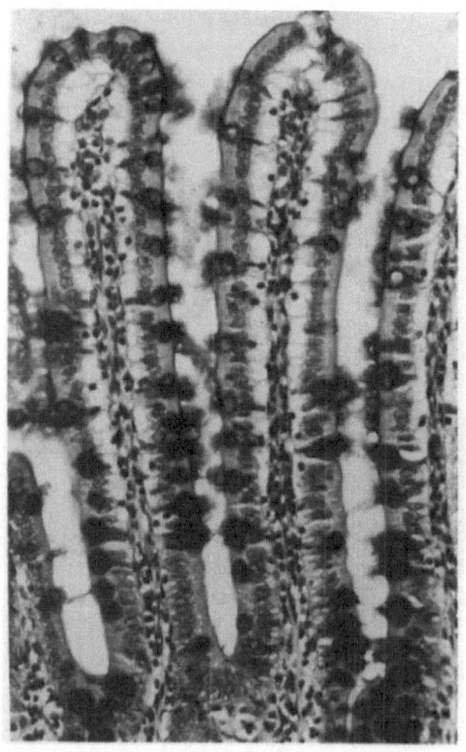

Fig. 15.   Goblet cell discharge and villus oedema following challenge
with 2 000 worms 30 minutes previously x 250.

DISCUSSION

Previous studies (Forstner, 1970; Forstner et al., 1973 a and b) have demonstrated a mucin glycoprotein in rat intestine with a molecular weight of 2×10^6 which was readily isolated from homogenates of intestinal scrapings or from intestinal washings by Sepharose 4B chromatography. By using similar methods we have also demonstrated a high molecular weight fraction (Fraction I) from Sepharose 4B chromatography which incorporates D-$(1-^{14}C)$ glucosamine and ^{35}S. The carbohydrate and protein content together with the staining properties of this fraction after polyacrylamide gel electrophoresis suggest that it is a glycoprotein closely resembling the mucin fraction identified and characterised by Forstner et at., 1973 a and b. Further support for this relationship is provided by the specificity for goblet cells of the antiserum raised against this fraction. Consequently it is reasonable to assume that Fraction I is predominantly soluble mucin.

Judging from the rate of incorporation of D-$(1-^{14}C)$ glucosamine into acid-precipitable material from intestinal secretions, *N. brasiliensis* has a profound effect on glycoprotein synthesis in the gut. This may be related both to the more rapid turnover of epithelial cells (Symons, 1965) and to increased rates of mucus synthesis. Although increased levels of incorporation were observed at all stages after infection. Consequently it seems likely that mucin turnover is maximal at about the time of worm expulsion which occurs between days 11 and 13 (Nawa and Miller, 1978). This is in good agreement with histological studies which show goblet cell numbers to be greatly increased at this time (Miller and Nawa, 1979).

It must be stressed that turnover studies of this type do not identify all of the products of the goblet cells and, in particular, those mucins which are less readily solubilised or are degraded. The rate of isotope incorporation may also be affected by qualitative changes in the composition of mucin. Furthermore, the effect of markedly increased rates of propulsion of intestinal fluids in parasitised gut (Castro et al., 1976) on the passage of intestinal mucus into the large bowel has yet to be assessed. Nevertheless, the increased radioactivity of the mucin fraction in parasitised rats at a stage when goblet cell differentiation is maximal would be consistent with an increased turnover of mucin at this time.

The presence of goblet cell mucin in the gut lumen of the parasites is not surprising since *N. brasiliensis* is thought to dwell and feed within the lumen of the jejunum rather than in the tissues (Symons, 1976). However, it is interesting to note that mucin was less readily detected in the worms later in infection. The parasites at this stage have been irreversibly damaged (Ogilvie and Hockley, 1968) and it is possible that they are less able to feed. Alternatively there may be an alteration in the solubility of the mucin. Both of these changes may have implications regarding the survival of parasite, but the relatively slow rate at which the worms are lost during spontaneous cure does not permit ready analysis of the events which cause worm expulsion.

This difficulty in assessing the functions of mucin during spontaneous cure led us to search for a model of rapid expulsion in which mucosal changes could be more readily visualised. Rapid expulsion of challenge infections from immune animals has been described for several host-parasite systems (Askenase, 1980). Of particular significance is recent work by Lee and Ogilvie (1980) who demonstrated that the exsheathed larvae of *Trichinella spiralis*, when injected intraduodenally into immune rats, are unable to penetrate the mucous barrier and are rapidly expelled. *In vitro* experiments have established that mucus, together with both specific and non-specific serum-derived factors, traps viable larvae (Lee and Ogilvie, 1980). These results indicate that mucus may play a primary role in preventing the establishment of challenge infections in immune gut.

There were a number of similarities between the system described by Lee and Ogilvie (1980) and the rapid expulsion phenomenon occurring in rats resistant to *N. brasiliensis*. Thus, the worms failed to penetrate between the villi and were eliminated within 4 hours of challenge, whereas they established between the villi within 30 minutes in normal control rats. The fact that the worms, as they moved posteriorly, were enveloped in viscid mucus would suggest *a priori* that mucus has a trapping function during the expulsion process. However, such observations must be treated with some caution since it is possible that the mucin is derived from the posterior half of the intestine and only envelopes the worms after they fail to establish in the jejunum.

Goblet cell changes were readily detected following a challenge dose of 1 000 - 2 000 worms when there was extensive discharge 30 minutes after challenge in immune rats. By contrast, goblet cell discharge was localised in the vicinity of the parasites in control rats. These observations suggest that although the mucous barrier may in itself prevent the establishment of small numbers (i.e. < 500) of parasites, the antigenic load with large numbers may be sufficient to trigger anaphylactic release of goblet cell mucins. Since it is now established that anaphylactic release of mucus can occur following oral immunisation and challenge with soluble antigens (Lake et al., 1980), our present work is directed to examining whether such events occur in immune rats challenged with *N. brasiliensis* .

ACKNOWLEDGEMENTS

We thank Judy Harriden, Graham Wallace and Jim Williams for technical assistance and Brian Easter for photographic assistance.

428

REFERENCES

Ackert, J.E. and Edgar, S.E., 1938. Goblet cells and age resistance to
    parasitism. J. Parasit. 24, 13.

Askenase, P.A., 1980. Immunopathology of parasitic diseases: Involvement
    of basophils and mast cells. Springer Seminars in Immunopathology
    2, 417.

Avrameas S., 1969. Coupling of enzymes to proteins with glutaraldehyde.
    Use of the conjuga tes for the detection of antigens and antibodies.
    Immunochemistry 6, 43.

Burstone, M.S., 1962. Enzyme Histochemistry. Academic Press, New York.

Castro, G.A., Badial-Aceves, F., Smith, J.W., Dudric, S.J., and
    Weisbrodt, N.W., 1976. Altered small bowel propulsion associated
    with parasitism. Gastroenterology 71, 620.

Dineen, J.K., Gregg, P., Windon, R.G., Donald, A.D. and Kelly, J.D., 1977.
    The role of immunologically specific and non-specific components of
    resistance in cross-protection to intestinal nematodes.   Int. J.
    Parasit. 7, 211.

Dobson, C., 1967. Changes in the protein content of the serum and
    intestinal mucus of sheep with reference to the histology of the
    gut and immunological response to *Oesophagostomum columbianum*
    infections. Parasitology 57, 201.

Dubois, M., Gilles, K.A., Hamilton, J.K., Rebers, P.A. and Smith, F., 1956.
    Colorimetric method for determination of sugars and related
    substances. Anal. Chem. 28, 350.

Etzler, M.E., 1979. Lectins as probes in studies of intestinal
    glycoproteins and glycolipids. Am. J. Clin. Nutr. 32, 133.

Forstner, G.G., 1970. $(1-^{14}C)$ glucosamine incorporation by subcellular
    fractions of small intestinal mucosa.   Identification by precursor
    labeling of three functionally distinct glycoprotein classes.
    J. Biol. Chem. 245, 3584.

Forstner, J.F., Jabbal, I. and Forstner, G.G., 1973b. Goblet cell mucin
    of rat small intestine. Chemical and physical characterisation.
    Can. J. Biochem. 51, 1154.

Forstner, J.F., Taichman, N., Kalnins, V. and Forstner, G., 1973a.
    Intestinal goblet cell mucus: isolation and identification by
    immunofluorescence of a goblet cell glycoprotein. J. Cell. Sci. 12,
    585.

Frick, L.P. and Ackert, J.E., 1948. Further studies on duodenal mucus as a factor in age resistance of chickens to parasitism. J. Parasit. 34, 192.

Graham, R.C., Jnr. and Karnovsky, M.J., 1966. The early stages of absorption of injected peroxidase in the proximal tubules of mouse kidney: ultrastructural cytochemistry by a new technique. J. Histochem. Cytochem. 14, 291.

Heyderman, E. and Neville, A.M., 1977. A shorter immunoperoxidase technique for the demonstration of carcinoembryonic antigen and other cell products. J. Clin. Path. 30, 138.

Lake, A.M., Bloch, K.J., Sinclair, K.J. and Walker, W.A., 1980. Anaphylactic release of intestinal goblet cell mucus immunology, 39, 173.

Lee, G.B. and Ogilvie, B.M., 1980. The mucus layer in intestinal nematode infections. 81st Ross Conference 'Mucosal Immune Systems' (in press).

Lowry, O.H., Rosebrough, N.J., Farr, A.L. and Randall, R.J., 1951. Protein measurement with the Folin phenol reagent. J. Biol. Chem. 193, 265.

Miller, H.R.P. and Nawa, Y., 1979. Immune regulation of intestinal goblet cell differentiation. Specific induction of nonspecific protection against helminths? Nouv. Rev. Fr. Hematol. 21, 31.

Nakane, P.K and Kawaoi, 1974. Peroxidase-labeled antibody a new method of conjugation. J. Histochem. Cytochem 22, 1084.

Nawa Y. and Miller, H.R.P., 1978. Protection against *Nippostrongylus brasiliensis* by adoptive immunisation with immune thoracic duct lymphocytes Cell. Immunol. 37, 51.

Ogilvie, B.M. and Hockley, D.J., 1968. Effects of immunity on *Nippostrongylus brasiliensis* adult worms: reversible and irreversible changes in infectivity, reproduction and morpholgy. J. Parasit. 54, 1073.

Ogilvie, B.M. and Love, R.J., 1974. Co-operation between antibodies and cells in immunity to a nematode parasite. Transplant Rev. 19, 147.

Symons, L.E.A., 1965. Kinetics of the epithelial cells and morphology of the villi and crypts in the jejunum of the rat infected by the nematode *Nippostrongylus brasiliensis*. Gastroenterology 49, 158.

Symons, L.E.A., 1976. Scanning electron microscopy of the jejunum of the rat infected by the nematode *Nippostrongylus brasiliensis*. Int. J. Parasit. 6, 107.

430

Uber, C.L., Roth, R.L. and Levy, D.A., 1980. Expulsion of *Nippostrongylus brasiliensis* by mice deficient in mast cells. Nature (in press).

Wakelin, D., 1978. Immunity to intestinal parasites. Nature (Lond.) 273, 617.

Wells, P.D., 1962. Mastcell, eosinophil and histamine levels in *Nippostrongylus*-infected rats. Exp. Parasit. 12, 82.

Wells, P.D., 1963. Mucin secreting cells in rats infected with *Nippostrongylus brasiliensis*. Expt. Parasit. 14, 15.

DISCUSSION

J. Clamp *(UK)*

 I don't know what the chemistry of mustard oil is but I presume it contains sulphydryl groups which give it its characteristic smell and so on, so presumably it is breaking down the disulphate linkages?

H. Miller *(UK)*

 This is just ordinary English mustard.

J. Clamp

 Does anyone know about the chemistry of mustard? I think it contains mercaptons.

K. Petzoldt *(FRG)*

 Is there any possibility that there are interactions between the components of the mucus and secreted mediators or components of cells under the mucus, for example, lymphokines?

H. Miller

 I think you would have to look at the lymphokines involved. The other possibility is that there are changes in the chemistry of the mucus as it is released. Certainly from our observations it is very soluble at 30 minutes but very insoluble at two hours after challenge. In this situation we wonder if there are, for example, some proteases affecting the composition of the mucus. We have been working on a mast cell protease which is present in atypical mast cells of the gut of the rat. We find that this protease is also present in goblet cells in immune rats. The protease is a very basic protein and presumably it just binds to the acid glycoprotein. How it gets there, we don't know. The possibility is that this might have some action on the mucus it-self as it is released and cause it to denature. Perhaps Professor Clamp would like to comment on that.

J. Clamp

I don't think you can talk about denaturation as far as mucus is concerned; you cannot denature mucus in that sense. But most proteases make mucus more soluble because they tend to attack in the naked peptide region. Once you break down the linkages then mucus becomes much more soluble.

Up until now most of us have been hypnotised into thinking that the only important component of mucus is the mucous glycoprotein I was talking about. However, it seems that there may be other proteins present in mucus which are important in modifying its properties. One of these might well be attacked specifically by this protease. You did mention that it does have unusual properties.

H. Miller

Woodbury suggests that it acts upon Type-4 collagen which is basement membrane. So presumably it will have some functional effect on the gut itself in terms of villus morphology.

J. Clamp

The explanation might be more simple. Very concentrated mucus is very difficult to make soluble. Cervical mucus, for example, in the progestational phase is very insoluble, but merely because it is very concentrated. If you shake it for long enough and heat it, it will eventually become soluble. The chains become tangled when it gets very concentrated so it is a time dependent process for the chains to untangle. All you mean by solubility is that it occupies the whole water volume and this takes time. It is not really insoluble, it is a gel; instead of being in the sol phase it is in the gel phase.

J. Soothill   (UK)

Do IgA antibodies to the worms develop, and if so do they sit on the surface of mucus bound to them by the glycoprotein component so that they are specifically wrapped round the worms?

H. Miller

That is certainly a possibility. I am not sure if anybody has actually analysed the IgA specific antibody against
Nippostrongylus. One of the problems with these parasites is their
antigenic complexity. But I am fairly sure that it has been
demonstrated against certain other helminth parasites. Perhaps
Dr. Bazin can comment on that.

H. Bazin   *(Belgium)*

It is quite difficult because you have non-specific binding of antibody.

H. Miller

Lee and Ogilivie have done experiments where they harvest
mucus by the mustard oil technique, either from normal or immune
rats. If they take it from immune rats they can demonstrate
that the *Trichinella* larvae are trapped in the mucus, on an *in
vitro* migration technique. However, if they take normal mucus,
and add normal serum to it, then that is equally as effective
in trapping the larvae. You get about 40% trapping. If you
heat and activate the normal serum then it is no longer effective. So there is a heat labile component in normal serum which
interacts within mucus to trap the larvae. To take it a stage
further, if you take normal mucus and add immune serum, you get
trapping. If you heat and activate the immune serum, that still
causes trapping. So there is a heat stable factor in immune
serum which presumably is antibody. But I am not sure whether
Lee and Ogilvie have classified the antibody that is heat stable
which will interact with the mucin and cause the trapping.

J. Clamp

One has to be awfully careful in adding things to mucus
because you can change its physical properties with a large
number of things. For instance if you add just plasma albumen
you can, in fact, change the composition of mucus and its
properties.

H. Miller

That is entirely feasible. One of the points about
parasitic infections is that in the rapid expulsion phenomenon
you can demonstrate concomitant expulsion of unrelated parasites.
Now, if you have a system whereby you get non-specific factors
released in serum which change the capacity of mucus to trap
worms, then this would be an obvious advantage to the host.

P. Brandtzaeg   (Norway)

I think I have seen some evidence that an excess of
absorbed iron is taken out through the goblet cells. Do you
know anything about the relationship of transferin and ferritin
to mucus?

H. Miller

I don't know anything about it. What about you, Professor
Clamp?

J. Clamp

Iron itself do you mean, or the whole ferritin molecule?

P. Brandtzaeg

Whether it is bound to a transferin or a ferritin - I am
not sure. I think both ferritin and transferin have been localised in the goblet cells by the immunoperoxidase technique.

J. Clamp

I have a feeling that one of the ways of regulating iron
levels in the body is the loss of ferritin from intestinal
cells. It is held there and is lost with the cells rather than
passing into the blood.

K.L. Morgan   (UK)

In the rapid expulsion phenomenon, where you take the
worms from a non-immune animal and put them into an immune animal, are they then killed?

H. Miller

No, they are not. In the period that we have looked at them some of them survive sufficiently to be able to migrate out of the mucus. We haven't looked at the ones that are trapped. The obvious thing to do is to transfer them back into normal animals and see whether they survive. I suspect they are not killed. The worms are very resistant little animals.

H. Bazin

If I remember correctly, when young rats are infected they have a chronic disease. In that case you have no mucus?

H. Miller

Young rats have a persistent infection. We have only done the goblet cell counts. We find that in this situation they do not develop the same number of goblet cells as adults, in fact significantly less than adults. But they are not expelling the worms either. So which comes first?

One thing we do find is that we are unable to immunise the young animals passively, as we can adult animals. We wanted to see if the defect we were detecting in young animals was related to the immune system or perhaps to the epithelium. So we transferred immune serum at the same dose rate. What we found in this situation was that the young animals do not expel the worms as efficiently as the adults. Also, we do not get goblet cell increases in the young animals to anything like the same extent as in the adult.

P. Bradtzaeg

We know that some patients with complete agammaglobulin-aemia, with no antibodies in the gut at all, have no gastro-intestinal disease - due to a normal cell mediated immunity. Is anything known about the number of goblet cells and mucin function in such patients?

H. Miller

I am not aware of anythinq. I would like to see how
agammglobulinaemic patients respond when they get parasitic
infections.

J. Soothill

Giardilamnia is a real problem in patients lacking immunoglobulin. I don't know how similar they would be to the sort
of systems you are talking about. The intestinal biopsies of
agammaglobulinaemic patients certainly have goblet cells.
Whether the numbers are normal or not I wouldn't know.

H. Miller

You would have to look at turnover of mucin.

J. Soothill

Yes, but I don't think that is feasible in humans is it?

H. Miller

I would think it would be difficult. But you could do
some work with intestinal biopsies *in vitro*. Certainly people
have looked at mucus synthesis.

G. Mayrhofer   *(UK)*

May I ask what the role of sulphate is thought to be in
mucus. The reason I ask is that I have been doing quite a lot
of staining of gut recently using Alcian blue. I have formed
the impression that the staining of the goblet cells changes
after infection which might be interpreted as being due to
sulphate.

H. Miller

Yes. I didn't mention that but certainly we seem to find
that during infection the mucins turn from fairly strongly
sulphated by histochemical criteria to more neutral glycoprotein.

J. Bienenstock   *(Canada)*

Does that mean that it is newer?

J. Clamp

Yes, there is some evidence that if you are rapidly synthesising the glycoprotein molecule, you don't have so many of the peripheral sugars. Sialic acid is always in a terminal position, as is fucose. A number of things can change it, certainly infections can, and position in the gut of course. The amount of sialic acid changes as you go down the gut, there is very little in the stomach and there is a great deal in the colon. The ratio of sialic acid to sulphate also changes in various levels of the gut. It is quite complicated.

J. Bienenstock

Does one find in patients or animals with diarrhoea that goblet cell numbers increase, regardless of the type of diarrhoea?

H. Miller

There is no diarrhoea in the rats that we look at. The level of infection that we are looking at is usually about 1 000 worms, so I can't comment at all.

J. Clamp

I don't know about chronic diarrhoea but patients who are chronic laxative takers have an increase in the goblet cell numbers. Presumably this is because of stimulation of the gut.

J. Hall   *(UK)*

May I ask where the goblet cells come from. What is the mechanism behind this rapid increase?

H. Miller

They are generated in the crypt from entero-blasts. No one quite knows what makes a cell differentiate into a goblet cell as opposed to an absorptive cell. One speculation is that

some sort of feedback mechanism operates. Supposing you have
a lot of immune complexes which are causing mucus release, does
mucus depletion, say in the crypt region, in some way influence
cells to differentiate into goblet cells? Is this a possibility?

H. Batten   (UK)

This may occur fairly quickly since young goblet cells
are known to be able to divide.

H. Miller

We have never looked at the division of goblet cells in
our system but I can say that I have never seen a goblet cell
in division on the villus.

H. Batten

No, I mean a crypt goblet cell.

H. Miller

In the crypt it is extremely difficult to count goblet
cells because they are so tightly packed together.

G. Mayrhofer

Is the normal mucous layer provided by the goblet cells?
I seem to remember in histology that there were things called
mucous neck cells.

H. Miller

Quite a lot of mucus is secreted in the stomach and that
is where your neck cells are. There will be some mucus secreted
in the Brunners gland but this will be a different quality.
Presumably, in animals that have gall bladders, there will be
some in the bile. Finally, there is the mucus secreted in the
small intestine. So, I think there would be a whole variety of
sources of mucin.

J. Clamp

It is interesting that the mucous neck cells are about the only mucus producing cells in the stomach which do contain sulphated glycoproteins. So they may produce a slightly different type of mucus.

R. Levinsky (UK)

Do you know if anyone has looked for IgA FC receptors on the mucous cell, which might trigger the release by this complex?

H. Miller

It is a thought I have had, and I have asked several people, including Per Brandtzaeg. Certainly, Per, I have asked you about secretory component in the goblet cells. Would you think the goblet cells might have a receptor for IgA?

R. Levinsky

I think it would be more likely to be FC actually to trigger the release of mucus by immune complex.

H. Miller

Yes, all right, but it would still be a receptor for the complex wouldn't it?

P. Brandtzaeg

I don't think we know the answer.

H. Miller

Have you ever done any experiments to try to remove the sialic acid from the goblet cells with neurominidase, for example, just to see whether there was any acid blocking, or hindrance .....

P. Brandtzaeg

I don't think there is any blocking by ethanol fixation.

J. Clamp

There is a lot of work - this is in respiratory mucus but it is under both nervous and hormonal control, so it is both cholinergic and andronergic. Also, some prostaglandins are quite powerful mucus releasers. So I don't think it has to be a direct effect; it could easily be mediated by some other mechanism.

H. Miller

Does prostaglandin E2 have any effect on mucus?

J. Clamp

I don't know about E2 particularly; the most powerful one is $F_2\alpha$.

Well, that concludes the session - our thanks to the speakers.

CLOSING SESSION

Chairman : J. Bienenstock

IMMUNOGLOBULIN SERUM LEVELS AND POPULATION OF INTESTINAL IgA PLASMA CELLS IN NORMAL AND IMMUNO-DEFICIENT (NUDE - NEONATALLY MU SUPPRESSED - NEONATALLY DELTA SUPPRESSED) RATS

H. Bazin, Bernadette Platteau and R. Pauwels

Experimental Immunology Unit, University of Louvain,
Clos Chapelle aux Champs 30, Brussels 1200

Department of Chest Diseases, Academic Hospital,
De Pintelaan 135, Ghent 9000

Belgium

ABSTRACT

Immunoglobulin serum levels and intestinal IgA containing cell populations of normal or immunodeficient rats have been studied in order to analyse the respective influences of thymus-independent and thymus-dependent natural antigen stimulation on the production of the different immunoglobulin isotypes and especially of IgA. It can be concluded from the results that the production of IgA molecules can be triggered by TI-1, TI-2 and TD antigens. However, under natural antigenic stimulation probably due to the intestinal flora, the synthesis of immunoglobulin is predominantly of the IgG and IgM classes, the IgA isotype being only a minor component.

INTRODUCTION

The presence of large numbers of plasma cells containing IgA in the *lamina propria* of adult mammals can be attributed to antigenic stimulation at the level of the intestinal mucosa. The microbial flora as well as food have been considered as the major stimuli for proliferation of IgA forming cells in the gut. However, studies of the axenic intestinal tract have clearly demonstrated that the normal microbial flora are the most important determining factors in the appearance of the intestinal IgA plasma cells.

The present study was performed in order to analyse the immunoglobulin (Ig) synthesis due to natural antigenic stimulations, and especially the appearance of the intestinal IgA cell population in normal and immunodeficient rats. The respective influences of the thymus-independent and the thymus-dependent antigens on such phenomena have been analysed.

MATERIALS AND METHODS

Animals

Outbred rats, having the Rnu mutation, were purchased from Proefdierencentrum, Leuven, and bred in our animal house, in very clean conventional conditions. Heterozygous females were mated with heterozygous male rats. Pregnant females were isolated before delivery and put into plastic isolators. The same standard conditions of sterility as those used for axenic rodents were applied. Sterile food, water and wood shavings were purchased from Usine d'Alimentation Rationnelle (Villemoisson sur Orge, France).

Suppression protocol

Rabbit anti-mu and anti-delta rat heavy immunoglobulin chains sera were raised by immunisation with purified monoclonal rat immunoglobulins obtained from LOU/C immunocytomas (Bazin et al., 1972; Bazin et al., 1973; Bazin et al., 1978). Monoclonal

IgM proteins of the IR202 and IR968 immunocytomas and monoclonal IgD proteins from the immunocytomas IR731, IR483 and IR504 were employed. The technique of immunisation has already been described in Bazin et al. (1974). Myeloma proteins were isolated from ascitic fluid as described in Rousseaux and Bazin (1979). Monospecificity of the antisera was obtained after appropriate absorptions with serum of germ free rats and the pseudoglobulin fraction of normal rat serum or normal rat serum checked as having very low IgD levels, respectively for the anti-mu and the anti-delta sera. Both antisera and the control normal rabbit serum were then absorbed with rat liver and kidney cells and were then shown not to bind to rat thymic cells by indirect immunofluorescence using a fluorescein isothiocyanate conjugated goat antiserum to rabbit IgA as developing reagent. Finally, the antisera were thoroughly dialysed against phosphate buffered saline (PBS) and sterilised by millipore filtration (0.22 micron filter).

At birth, each litter was divided into two groups, one being injected either with the anti-mu or with the anti-delta sera and the other with the normal rabbit serum. The rats were injected every other day, from day 0 to day 10, and three times a week from day 10 to the end of the experiments. The doses during the first ten days were 0.2 ml/injection/animal and from day 10 on, the doses were increased to 0.3 ml.

Determination of immunoglobulin serum levels

The serum IgM, IgA, IgG1, IgG2a, IgG2b and IgG2c levels were determined by single radial immunodiffusion. IgD and IgE serum concentrations were obtained by radio-immuno-assays as described by Bazin et al. (1978) and Pauwels et al. (1977). Serum samples were analysed separately. IgM, IgA, IgD, IgE, IgG1, IgG2a, IgG2b and IgG2c standards were LOU/C monoclonal purified proteins (Rousseaux and Bazin, 1978; Bazin et al., 1978) of the same isotype but different from those used for raising the antisera. Antisera were raised as already described in Bazin et al. (1974).

Immunofluorescence

Staining for IgA was carried out as previously described (Mayrhofer et al., 1976). Tissues were prepared in paraffin wax, sectioned and then dewaxed and incubated with a fluorescein isothiocyanate conjugate of goat antibodies anti rat alpha chain. They were examined for fluorescence with a Leitz Ortholux microscope equipped with an Osram HG200 mercury lamp.

RESULTS AND DISCUSSION

Nude rats

The IgA serum levels of nude mice have been found to be lower than in their control animals (Salomom and Bazin, 1972; Luzzati and Jacobson, 1972; Bloemmen and Eyssen, 1973; Pritchard et al., 1973). However, such a result has not been confirmed in nude rats (Bazin et al., 1980). In Tables 1 and 2, the results obtained with groups 2 and B respectively are in agreement with those found for nude mice. Such a discrepancy is probably correlated to the antigenic stimulation to which the animals were submitted. Nevertheless, these results show that the rat IgA immune responses are at least partially thymus-independent.

We found the IgA population of the intestinal tract to be inferior in the nude to that of the control rats but clearly developed and showing that the intestinal IgA production is partially thymus-independent (Figures 1 and 2).

Mu suppressed rats

The isotypic suppression of all immunoglobulin classes by repeated anti μ serum injections has already been described in the mouse and in the chicken species for IgM, IgA, IgE and IgG classes (Manning, 1975; Manning et al., 1976). These observations have been confirmed in the rat species and extended to the IgD class and to four IgG subclasses: IgG1, IgG2a, IgG2b and IgG2c (Bazin et al., 1978). The present data given in Table 1 are in accordance with our previous results (Bazin et al., 1978; Bazin et al., 1980). As compared to group 1 which can be taken

TABLE 1

IMMUNOGLOBULIN SERUM LEVELS OF 55 DAYS OLD NUDE RATS AND THEIR CONTROLS, SUPPRESSED OR NOT BY ANTI RAT MU IMMUNOGLOBULIN HEAVY CHAIN SERUM INJECTIONS.

Group	Rats	Injected with	Number of animals	Immunoglobulin isotypes							
				IgM mg/ml	IgD ng/ml	IgA µg/ml	IgE ng/ml	IgG1 mg/ml	IgG2a mg/ml	IgG2b mg/ml	IgG2c mg/ml
1	Rnu/+	Normal rabbit serum	4	.7±.1[+]	372±39	60±5	692±288	ND[++]	1.3±.3	1.2±.4	1.1±.2
2	Rnu/Rnu	Normal rabbit serum	2	1.2±.1	107±107	30±.0	20±11	ND	0.0±.0	.1±.0	4.8±4.5
3	Rnu/Rnu	Rabbit serum anti-mu chain	6	0.0±.0	399±260	0.0±.0	29±17	ND	0.0±.0	0.0±.0	0.0±.0

+ mean ± standard error of the mean

++ not done

TABLE 2

IMMUNOGLOBULIN SERUM LEVELS OF 55 DAYS OLD NUDE RATS AND THEIR CONTROLS, SOME OF THESE ANIMALS HAVING BEEN SUPPRESSED BY ANTI RAT DELTA IMMUNOGLOBULIN HEAVY CHAIN SERUM INJECTIONS.

Group	Rats	Injected with	Number of animals	Immunoglobulin isotypes							
				IgM mg/ml	IgD ng/ml	IgA µg/ml	IgE ng/ml	IgG1 mg/ml	IgG2a mg/ml	IgG2b mg/ml	IgG2c mg/ml
A	Rnu/+	Normal rabbit serum	7	1.2±.1[+]	1195±294	37±4	162±66	.8±.1	.7±.3	2.9±.3	5.1±2.4
B	Rnu/Rnu	Normal rabbit serum	10	1.1±.1	390±235	13±1	54±47	.2±.2	.0±.0	1.3±.3	6.5±.3
C	Rnu/Rnu	Rabbit serum anti-delta chain	8	1.3±.2	73±53	50±6	5±4	.9±.2	.2±1	2.7±.3	12.6±1.9

+ mean ± standard error of the mean

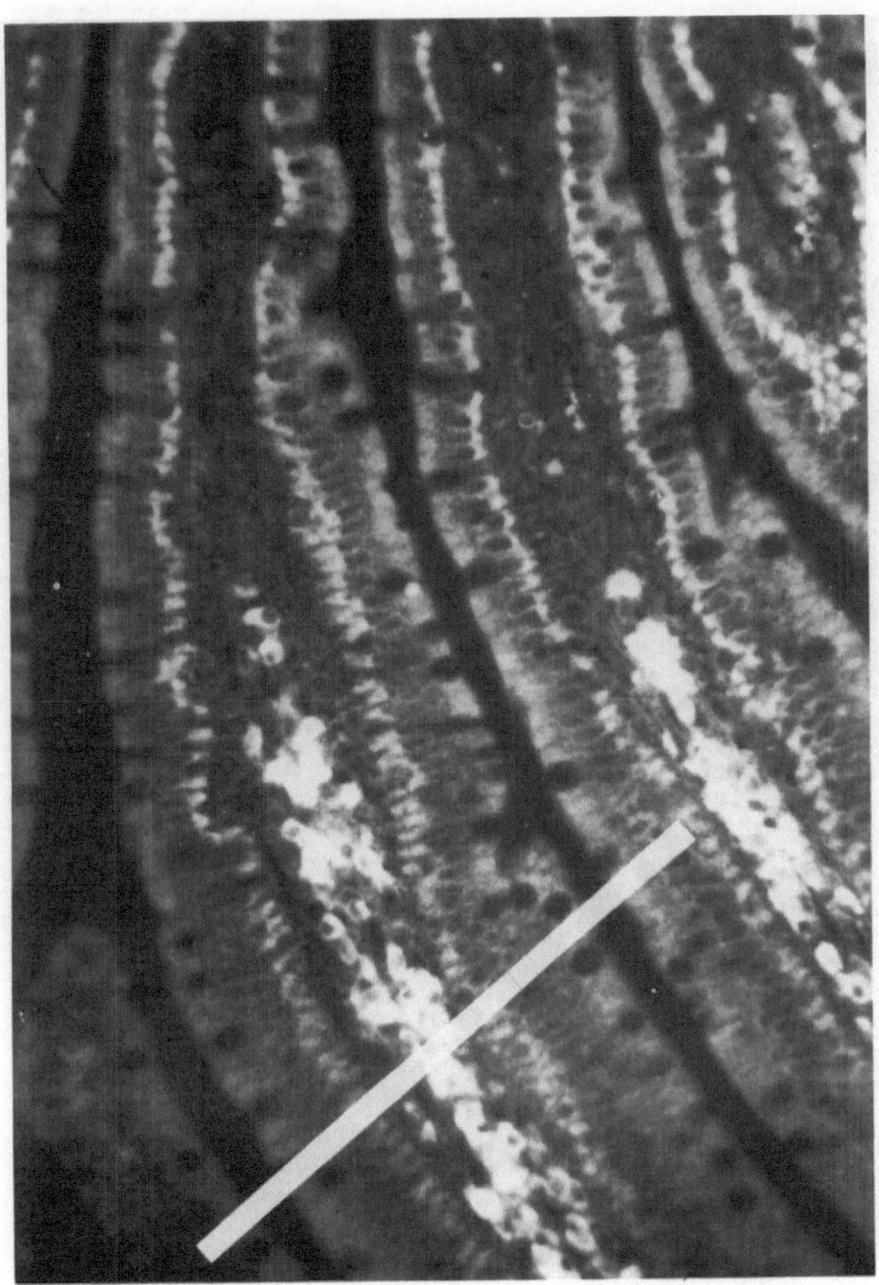

Fig.1. IgA containing plasma cells in the jejunal mucosa of a normal, non-suppressed rat.

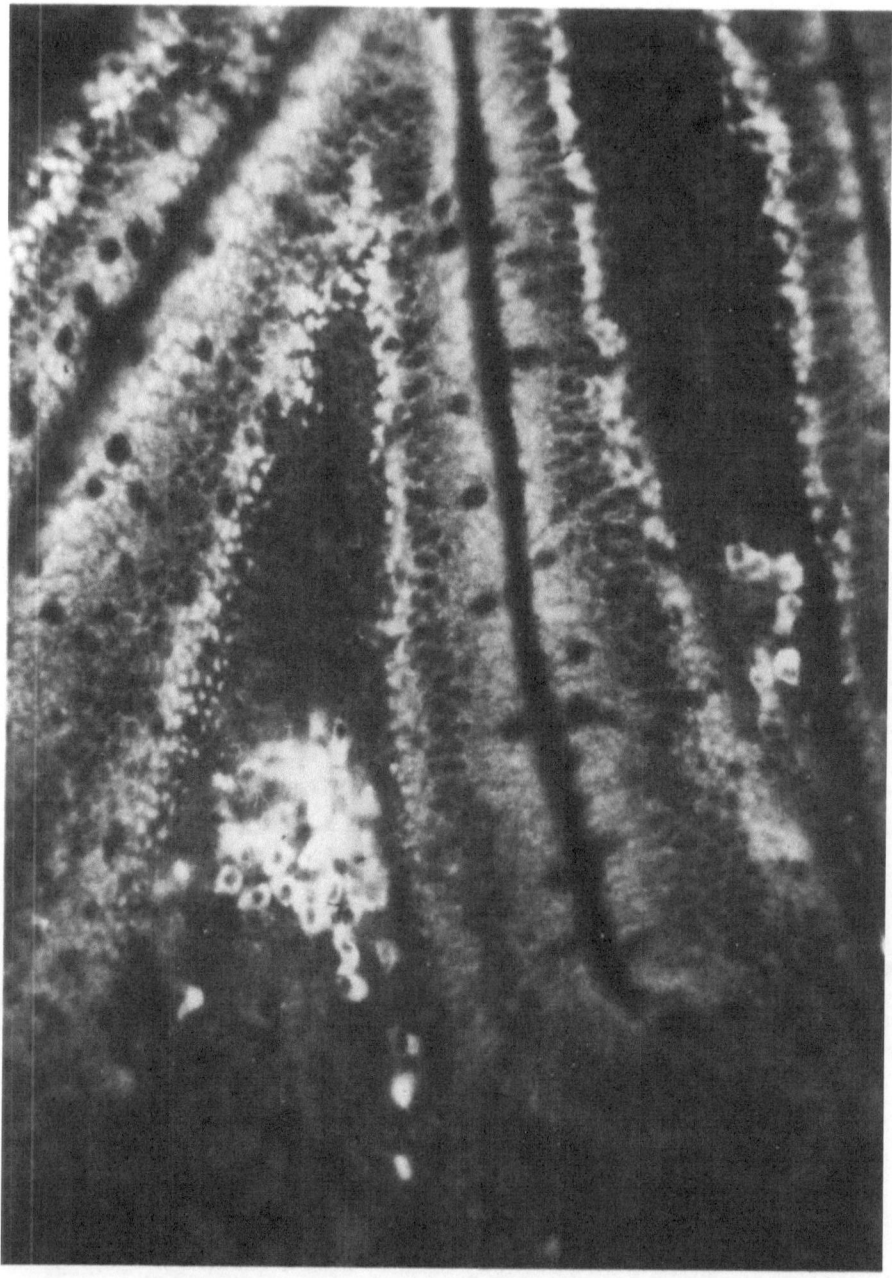

Fig.2. IgA containing plasma cells in the jejunal mucosa of a nude, non-suppressed rat.

as a control, group 3 shows a very small production of immuno-globulin, not demonstrable by the radial immunodiffusion tech-nique, but only by radio-immuno-assay.

The mu suppressed rats had very few, if any, intestinal IgA plasma cells. Figure 3 gives an example of this great depletion. Compared with the mu suppressed group, the control, in this experiment had a normal IgA cell population in its *lamina propria*. Such results are in agreement with those of Lawton et al.(1972) which were obtained in mice.

Delta suppressed rats

The effects of the delta suppression on the immunoglobulin synthesis have been reported: the IgD and the IgE productions were found to be clearly diminished. The different IgG sub-classes were more or less affected, except the IgG2c serum level which was generally increased. The IgM and IgA syntheses were both slightly diminished with respect to their serum levels but significantly so at the lymphocyte membrane level (Bazin et al., 1978). Our present results concern the effects of delta suppression on nude rats. The delta suppressed nude animals showed a clear diminution of their IgD and IgE serum levels but an increase in the IgG2b and IgG2c levels. From immunofluor-escence, it was clear that the intestinal IgA forming population was smaller than that found in the control animals (group A) but comparable to that found in the nude non-suppressed rats (group B), (Figures 2 and 4).

CONCLUSION

Antigens have been divided into three classes: thymus-independent - 1 (TI-1), thymus-independent - 2 (TI-2) and thymus-dependent (TD) (Mosier et al., 1977). The difference between class 1 and class 2 of thymus-independent antigens has been demonstrated by using CBA/N mouse strain (Mosier et al., 1977; Mond et al., 1978). The absence of adult type IgD bearing lymphocytes which can respond to TI-2 antigens seems to be the basis of the CBA/N genetic defect (Mosier et al., 1977; Mond et

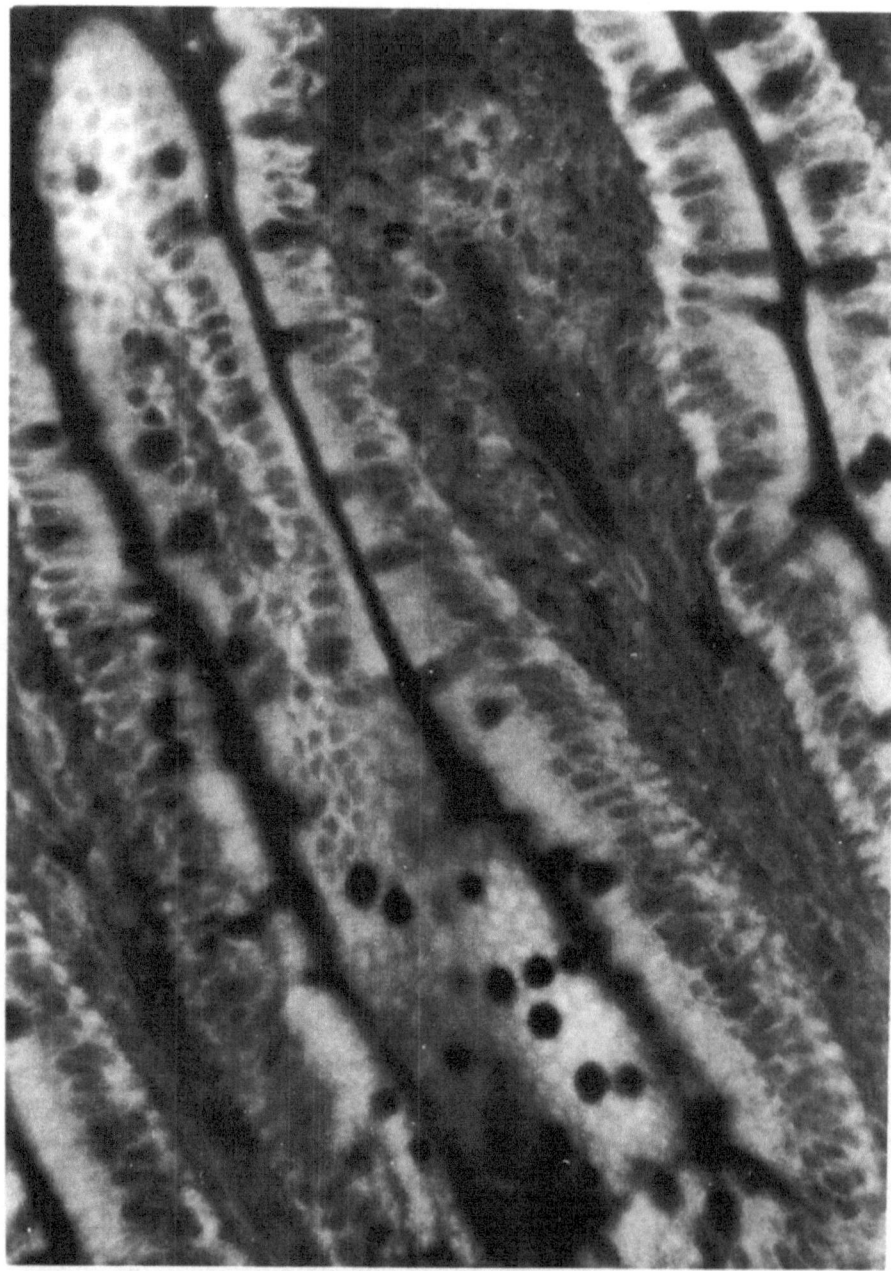

Fig. 3. IgA containing plasma cells in the jejunal mucosa of a nude, mu depressed rat

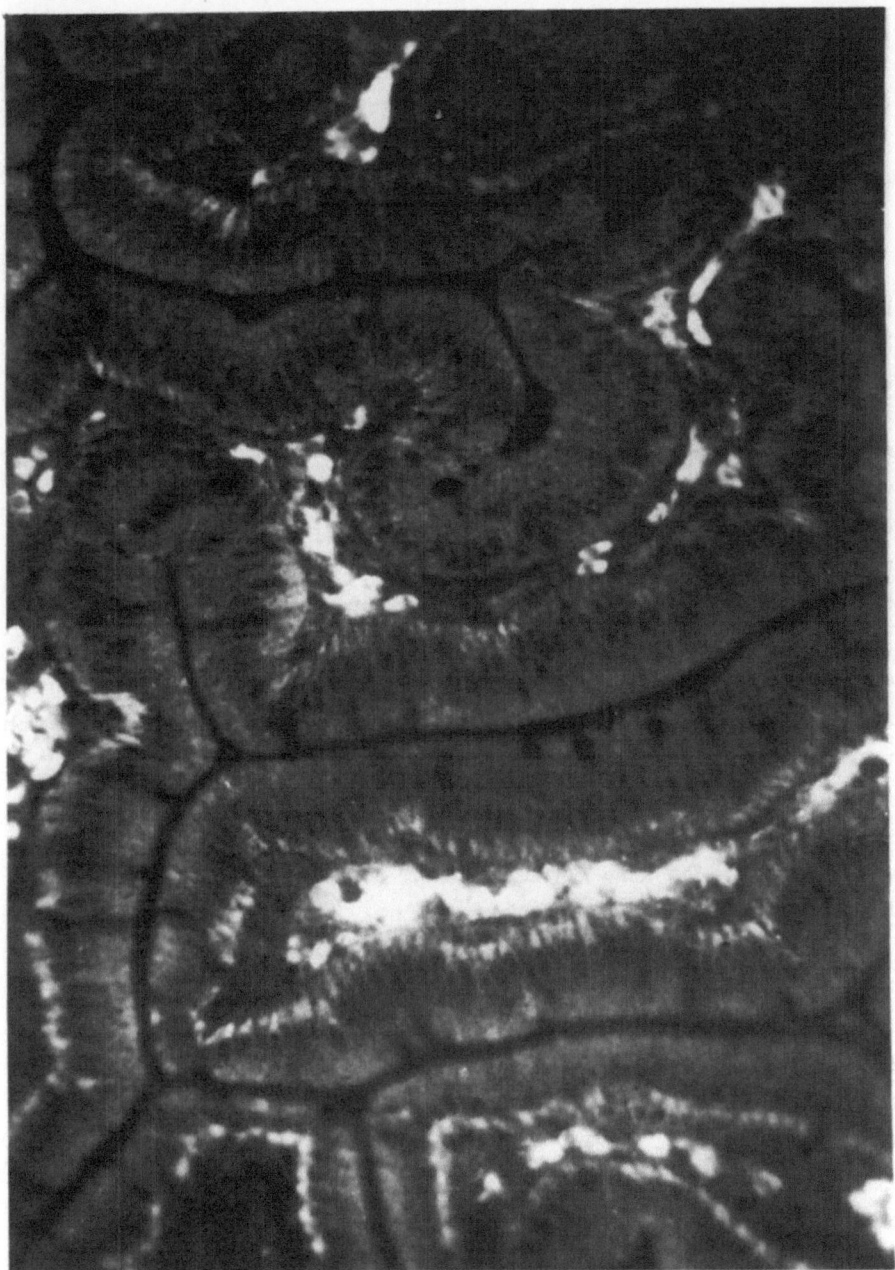

Fig.4. IgA containing plasma cells in the jejunal mucosa of a nude, delta-depressed rat

al., 1978; Zitron et al., 1977; Fidler et al., 1980; Vitetta et al., 1977; Mosier et al., 1977; Scott et al., 1977). In fact, it is more a delay in the appearance of the IgD receptors than a real absence (Fidler et al., 1980). Nevertheless, as this antigen classification seems correct, at least for the rat and mice species (Der Balian et al., 1980), it is quite probably equally correct in the case of other species.

It can be suggested that the immunoglobulin production in response to the stimuli of the different classes of natural antigens is such as shown in Table 3. All animals having been kept in the same experimental conditions, it is possible to distinguish, at least as a hypothesis, the relative part of the immunoglobulin serum levels due to the different classes of antigens: immunoglobulin production in response to TI-1 antigens: group III of Table 3, TI-2 antigens: group III subtracted from group II, TD antigens: group II subtracted from group I. Such calculations certainly oversimplify the problem. However, they lead to a distribution of immunoglobulin by IgG subclasses (Table 4) which seem more or less in accordance with the data published by Der Balian et al., (1980), using a completely different approach. TI-1 and TI-2 antigens induce the synthesis of much more IgG2b and IgG2c than IgG1 or IgG2a immunoglobulins. On the contrary, TD antigens induce a production of IgG1, IgG2a and IgG2b but few, if any, IgG2c molecules (Table 4). In the results of Der Balian et al. (1980), TD antigens are poor inducers of IgG2b synthesis. On the contrary, our present results show a clear and important IgG2b synthesis in response to TD antigen stimulations. Such a discrepancy could be due to the antigens used which are limited to ovalbumin, keyhole limpet haemocyanin and their dinitrophenyl and azobenzene-arsonate conjugates in the studies of Der Balian et al. (1980) and probably to a large array of antigens in our case. However, the at least partial coincidence of both these results can be considered as a support for the hypothesis given in Table 3.

TABLE 3

THEORETICAL IMMUNE RESPONSES IN NORMAL OR IMMUNODEFICIENT RATS IN RELATION
TO THE DIFFERENT CLASSES OF ANTIGENS

Group	Rats	Injected with	Antigenic classes		
			TI-1	TI-2	TD
I	Rnu/+	Normal rabbit serum	+	+	+
II	Rnu/Rnu	Normal rabbit serum	+	+	-
III	Rnu/Rnu	Anti-delta serum	+	-	-

TABLE 4

IgG SUBCLASS DISTRIBUTION OF RAT IMMUNOGLOBULIN TO NATURAL ANTIGENIC
STIMULATION, BY ANTIGENIC CLASS.

Antigenic classes	Immunoglobulin subclasses			
	IgGl	IgG2a	IgG2b	IgG2c
TI-1	4	O	7	88
TI-2	2	1	27	71
TD	22	23	55	O

Table 5 gives the distribution (in percentage and by class
of antigens) of the immunoglobulin serum levels obtained with
the same hypothesis. In all antigenic classes, the IgG isotype
is strongly predominant as compared to all other classes of
immunoglobulin but the IgM isotype is also well represented, at
least in the case of stimulation by TI-1 antigens. The Iga class
is poorly represented in response to TI-2 antigens, somewhat better
in response to TI-1 antigens and is well represented in response
to TD antigens. However, when the respective percentages of
immunoglobulin induced by each antigenic class, in the con-
stitution of the total Ig serum level (group A of Table 2), are
taken into account, TI-1 and TD antigens both induce about the
same quantity of IgA circulating molecules (0.024 mg/ml of IgA

456

TABLE 5

ISOTYPE DISTRIBUTION, IN PERCENTAGE, OF RAT IMMUNOGLOBULIN TO NATURAL
ANTIGENIC STIMULATIONS, BY ANTIGENIC CLASSES.

Antigenic classes	Percentage of immunoglobulin isotypes by antigenic classes					Total circulating immunoglobulins
	IgM	IgD	IgA	IgE	IgG	
TI-1	18.1	–	0.4	–	81.5	5.24 (48%) +
TI-2	4.7	–	–	–	95.3	4.05 (37%)
TD	3.9	–	1.3	–	94.7	1.53 (14%)

+ in mg/ml and between brackets, percentage of immunoglobulin induced by
each antigenic class. The total immunoglobulin serum level considered
as 100% being of 10.83 mg/ml (group A of Table 2).

serum level). However, much less IgA than IgM or IgG molecules
are synthesised in response to antigens of the three classes.
IgD and IgE serum levels are very low and their production in
response to antigenic stimulations is always very low in quantity and difficult to evaluate. It must be emphasised that the
serum level of each class of immunoglobulin is not clearly
correlated to its own synthesis, as the catabolism of each Ig
isotype is different. Moreover, the biological roles of each
Ig isotype are also variable and their physiological importance
cannot be considered to be directly linked to their serum levels.

The classification of antigens in three groups offers a
new possibility of analysing the immune responses and particularly the immunoglobulin synthesis due to natural antigenic
stimulations. Our present experiments have shown that the IgA
synthesis can be triggered by antigens belonging to the three
classes: TI-1, TI-2 and TD. Nevertheless, the synthesis of
the IgA isotype and the others seems strongly dependent on the
class of antigens which stimulates their production.

ACKNOWLEDGEMENTS

This work has been supported by the NIH (USA), grant No.
RO1 AI 12840, by the FRSM (Belgium), grants No. 3.4518 and
3.9005.78, and the Radiation programme of the Commission of the
European Communities, contract 250.77.1.BIO B, contribution No.
1713. We thank Mrs. Geraldine F. Johnson for her help in pre-
paring the manuscript.

REFERENCES

Bazin, H., Beckers, A., Deckers, C. and Moriame, M., 1973. Transplantable
immunoglobulin-secreting tumors in rats. V. Monoclonal immunoglobulins
secreted by 250 ileocecal immunocytomas of the LOU/Wsl rats. J. Natl.
Cancer Inst., 51: 1359.

Bazin, H., Beckers, A. and Querinjean, P., 1974. Three classes and four
subclasses of rat immunoglobulins: IgM, IgA, IgE and IgG1, IgG2a,
IgG2b, IgG2c. Eur. J. Immunol., 4: 44.

Bazin, H., Beckers, A., Urbain-Vansanten, G., Pauwels, R., Bruyns, C.,
Tilkin, A.F., Platteau, B. and Urbain, J., 1978. Transplantable IgD
immunoglobulin-secreting tumors in rat. J. Immunol., 121: 2077.

Bazin, H., Capron, A., Capron, M., Joseph, M., Dessaint, J.P. and Pauwels, R.,
1980. Effect of neonatal injection of anti-μ antibodies on immunity
to schistosomes (S. mansoni) in the rat. J. Immunol., 124: 2373.

Bazin, H., Deckers, C., Beckers, A. and Heremans, J.F., 1972. Transplantable
immunoglobulin-secreting tumors in rat. I. General features in
LOU/Wsl strain rat immunocytomas and their monoclonal proteins. Int.
J. Cancer, 10: 568.

Bazin, H., Platteau, B., Beckers, A. and Pauwels, R., 1978. Differential
effect of neonatal injections of anti-mu or anti-delta antibodies on
the synthesis of IgM, IgD, IgE, IgA, IgG1, IgG2a, IgG2b, and IgG2c
immunoglobulin classes. J. Immunol., 121: 2083.

Bazin, H., Platteau, B., Pauwels, R. and Capron, A., 1980. Immunoglobulin
production in nude rats with special attention to the IgE isotype.
Ann. Immunol. (Inst. Pasteur), 131 C: 31.

Bloemmen, J. and Eyssen, H., 1973. Immunoglobulin levels of sera of
genetically thymusless (nude) mice. Eur. J. Immunol., 3: 117.

Der Balian, G., Slack, J., Clevinger, B., Bazin, H. and Davie, J.M., 1980.
Subclass restriction of murine antibodies. III. Antigens which
stimulate IgG3 in mice stimulate IgG2c in rats. J. Exp. Med., 152: 209.

Fidler, J.M., Morgan, E.L. and Weigle, W.O., 1980. B lymphocyte differentiation in the CBA/N mouse: a delay in maturation rather than a total
arrest. J. Immunol., 124: 13.

Lawton, A.R., Asofsky, R., Hylton, M.B. and Cooper, M.D., 1972. Suppression
of immunoglobulin class synthesis in mice. I. Effects of treatment
with antibody to μ-chain. J. Exp. Med., 135: 277.

Luzzati, A.L. and Jacobson, E.B., 1972. Serum immunoglobulin levels in
nude mice. Eur. J. Immunol., 2: 473.

Manning, D.D., 1975. Heavy chain isotype suppression: a review of the immunosuppressive effect of heterologous anti-Ig heavy chain antisera. J. Reticuloendothel., 18: 63.

Manning, D.D., Manning, J.K. and Reed, N.D., 1976. Suppression of reaginic antibody (IgE) formation in mice by treatment with anti-mu antiserum. J. Exp. Med., 144: 288.

Mayrhofer, G., Bazin, H. and Gowans, J.L., 1976. Nature of cells binding anti-IgE in rats immunized with *Nippostrongylus braziliensis*: IgE synthesis in regional nodes and concentration in mucosal mast cells. Eur. J. Immunol., 6: 573.

Mond, J.J., Sher, I., Mosier, D.E., Baese, M. and Paul W.E., 1978. T-independent responses in B cell-defective CBA/N mice to *Brucella abortus*. Eur. J. Immunol., 8: 459.

Mosier, D.E., Mond, J.J. and Goldings, E.E., 1977. The ontogeny of thymic independent antibody responses *in vitro* in normal mice and mice with an X-linked B cell defect. J. Immunol., 119: 1874.

Mosier, D.E., Zitron, I.M., Mond, J.J., Ahmeda, Sher, I. and Paul, W.E., 1977. Surface immunoglobulin D as a functional receptor for a subclass of B lymphocytes. Immunol. Rev., 37: 89.

Pauwels, R., Bazin, H., Platteau, B. and Van der Straeten, M., 1977. The measurement of total serum IgE levels in rats. J. Immunol. Meth., 18: 133.

Pritchard, H., Riddaway, J. and Micklem, H.S., 1973. Immune responses in congenitally thymusless mice. II. Quantitative studies of serum immunoglobulins, the antibody response to sheep erythrocytes and the effect of thymus cell grafting. Clin. Exp. Immunol., 13: 125.

Rousseaux, J. and Bazin, H., 1979. Rat immunoglobulins. Vet. Immunol. Immunopathol., 1: 61.

Salomon, J.C. and Bazin, H., 1972. Low levels of some serum immunoglobulin classes in nude mice. Rev. Eur. Et. Clin. Biol., 27: 880.

Scott, D.W., Layton, J.E. and Nossal, G.J.V., 1977. Role of IgD in the immune response and tolerance. I. Anti delta pretreatment facilitates tolerance induction in adult B cells *in vitro*. J. Exp. Med., 146: 1473.

Vitetta, E.S., Cambier, J.C., Ligler, F.S., Kettman, J.W. and Uhr, J.W., 1977. B cell tolerance. IV. Differential role of surface IgM and IgD in determining tolerance susceptibility of murine B cells. J. Exp. Med., 146: 1804.

Zitron, I.M., Mosier, D.E. and Paul, W.E., 1977. The role of surface IgD in the response to thymic-independent antigens. J. Exp. Med., 146: 1707.

THE EXPERIMENTAL BASIS FOR ORAL IMMUNISATION AGAINST CHOLERA

N. F. Pierce

The Departments of Medicine of Johns Hopkins
University School of Medicine and Baltimore City
Hospitals, Baltimore, Maryland 21224, USA.

ABSTRACT

For nearly a century cholera immunisation has been given parenterally, with very limited success. Experimental vaccines have varied in antigenic composition, but not in route of administration. Recent studies on immunologic defence of the gut emphasise the role of intraluminal (secretory) antibody in protection against non-invasive pathogens, such as V. cholerae, and permitted detailed comparison of the effectiveness of parenteral or local (oral) immunisation in stimulating protective responses.

Parenteral immunisation may provide brief protection by stimulating high, but transient, levels of serum IgG antibody, which enters the gut passively and inefficiently. Under some conditions, parenteral immunisation may also stimulate the mucosal IgA immune system, but this effect is followed by long-lasting suppression of the mucosal IgA response and cannot be repeated. In contrast, the enteric mucosal immune system appears designed for efficient response to mucosal antigens and protection of mucosal surfaces. This design includes specialised mechanisms for sampling of mucosal antigens, cellular traffic patterns which disseminate immunologic memory to distant mucosae but focus the specific antibody response at the site of antigen exposure, and the production of secretory IgA antibody which is efficiently secreted to the mucosal surface. Some features of antigens which favour mucosal immunogenicity have been identified and long-lasting memory in this system has been observed. Oral immunisation with killed or living bacterial antigens has been shown to evoke relatively long-lasting protection against mucosal infection.

Present evidence strongly favours oral immunisation with appropriately selected antigens as the best approach to immunoprophylaxis of cholera and related enteric infections.

INTRODUCTION

For nearly 100 years, attempts to immunise against cholera have relied upon parenteral vaccines. These have included a killed *Vibrio cholerae* vaccine (Oseasohn et al., 1965), and experimental trials of a purified LPS vaccine (Benenson et al., 1968) and an adjuvanted toxoid vaccine (Curlin et al., 1975). Although each evoked high titres of serum antibody, none was protective for more than a few months. Most efforts to improve these results have focused on novel or more potent antigens and the use of adjuvants in the hope that parenteral immunisation could stimulate higher titres of serum antibody and cause lasting protection.

Now, two lines of evidence suggest that the goal of immunisation should be stimulation of an immune response in intestinal lymphoid tissue and that this may be best done by giving antigen orally. First, it is known that *Vibrio cholerae* is non-invasive; it causes diarrhoea by colonising the small intestine and secreting a protein enterotoxin which acts directly upon intestinal epithelium to stimulate electrolyte secretion. Any immunologic defence against this process would have to work at the mucosal surface or within the bowel lumen. Secondly, lymphoid tissue closely associated with mucosal surfaces appears to play a major role in their defence. A major product of this system is IgA antibody which is stimulated by absorbed antigens and actively secreted to the mucosal surface.

Support for the possible effectiveness of oral immunisation against cholera also comes from evidence that enteric exposure to *Vibrio cholerae* or its products causes substantial immunity to cholera. In cholera endemic areas, multiple accidental ingestions of *Vibrio cholerae* cause an age-related acquisition of immunity (Mosley, 1969). Studies in volunteers show that persons convalescent from a single episode of induced cholera are highly protected against rechallenge for at least two to four years (Cash et al., 1974; Levine, M.M., unpublished). Although the mechanism of protection in these instances is unknown, stimulation of effective mucosal immunity by absorbed enteric antigens is an attractive possibility.

Despite the above observation, uncertainty remains as to the best means of stimulating a mucosal immune response, and basic features of the response are less well understood than are those of systemic immune responses. For example, although the enteric immune system seems especially designed to respond to locally applied antigens (Walker and Isselbacher, 1977), the simple feeding of protein antigens, even for prolonged periods, has often caused only modest local IgA responses (Crabbé et al., 1969). Moreover, reports that a mucosal IgA response may be either primed (Pierce et al., 1978) or boosted (Svennerholm et al., 1977) by parenteral immunisation suggest alternate approaches to achieving mucosal protection.

The purpose of this paper is to review our recent studies of basic features of the mucosal immune system which are relevant to the stimulation of local immunity. The effects of parenteral and oral antigen on the enteric immune system are compared. The nature of protection which follows either of these approaches is considered. The results strongly favour oral immunisation as the most likely means to achieve optimal immunity to cholera.

MATERIALS AND METHODS

The studies were performed in rats or dogs using techniques and antigens described in detail elsewhere (Pierce and Gowans, 1975; Pierce et al., 1977; Pierce, 1978). Immunisation was with purified cholera toxin or toxoid, or a combination of crude toxoid and toxin. Parenteral immunisation used only the purified toxoid; oral or intra-intestinal immunisation used purified cholera toxin, the crude toxoid/toxin combination, or purified toxoid.

The enteric immune response to cholera toxin was studied directly in rats using a fluorescent antibody technique to detect and enumerate antitoxin-containing plasma cells (ACC) in the lamina propria of frozen sections of intestine (Pierce and Gowans, 1975); such cells were mostly of the IgA class (Pierce and Gowans, 1975). In some studies, sensitised lymphoid cells (thoracic duct lymphocytes or spleen cells) were obtained from immune donors by standard methods, washed, and given intravenously to immune or non-immune syngeneic recipients. Thiry-Vella loops of jejunum were constructed in rats as described elsewhere (Husband and Gowans, 1978).

Protection against cholera-like diarrhoea due to oral challenge with living *Vibrio cholerae* was studied in dogs (Pierce et al., 1977). Non-immune controls were challenged with each group of immunised dogs, the inoculum being 100 ml containing 10^9 *Vibrio cholerae* per ml. Protection of immunised dogs is expressed as the percent protection against severe or lethal diarrhoea when compared with concurrently challenged non-immune controls. Some studies involved dogs with chronic Thiry-Vella loops of jejunum. Loop washings were used to measure directly antitoxic antibody in the intestinal lumen (Pierce et al., 1978).

RESULTS AND DISCUSSION

Protection by parenteral immunisation

The aim of initial studies was to determine the extent to which parenteral immunisation could protect against experimental cholera and the mechanism of such protection.

Dogs given two parenteral doses of cholera toxoid developed high serum antitoxin titres and were substantially protected (77% protection) against challenge with living *Vibrio cholerae* 14 days after immunisation; however, serum antitoxin titres had fallen by 80% and protection had disappeared when the interval between immunisation and challenge was increased to 133 days. In individual parenterally

immunised dogs, protection correlated closely with the serum
antitoxin titre at the time of challenge (Pierce et al., 1977).
These observations suggested that protection of parenterally
immunised dogs was due to serum-derived antibody. This was
confirmed by showing that there was no detectable mucosal
antitoxin response in jejunal biopsies from parenterally
immunised dogs (Pierce et al., 1977) and that transfusion of
non-immune dogs with hyperimmune serum from parenterally
immunised donors caused protective levels of IgG antitoxin to
appear in jejunal washings (Pierce and Reynolds, 1974).

These results resemble the brief protection observed in
humans immunised parenterally with bacterial or toxoid vaccines
and suggest that such protection may also be due largely to
high, but transient, peaks of serum antibody which reach the
gut by inefficient passive processes (McCleery et al., 1970).
They directly support the notion that immunity to cholera,
induced by parenteral immunisation, is likely to be short-lived
at best.

Stimulation of the enteric immune system by local immunisation.

Since parenteral immunisation caused neither lasting
protection against cholera nor a detectable mucosal immune
response, further studies were aimed at determining how such
a response could best be produced and at describing basic
features of the response which would be relevant to vaccine
development.

Antigen features which enhance stimulation of the mucosal immune system.

Stimulation of an enteric immune response by local antigen
requires that the antigen be absorbed intact and then trapped
in gut associated lymphoid tissue, i.e. the Peyer's patches or
mesenteric lymph nodes, where stimulation of IgA-committed
lymphocytes occurs (Husband and Gowans, 1978; McWilliams et al.,
1977). However, antigen features which promote these events
have not been thoroughly studied. Many proteins stimulate only

modest mucosal immune responses, even when large amounts are fed for prolonged periods. Cholera toxin proved to be an exception; sequential doses of a few micrograms of this protein evoked vigorous mucosal immune responses in rats (Pierce, 1978).

Two features of cholera toxin appeared to account for its effectiveness. The first was the ability of its antigenic B sub-unit to bind avidly to ganglioside receptors present in almost all mammalian cell membranes. This feature appeared to facilitate trapping of absorbed toxin, or its B sub-unit, by lymphoid cells in Peyer's patches or mesenteric lymph nodes (Pierce, 1978). This proved especially advantageous when attempting to evoke a primary mucosal immune response, perhaps because antigen trapping was poorest in unprimed lymphoid tissue. As a result, either cholera toxin or its B sub-unit were much more effective as mucosal priming antigens than was an inactivated toxoid which had lost the membrane-binding property (Pierce, 1978). The second was the ability of the holotoxin to stimulate intracellular synthesis of 3', 5' cyclic AMP by activation of adenylate cyclase through the action of its A sub-unit. This appeared to enhance directly lymphocyte responsiveness to this antigen and thus had a self-adjuvanting effect; it is known that cyclic nucleotides actively modulate lymphocyte function (Ishizuka et al., 1971). This feature of cholera toxin enhanced both primary and secondary types of mucosal antitoxin responses (Pierce, 1978).

The studies described above support the view that antigen properties which promote absorption and interaction with mucosa-associated lymphoid tissue favour stimulation of a mucosal immune response. Antigens with such properties would be especially attractive as possible oral or topical immunising agents. Examples of such antigens might include:

1. naturally occurring cell-adherent antigens such as cholera toxin or bacterial surface antigens involved in mucosal adherence,

2.   non-adherent antigens modified so as to render them
       cell-adherent,

3.   attenuated live bacteria which colonise the mucosa and
       there release adherent (and non-adherent) antigens in
       concentrations which favour absorption.

The above studies also suggest one means of adjuvanting a
specific mucosal immune response, i.e. by raising cyclic
nucleotide levels in mucosal lymphoid tissue concurrently with
antigen administration. Other approaches to enhancement of a
mucosal immune response by adjuvants may be possible, but
remain to be demonstrated.

Dissemination of immunologic memory in the mucosal immune system.

Repeated applications of cholera toxin to intestinal
mucosa provoked distinct primary and secondary types of mucosal
antitoxin responses of the IgA class. Thus, a single toxin
application caused a modest local antitoxin response which
peaked two to three weeks later, whereas a second application
caused a 10 - 20 fold greater response which peaked after five
days (Pierce, 1978). With this observation, detailed studies
of the features of these responses became possible.

By restricting the application of cholera toxin to a
single mucosal site, it was shown that priming for a mucosal
immune response included distant non-exposed mucosae. For
example, rats primed intracolonically showed local secondary-
type mucosal antitoxin responses when challenged not only in
the colon, but also in the duodenum or trachea (Figure 1). It
was also noted that the secondary response was restricted
largely to the challenge site (Figure 1) and was greatest when
priming and challenge were at the same site (Figure 2). These
latter two observations will be discussed later.

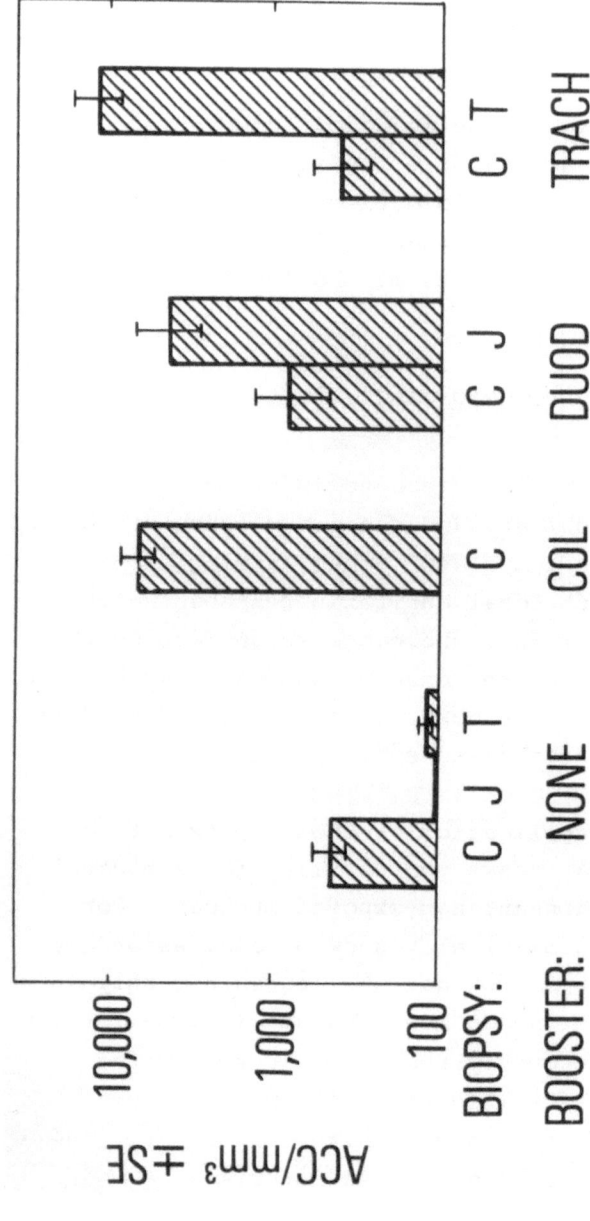

Fig. 1. Dissemination of mucosal priming to cholera toxin. All rats were primed in the colon with cholera toxin (12.5 μg). The booster dose toxin (12.5 μg) was given on day 14 in the colon (COL), duodenum (DUOD), or trachea (TRACH). Biopsies of colon (C), jejunum (J) and trachea (T) were taken 5 days later. ACC= antitoxin containing plasma cells in the lamina propria. Each geometric mean is data from at least 6 rats.

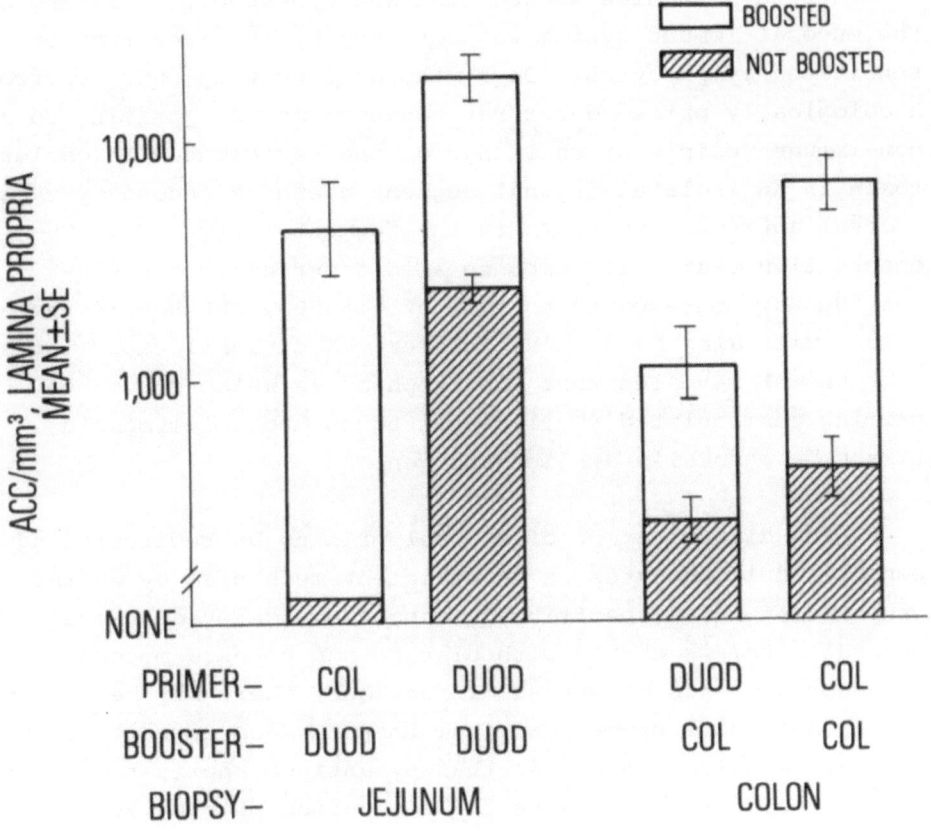

Fig. 2. Comparison of secondary mucosal antitoxin responses in rats primed and boosted at the same or different enteric sites. Priming and boosting doses of cholera toxin (12.5 µg) were injected into the duodenum (DUOD) or ascending colon (COL) with a 14 day interval. Intestinal biopsy was 5 days later. At least 7 rats were used for each geometric mean.

Further studies showed that antigen-specific priming of the mucosal immune system was conveyed by the migration of sensitised lymphocytes. Thus, thoracic duct lymphocytes from a colonically primed donor rat conveyed mucosal priming to a non-immune recipient; challenge of the recipient with cholera toxin in an isolated jejunal segment caused a secondary-type mucosal antitoxin response in the segment (Figure 3). The observation that this response also occurred in the non-contiguous, non-exposed portion of jejunum, but not in the colon, will also be discussed later. Additional experiments (not shown) revealed that the lymphocytes which conveyed priming recirculated until recruited to mucosal lymphoid tissue by mucosally applied antigen.

The dissemination of mucosal priming by recirculating sensitised lymphocytes is an efficient mechanism by which preparation for a specific IgA response, achieved at one mucosal site, is shared with distant non-exposed mucosae. For immunoprophylaxis of mucosal infections, there may be instances in which it will prove practical to prime non-enteric mucosae by oral immunisation rather than by antigen application to the site to be protected. Nevertheless, since priming is greatest at the exposed site, it would seem best to deliver the priming dose of antigen to the surface to be protected, if possible. In the case of cholera, this would be the small bowel.

'Focusing' of the specific mucosal IgA antibody response.

It was noted above that the secondary mucosal immune response was greater at the boosted mucosal site than at distant non-boosted sites (Figure 1) and that the greatest secondary response was achieved when priming and challenge were at the same site (Figure 2). This 'focusing' of specific IgA-producing plasma cells at, or near, the site of secondary antigenic challenge was shown to be due to at least three related events. First, the antigen-sensitised, recirculating IgA memory cells, referred to above, were recruited by mucosally applied antigen to the lymphoid tissue associated with the challenge site; in

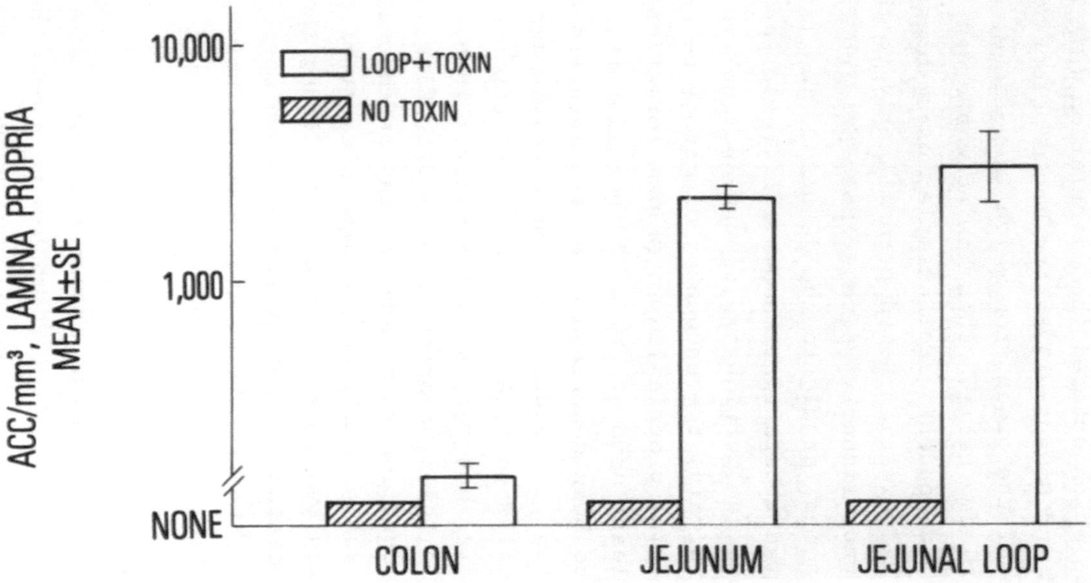

Fig. 3. Transfer of mucosal priming by immune thoracic duct lymphocytes. Thoracic duct lymphocytes were collected 14 days after intracolonic priming of donor rats with cholera toxin (12.5 μg). Non-immune rats with previously constructed Thiry-Vella loops of jejunum received 5 x 10⁸ washed lymphocytes i.v. and 12.5 μg cholera toxin was placed in the jejunal loop; controls received lymphocytes but no cholera toxin. Biopsy of the jejunal loop, jejunum excluded from the loop, and colon was 5 days later. At least 5 rats were used for each geometric mean.

the small intestine, this includes the lamina propria, and the Peyer's patches and/or the draining mesenteric lymph nodes (Pierce, N.F., unpublished). Secondly, the encounter with antigen in Peyer's patches or mesenteric lymph nodes led to transformation and division of the B memory cells, one product being IgA plasmablasts which entered the circulation (Pierce and Gowans, 1975; Husband and Gowans, 1978) and homed selectively to the lamina propria of the organ from which they arose, where they appeared as IgA plasma cells. This homing was organ-specific but antigen-independent. For example, plasmablasts arising from colonic immunisation homed predominantly to the colon (Pierce, N.F., unpublished), whereas those arising from jejunal immunisation homed largely to the jejunum. The latter process accounts for the substantial mucosal antitoxin response observed in the non-boosted portion of jejunum, but not in the colon, in Figure 3. Thirdly, the encounter of memory cells with antigen in the lamina propria led to *in situ* formation of IgA plasma cells, at least some of which did not migrate. This process, which has also been described by others (Husband and Gowans, 1978), accounted for about 30% of the specific IgA plasma cells at the challenge site and caused the response at that site to be modestly, but consistently, greater than at non-challenged sites in the same organ (Figure 3). Finally, the greater local response observed when priming and boosting were at the same site was probably due to a complement of sensitised non-migrating lymphocytes which arose during the primary response and remained in the lymphoid tissue associated with that site, thus apparently giving that site the unique benefit of both recirculating and resident populations of sensitised lymphocytes.

'Focusing' of the local immune response at, or near, the site of mucosal exposure to antigen, which has been observed by others (Ogra and Karzon, 1969; Husband and Gowans, 1978), has obvious advantages for mucosal defence. Since this effect is due to events initiated by secondary antigenic challenge and since the site of maximum response is determined by the site of challenge, it is logical that, as with priming, booster immunisation(s) be delivered to the mucosal surface to be protected so that a maximum local immune response is achieved.

Duration of priming in the mucosal immune system.

A single enteric exposure to cholera toxin caused relatively long-lasting priming of the mucosal immune system. Rats challenged enterically with a standard booster dose at intervals up to 32 weeks after priming showed large, undiminished secondary-type mucosal antitoxin responses (Pierce, 1978); longer intervals were not examined. The duration of immunologic memory in the mucosae of longer-lived animals or man is unknown, but may be an important determinant of the duration of protection achieved by mucosal immunisation.

Modulation of the mucosal immune response by parenteral antigen

Although, as described earlier, parenteral immunisation did not evoke a protective mucosal immune response in previously non-immunised dogs, it remained possible that it had modulating effects, either stimulatory or suppressive, on the mucosal immune system. Further studies explored these possibilities.

Stimulation of the enteric immune response by parenteral antigen.

The aim of these studies was to determine the conditions under which parenteral antigen could stimulate a specific mucosal IgA immune response. It seemed important to know whether such a response could be primed and/or boosted by parenteral antigen, and whether a booster effect could be achieved repeatedly.

Studies in rats showed that cholera toxoid given parenterally could either prime for, or boost, an enteric mucosal antitoxin response, but, as previously noted in dogs, it could not do both; at least one intestinal application of cholera toxin was required to achieve a vigorous mucosal immune response (Table 1). Moreover, parenteral priming occurred only when toxoid was given i.p. and required Freund's adjuvant to be maximally effective (Pierce and Koster, 1980), and parenteral boosting was also most effective by the i.p. route (Table 2). It was also shown that parenteral boosting after local priming could not be repreated, the second parenteral injection having little, if any, mucosal booster effect (Table 2). Related studies in dogs showed that aluminium-adjuvanted toxoid given i.m. primed for an enteric antitoxin response, but the priming effect was relatively weak, multiple enteric boosters being required to evoke a substantial mucosal antitoxin response (Pierce et al., 1978).

TABLE 1

PRIMING OR BOOSTING OF THE ENTERIC IMMUNE RESPONSE BY PARENTERAL CHOLERA TOXOID IN RATS

Immunisation route		ACC/mm^3 in jejunum ‡	
Primer*	Booster†	Boosted	Not boosted
i.p.	Duodenum	8 000 §	670
		(1.2)	(1.2)
Oral	i.p.	5 000	200
		(1.1)	(1.4)
i.p.	i.p.	570	670
		(1.5)	(1.2)

* Priming was with purified toxoid, 100 µg plus Freund's complete adjuvant, given i. p., or a combination of crude toxoid and toxin, 600 mg, in drinking water over an 8 - 16 day period.

† Boosting was on day 14. Purified toxoid was given i. p. (100 µg) or into the duodenum (1 mg).

‡ Antitoxin-containing plasma cells in jejunal lamina propria 5 days after boosting, or 19 days after priming if no booster was given.

§ Geometric mean ($\overset{x}{\div}$ SE), n = 8 rats for each mean.

TABLE 2

EFFECT OF REPEATED PARENTERAL BOOSTING ON THE ENTERIC IMMUNE RESPONSE OF COLONICALLY PRIMED RATS

Immunisation		ACC/mm^3 in	
Primer*	Booster(s)†	jejunum‡	
Colon	i.p.	4 900§	(1.4)
Colon	s.c.	490	(1.4)
Colon	none	100	-
Colon	i.p., i.p.,	210	(1.4)
Colon	i.p., none	100	-

* Priming was with purified cholera toxin, 12.5 μg, given into the ascending colon.

† Boosting was at 14 day intervals after priming. Purified toxoid, 100 μg, was given i.p.

‡ Antitoxin-containing plasma cells in jejunal lamina propria 5 days after boosting, or 19 days after last immunisation if final booster was omitted.

§ Geometric mean ($\overset{x}{\underset{\div}{}}$ SE), n = 5 - 7 rats for each mean. Biopsies in which no ACC were seen were assigned a value of $100/mm^3$, which is the lower limit of the sensitivity of the assay, for calculation of geometric means.

Taken together, the above observations support the notion that parenteral immunisation is an inefficient means of stimulating a mucosal immune response, at least in rats. This is probably because it is difficult to deliver, by any parenteral route, an adequate antigenic stimulus to IgA-committed lymphocytes, which are sequestered largely in gut-associated and other mucosa-associated lymphoid tissue (Gearhart and Cebra, 1979). This difficulty appears to be compounded by prior parenteral immunisation which may cause increased trapping of injected antigen by sensitised systemic lymphoid tissue and, thus, further restrict its availability to distant mucosa-associated sites. Consistent with this view was the observed inability to boost parenterally the mucosal antitoxin response in animals previously primed or boosted parenterally.

Suppression of the enteric immune response by parenteral antigen.

It is known that local intestinal immunisation stimulates immune mechanisms which suppress the systemic immune response to the same antigen given parenterally (Thomas and Parrott, 1974). Little attention has been given, however, to the possibility that the opposite might also be true, i.e. parenteral immunisation might suppress the mucosal immune response to locally applied antigen. This possibility was raised by the observation in rats that an increased booster dose was required when the interval between i.p. priming with toxoid and Freund's adjuvant and enteric boosting with cholera toxin was greater than two weeks; for example, the enteric booster dose required to evoke similar mucosal antitoxin responses was almost 1 000-fold greater at eight weeks than at two weeks after i.p. priming (Pierce, N.F., unpublished).

Further studies in rats showed that parenteral immunisation with cholera toxoid, but not with unrelated antigens, did cause substantial suppression of the enteric immune response to cholera toxin and that this suppressive effect was independent of any priming effect (Pierce and Koster, 1980). Thus, rats given toxoid either i.p. or s.c. showed impaired mucosal antitoxin responses when an otherwise effective intestinal immunisation sequence with cholera toxin was begun two weeks later (Table 3). Suppression of the response to enteric boosting was also seen when parenteral toxoid was given two weeks after enteric priming and two weeks before enteric boosting with cholera toxin (Pierce and Koster, 1980).

TABLE 3

SUPPRESSION OF THE ENTERIC IMMUNE RESPONSE BY PARENTERAL CHOLERA TOXOID
IN RATS

Parenteral toxoid given before enteric priming *	ACC/mm^3 in jejunum †
None	9 900 ‡ (1.3)
Plain toxoid, i.p.	1 400 (1.7)
Toxoid plus aluminum hydroxide, s.c.	600 (1.9)

* Enteric immunisation was with a combination of crude toxoid and crude
toxin; two doses were given into the duodenum with a 14 day interval.
Parenteral toxoid, 40 μg, was given 14 days before the first enteric
immunisation.

† Antitoxin-containing plasma cells in jejunal lamina propria 5 days
after the second duodenal immunisation.

‡ Geometric mean ($\overset{x}{\div}$ SE), n = 8 - 14 rats for each mean.

The means by which parenteral immunisation with toxoid
suppressed the mucosal immune response to cholera toxin are
only partly understood. Suppression was independent of
mucosal priming since it occurred when parenteral antigen was
given by routes which did not cause detectable priming, for
example s.c. or i.v.. Thus, suppression did not appear to
require the encounter of antigen with IgA-committed lymphocytes
and was not simply a regulatory consequence of mucosal priming.
In other studies, adoptive transfer of spleen cells from
parenterally primed donors transferred the suppression and
suggested that it was, at least partly, cell-mediated (Figure 4).
On the other hand, the transfer of hyperimmune serum from
parenterally immunised donors was also highly suppressive
(Figure 5). This suppression was caused by antitoxic antibody,
did not involve interference with antigen absorption from the
gut, and might contribute to suppression of the enteric immune
response in animals given multiple parenteral immunisations
(Pierce, 1980).

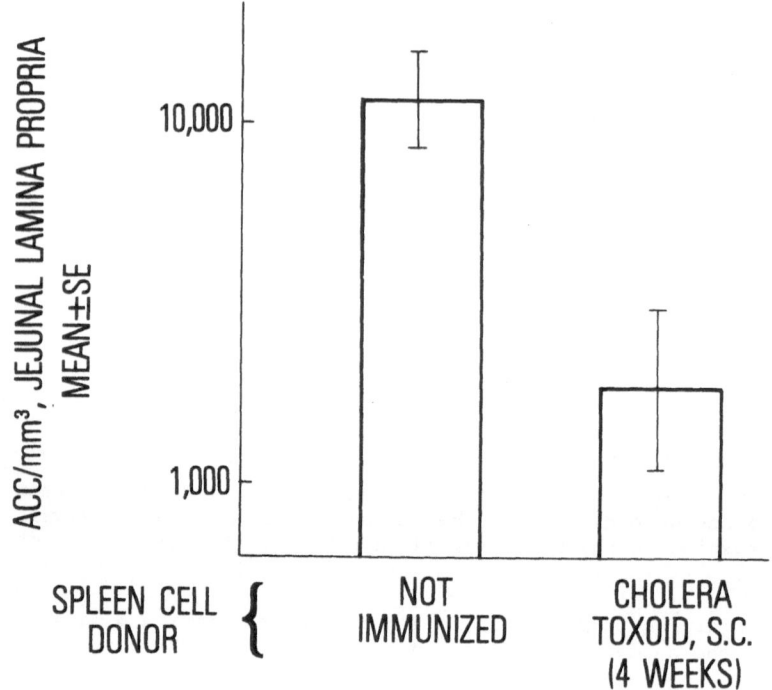

Fig. 4.   Suppression of mucosal antitoxin response by immune spleen cells.
Spleen cells were harvested 4 weeks after s.c. priming of donor
rats with cholera toxoid (40 μg); control cells were from non-
immune donors.   Non-immune rats received 1.5 x 10^8 washed spleen
cells i.v. and 10 μg cholera toxin intraduodenally.   The intraduodenal dose of toxin was repeated 14 days later and jejunal
biopsies were obtained after 5 more days.   Each mean is data from
at least 6 rats (source: Koster, F.T. and Pierce, N.F.,
unpublished).

479

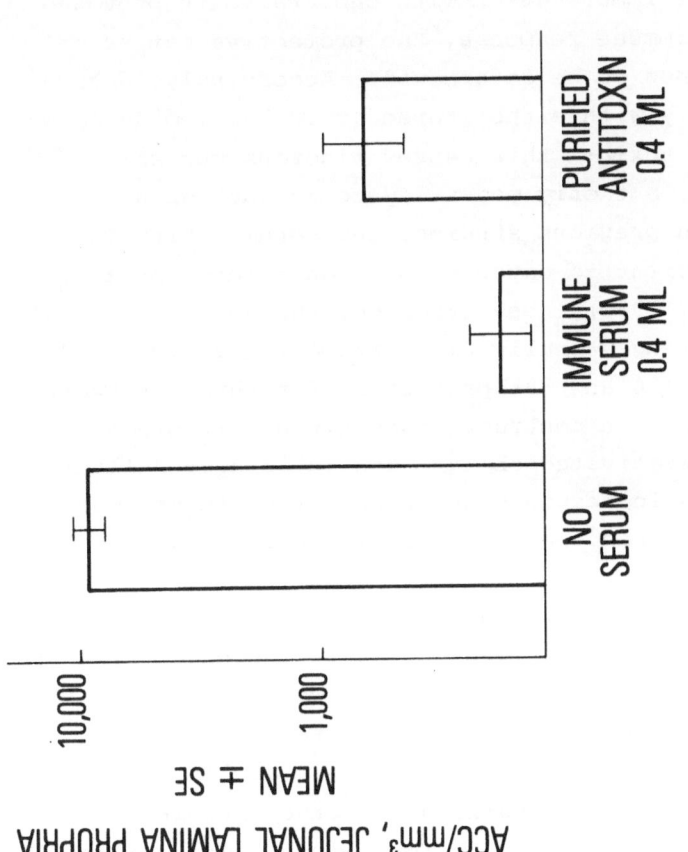

Fig. 5. Suppression of mucosal antitoxin response by serum antitoxin. Immune serum was from rats primed i.p. with cholera toxoid (25 μg) plus Freund's complete adjuvant, boosted i.v. 6 weeks later with toxoid (50 μg), and bled 8 - 12 days after boosting. Purified antitoxin was obtained from this serum by absorption to, and elution from, a toxoid-Sepharose affinity column as described (Pierce and Gowans, 1975). Non-immune rats received immune serum (0.4 ml), or purified antitoxin from 0.4 ml of serum, i.p. one day before intraduodenal priming with cholera toxin (12.5 μg). Boosting with intraduodenal toxin (12.5 μg) was 14 days later; jejunal biopsies were taken 5 days after boosting. Each geometric mean is data from at least 8 rats.

Suppression of the mucosal immune response, if it occurs in man, would provide a compelling reason to avoid parenteral immunisation for superficial mucosal infections such as cholera. Even apparent benefits of parenteral immunisation, such as priming for, or boosting of, a mucosal immune response may be outweighed by the undesirable suppressive effects which ensue.

PROTECTION AFTER LOCAL IMMUNISATION

Although local immunisation with cholera toxin provoked a vigorous mucosal immune response, the protective nature of this response remained to be determined. Accordingly, dogs were immunised orally with either three or twelve 100 µg doses of purified cholera toxin; this caused vigorous mucosal antitoxin responses, but only modest systemic antitoxin responses. Based on previous studies, the serum antitoxin titres were insufficient to cause protection (Pierce et al., 1977; Pierce et al., 1980). Nevertheless, the dogs were highly protected when challenged orally with live *Vibrio cholerae* 21 days after the last dose (76 and 88% protection for three or twelve doses, respectively). In contrast, dogs given multiple oral doses of purified inactivated cholera toxoid developed little or no mucosal antitoxin response and were not protected when similarly challenged (Pierce et al., 1977; Pierce et al., 1978).

Protection occurred only in dogs in which a vigorous mucosal antitoxin response had been evoked. The exact role of antitoxic antibody in mediating protection was, however, uncertain since the peak mucosal antitoxin response, which occurred five days after antigen feeding, had declined by at least 95% when the dogs were challenged. Other studies in dogs suggest that protection due to local immune mechanisms lasts nearly a year (Pierce et al., 1977).

The duration of protection conferred by mucosal immunisation and the exact means by which it is prolonged are important questions requiring further study. Nevertheless, these studies and the demonstration of lasting immunity to cholera in previously challenged volunteers, described earlier, strongly support the view that the mucosal immune system is able to provide relatively long lasting protection, once effectively stimulated, and that such protection outlasts that achieved by vigorous parenteral immunisation.

CONCLUSIONS

The observations reviewed here strongly support the view that immunity to cholera and related mucosal infections will be best achieved by oral immunisation with materials selected for their ability to promote a mucosal immune response. Specific conclusions which deserve emphasis are as follows:

1. The brevity of mucosal protection which follows vigorous parenteral immunisation and the suppressive effects it exerts on the mucosal immune system argue against the use of parenteral vaccines to prevent cholera or related mucosal infections, a possible exception being circumstances in which brief protection is the only objective.

2. Antigens selected for use as mucosal immunogens, whether living or non-living, should be those shown to be especially effective at promoting a mucosal immune response. Antigen features which favour stimulation of a mucosal immune response differ, at least in part, from those which promote a systemic immune response. Thus, antigens which are effective immunogens when given parenterally will not necessarily be effective when given orally.

3. Local immunisation of the gut should involve antigen delivery to the mucosal surface to be protected, since the mucosal immune response is greatest at the site of antigen exposure. In the case of cholera, this would be the small bowel.

4.   The responsiveness of the mucosal immune system to
     repeated local applications of selected antigens and
     the relatively long lasting protection which ensues
     strongly favour oral immunisation for optimal protection
     against cholera. In endemic areas, oral immunisation
     should be aimed at young children, the most susceptible
     population. Subsequent accidental ingestion of *Vibrio
     cholerae* may serve to reinforce and prolong vaccine-
     induced mucosal immunity.

ACKNOWLEDGEMENTS

Research space was generously provided by the Gerontology
Research Center of the National Institute of Aging, National
Institutes of Health, under its Guest Scientist Program.

This work was supported by Research Contract No. 1 AIO2051
and Research Grant No. 1 PO1 AI14480 from the National
Institute of Allergy and Infectious Diseases, National
Institutes of Health.

REFERENCES

Benenson, A.S., Mosley, W.H., Fahimuddin, M. and Oseasohn, R.O., 1968.
Cholera vaccine field trials in East Pakistan. 2. Effectiveness
in the field. Bull. Wld. Hlth. Org. 38, 359.

Cash, R.A., Music, S.I., Libonati, J.P., Craig, J.P., Pierce, N.F. and
Hornick, R.B., 1974. Response of man to infection with *Vibrio
cholerae*. II. Protection from illness afforded by previous disease
and vaccine. J. Infect. Dis. 130, 325.

Crabbé, P.A., Nash, D.P., Bazin, H., Eyssen, H. and Heremans, J.F., 1969.
Antibodies of the IgA type in intestinal plasma cells of germ-free
mice after oral or parenteral immunisation with ferritin.
J. Exp. Med. 130, 723.

Curlin, G., Levine, R., Aziz, K.M.A., Rahman, M.A.S.M. and Verwey, W.F.,
1975. Field trial of cholera toxoid. In: Proc. 11th US - Japan
Cholera Conf. 314. US Department of Health Education and Welfare.

Gearhart, P.J. and Cebra, J.J., 1979. Differentiated B lymphocytes:
potential to express particular antibody variable and constant
regions depends on site of lymphoid tissue and antigen loan.
J. Exp. Med. 149, 216.

Husband, A.J. and Gowans, J.L., 1978. The origin and antigen-dependent
distribution of IgA-containing cells in the intestine.
J. Exp. Med. 148, 1146.

Ishizuka, M., Braun, W. and Matsumoto, T., 1971. Cyclic AMP and immune
responses. 1. Influence of poly A : U and cAMP on antibody
formation *in vito* J. Immunol 107, 1027.

McCleery, J.L., Kraft, S.C. and Rothberg, R.M., 1970. Demonstration of
antibody in rabbit feces after active or passive parenteral
immunisation. Digestion 3, 213.

McWilliams, M., Phillips-Quagliata, J.M. and Lamm, M.E., 1977. Mesenteric
lymph node B lymphoblasts which home to the small intestine are
precommitted to IgA synthesis. J. Exp. Med. 145, 866.

Mosley, W.H., 1969. The role of immunity in cholera. A review of
epidemiological and serological Studies. Texas Reports on Biology
and Medicine 27 (supplement 1), 227.

Ogra, P.L. and Karzon, D.T., 1969. Distribution of poliovirus antibody in
serum, nasopharynx and alimentary tract following segmental
immunisation of lower alimentary tract with polio vaccine. J. Immunol.
120, 1423.

484

Oseasohn, R.O., Benenson, A.S. and Fahimuddin, M., 1965. Field trial of cholera vaccine in rural East Pakistan. Lancet i, 450.

Pierce, N.F., 1978. The role of antigen form and function in the primary and secondary intestinal immune responses to cholera toxoid and toxin in rats. J. Exp. Med. 148, 195.

Pierce, N.F., 1980. Suppression of the intestinal immune response to cholera toxin by specific serum antibody. Infect and Immun. in press.

Pierce, N.F., Cray, W.C. Jr. and Engel, P.F., 1980. Antitoxin immunity to cholera in dogs immunised orally with cholera toxin. Infect. and Immun. 27, 632.

Pierce, N.F., Cray, W.C. and Sircar, B.K., 1978. Induction of a mucosal antitoxin response and its role in immunity to experimental canine cholera. Infect and Immun. 21, 185.

Pierce, N.F. and Gowans, J.L., 1975. Cellular kinetics of the intestinal immune response to cholera toxoid in rats. J. Exp. Med. 142, 1550.

Pierce, N.F. and Koster, F.T., 1980. Priming and suppression of the intestinal immune response to cholera toxoid/toxin by parenteral toxoid in rats. J. Immunol. 124, 307.

Pierce, N.F. and Reynolds, H.Y., 1974. Immunity to experimental cholera. I. Protective effect of humoral IgG antitoxin demonstrated by passive immunisation. J. Immunology 113, 1017.

Pierce, N.F., Sack, R.B. and Sircar, B.K., 1977. Immunity to experimental cholera. III. Enhanced duration of protection after sequential parenteral-oral administration of toxoid to dogs. J. Infect. Dis. 135, 888.

Svennerholm, A.M., Holmgren, J., Hanson, L.A., Lindblad, B.S., Quereshi, F. and Rahimtoola, R.J., 1977. Boosting of secretory IgA antibody responses in man by parenteral cholera vaccination.
Scan. J. Immunol. 6, 1345.

Thomas, H.C. and Parrott, D.M.V., 1974. The induction of tolerance to a soluble protein antigen by oral administration. J. Immunol. 27, 631.

Walker, W.A. and Isselbacher, K.L., 1977. Intestinal antibodies.
New Engl. J. Med. 297, 767.

SHORT COMMUNICATION

J. Bienenstock   *(Canada)*

As you know, Professor Pierce is unfortunately unable to
be with us today although we have his paper. In place of
Professor Pierce there will be three short presentations, one
from myself and the others from Professor Bohl and Dr. Williams
Smith.

Professor Pierce has a particular interest in cholera and
has made a number of observations which relate to how best to
immunise humans against cholera. This is a major problem in
Third World areas. He is also trying to derive information
which will help in the design of vaccines to prevent diarrhoeal
disease.

He initially demonstrated, quite unequivocably, that, in
the rat, parenteral immunisation primed the IgA system, at
least as judged by IgA cells in the intestine, for an oral
booster. This combination of parenteral priming and oral boosting was far better for the gut in terms of IgA antibody, producing in local plasma cells, directed against the organisms.
The parenteral priming however was via the peritoneum, that is
IP, and obviously is not a very practical route. Furthermore,
if one tries to avoid the peritoneal priming and uses subcutaneous priming, one does not get the same good boosting of the
mucosal IgA system.

The second important thing, in my view, that Professor
Pierce showed very clearly, was that as far as immunogenicity
of cholera preparations was concerned, it appeared necessary
for the cholera toxin to be able to combine with its known
receptor on the epithelial cell surface. If this did not occur
then the molecule was less immunogenic. So, receptor binding
of antigen to the epithelial cell or beyond, in the mucosa, was
necessary to get a satisfactory IgA response. This is a very
important observation because when you are talking about design

of vaccines and how best to produce immunity, you have to take
into consideration how best to get _it_, whether it is the bacteria,
virus or antigen, close to and onto the epithelial cell in the
intestine. Whether that is an epithelial cell over a Peyer's
patch or elsewhere, is very unclear. We know very little about
the processing of antigen in and at the mucosal level.

This is a terrible problem if one is talking about the
design of vaccines. I will say at this stage that I really do
not consider that it is possible with the current knowledge to
be able to design a vaccine and guarantee a certain result.
The state of the art is just not at that level at present.

We can list some issues that all this raises:

> Type of antigen
> Route
> Dose
> Vehicle.

On the question of the type, or the chemical nature, of
the antigen, I would remind you that bile and dead bacterial
vaccines have been used together very effectively. It may be
that bile which contains mucolytic agents and a variety of
things which help neutralise acidity in the stomach, may have
allowed the antigen through the stomach and close to the epithelial cell, one way or the other.

The route: again I talk about parenteral priming versus
oral priming, or oral priming versus secondary oral priming.
Again, Pierce's more recent data show that he can immunise very
effectively and effect resistance to subsequent challenge by
oral immunisation with killed, or molecular forms of the cholera
toxin as a priming and a secondary response, providing that the
timing is right and providing that he manipulates it correctly.

This takes me to the very important point that it really
does not matter what mechanism you stimulate or measure IgG1,

cell mediated immunity, or whatever, the end point must be
protective if the vaccine is to be useful.

I do not think there is any point in spending too much
time in out-thinking the body and presuming that IgA really is
the most important defence mechanism. I will be a little
controversial here and say that there is no direct evidence
whatsoever to support that statement. There is indirect evidence to support it but no direct evidence.

Now, the dose: depending on the dose, which appears to be
very important, you can, in fact, get very good mucosal resistance following mucosal presentation of antigen. The dose must
include the vehicle because one of the major problems in dose
is that you have to get it past the stomach. If you present it
into the intestine, for example, and bypass the stomach, you
can produce very effective immunisation procedures. So the
vehicle is important and it may simply be a question of an
antacid in man or a buffer in animals, or some mechanism to get
it through the stomach.

The next question to take into account is that of previous
exposure. If you have been previously exposed and you have, in
fact, been primed, then a subsequent challenge by any route will
produce a boosting effect. So, if the organism with which you
are dealing is prevalent in the environment, and not eradicated,
then it would not be at all surprising that parenteral immunisation would produce quite satisfactory mucosal immune type responses. It is necessary to bear that in mind because when you
talk to some of the vaccine producers, in man, you say, mucosal
immunity, and they say, forget it, because we can immunise
against mumps with a parenteral immunisation perfectly adequately.
They can give you many examples of this approach - effective
parenteral immunisation producing apparent mucosal immunity.

There is another thing which has come out of this meeting.
Many of you talk about IgG; we know about IgG1 being a very
selectively concentrated antibody in bovine mammary secretions.

We talk about IgA - it seems to me that we know an awful lot
more about IgA at the present time than we know about IgG1 We
know very little about the traffic of IgG1 we know very little
about what it does and about the mechanism of selective transport in comparison to the level of sophistication that Hall and
Vaerman have brought us with regard to the hepatocyte and its
transport system. IgG1 may be just as important as a defence
mechanism in the bovine as is IgA in other species. If it is a
predominant immunoglobulin in cow then we have to assume that
it is there for a good purpose - it has been there for a long
time. We ought to be not unhappy that some of our immunisation
procedures are producing good antibody in a class other than the
one about which we have this preconceived idea, namely IgA. So
I think a lot more work ought to be done in regard to that.
Some of the questions that Bazin's work raised are the relationships between these various immunoglobulins. At the moment, in
mouse physiology it seems fairly clear that you start with an
IgM bearing cell which may turn into something else as it goes
down the line. If we are talking about a special mucosal population of B cells, this raises the question as to where and at
what point that commitment occurs.

Cebra has the idea that if you stimulate sufficiently
often almost any B cell on its travels through the body will
eventually turn into an IgA producing cell. You just keep going.
It is the old Cooper idea that you keep pushing with antigen and
it will do it. This may or may not be right. My own feeling
(and there is no information in this) is that, in fact, in the
bone marrow, at some point, there is a commitment to a mucosa
seeking population of cells, and that that population of cells,
in its traffic through the body, can be recruited by the suitable
presentation of antigen to that mucosa. So, I don't think that
we should consider only IgA in the mucosa but also IgM and IgG.
That would make it easier to explain some of the known observations of IgA deficiency in man in which you get almost total
repopulation with the IgM group of cells.

The practical relevance of this is that when we are trying to recruit a population of cells we still do not fully understand what route to take and where best to present antigen in order to recruit a cell population of whatever class into the bowel.

So, many questions arise. The message at the moment appears to be that you can immunise mucosal tissue, such as the gut, by suitably presenting the antigen, or modifying the antigen. Here, the work of Dr. Morein is relevant, the work on virosomes and liposomes, and the issue of lipids and lipid conjugation, being able to take that antigen, somehow present it in a form that is well recognised by the gut, and produce good mucosal immunity. This is a very nice piece of work and I think we are going to hear a lot more about manipulation of chemical structure. The binding, or bringing together, of that antigen with the epithelium seems very important too. The amount appears important, as well as the question of adjuvant which has hardly been mentioned. The only thread that runs through our discussion on antigens, are factors that seem to cause changes in epithelial cell physiology and allow antigen access.

The last thing I will mention is the question of cell traffic. It seems fairly clear that there are cells which can arise in Peyer's patches with fairly advanced differentiation which migrate via the mesenteric lymph node to the thoracic duct into the blood, and at some point will end up in mucosal tissue, not only of the gut, but also other tissues such as the mammary gland, and, for example, the mucosa of the lung. This traffic seems to be reasonably well established both in theoretical and practical terms.

The other question is whether the reverse type of flow occurs. My feeling is that there are so many more cells that are coming from the Peyer's patches that can be stimulated in the gut and seeded by thoracic duct blood into the rest of the body, that the contribution of a priming into the lung, and an attempt to do this in reverse, is just practically not going

to work, because you are just not going to see a large number
of cells - it is inconceivable that you will. If, on the other
hand, you do it this way, I would expect you would then get
cells in the bowel, very few in number, ready potentially to be
stimulated by antigen that would then come in. If they don't
meet antigen, those cells will then go on and do whatever they
do, emigrate or die. If they meet antigen, then they will stay
there and potentially they will proliferate and the whole cycle
will then proceed.

So, if you try to manipulate this system, the issue is -
where does antigen normally present itself with the normal route
of entry of that particular organism or antigen, and then where
can you maximise contact with that particular antigen again?
If you think of this for a particular organism you might manipulate the system in different ways but you should bear in mind
the numbers game which certainly suggests that the gut is the
prime tissue in contact with the most quantitatively large
amount of antigen.

SHORT COMMUNICATION

E. Bohl   *(USA)*

   As you may know, *E. coli* is a very serious infection in
the newborn animal, resulting in severe diarrhoea, usually
dehydration, and quite often death. Following our work with
TGE in developing some immunological concepts, we decided to
apply them to coli bacillosis.

   We exposed pregnant swine to large numbers of live *E. coli*
simply by growing the organism in milk and pouring the cultured
milk onto the feed. The antigenic stimulation of the gut we
hoped would produce IgA antibodies. We compared this with
intramuscular injection either of live or killed organisms of
the same serotype. The experiment was performed with three or
four different groups of sows and we got much better protection
in the pigs that were suckling the orally vaccinated sows, in
contrast to the pigs that were suckling sows which had been
intramuscularly injected with either dead or live *E. coli.*

   This substantiated the work with TGE and led to the
development of field trials. Dr. Kohler in our laboratory then
devised a rather simple way in which veterinarians could prop-
agate the *E. coli* in great numbers and feed them in a practical
way to swine. The general procedure has been this: the pathogenic *E. coli* is isolated from involved pigs on a particular farm.
The pathogenic *E. coli* is then used to inoculate the milk, usually
in quarter gallon containers, using pasteurised or reconstituted
skimmed milk. The local herdsman or the veterinarian can do this
after he has been supplied with the organism. This is fed to
swine on that particular farm for three consecutive days, using
about 200 ml of the cultured milk per animal. This is done
about three weeks before expected farrowing. This procedure has
been followed very extensively in the Mid-West in the last four
or five years. Dr. Kohler has obtained much reliable information on the efficacy of this procedure and the results we get
back are very good. Many veterinarians will say that they have
been able to control newborn pig diarrhoea by this technique.

We know for a fact that this *E. coli* diarrhoea is the principal cause of baby pig scours in the Mid-West of the United States.

Some of you will no doubt put forward the view that this is a very crude way of doing things and will tend to perpetuate an infectious agent. However, you must bear in mind that we only use the agent that has been isolated from that same farm. We are perpetuating it rather more than it would have been perpetuated on that farm but probably not to a degree where it would be more apt to spread to other farms.

So this technique is being used very effectively if we can judge by the results that we are getting from the field, giving high levels of protection and no undesirable side effects.

DISCUSSION

B. Morein   *(Sweden)*

It is not so difficult to control newborn pig diarrhoea.
By parenteral injection it works, at least in Sweden. But what
happens is that the piglets get the same disease after about
two or three weeks, it just delays it. We find this is a common
occurrence. I am not a practitioner but I understand they can
solve about 80% of the problem by using mixed vaccines, and
immunise the sow. They do get exactly the same pattern two or
three weeks afterwards but it is not so serious at that stage.
Not all of them get it later but some do.

SHORT COMMUNICATION

H. Williams Smith   *(UK)*

I don't think anyone would doubt that what Ed Bohl has
said is correct, that you would get very good immunity by using
the procedure he has described. The question is whether it is
a desirable thing to do or not. Of course, he is talking about
a method of control in which you are presenting animals with
very large numbers of pathogenic organisms at a time when they
are not susceptible to the clinical disease themselves. The
opposite side of that spectrum is the way in which we control
diseases like foot and mouth and swine fever in this country
on a national basis whereby our aim is to keep a parasite away
from the host on a national boundary scale. If infection does
occur, we follow a slaughter policy and for diseases like foot
and mouth in this country it has worked tolerably well. With
swine fever it has worked remarkably well; this is because
swine fever virus does not last long outside the body and it is
not highly infectious.

We have also tried this policy with other diseases such
as Newcastle disease and here we have failed dismally. We are
now in the situation where we have to vaccinate all our chickens
continuously which is a very unpleasant situation.

That is on a national basis. On a local basis, many farmers try to control disease by preventing the parasite coming on
to the farm. Many farmers are highly successful in so doing as
regards many diseases. However, there is one disease which
really presents them with a problem and this is *E. coli*. It is
considered in this country, and I see no reason to doubt it,
that *E. coli* is the most important single cause of loss to the
pig industry. Looking at the natural history of *E. coli* diarrhoea
in piglets, a farm may be free of disease for a long time and
then suddenly the farmer may decide to buy a few pigs in. This
is a very dangerous thing to do because he may well bring a
serotype onto the premises which is not already there. The
natural history then would be for him to have a few outbreaks

of neonatal diarrhoea to start off, then an increasing number of them, then a slow decrease. The whole process would probably take about four to six months, the end point being not that the parasite has disappeared from the environment but that a herd immunity has developed.

The immunity develops naturally and you can encourage it by keeping your sows as close together as you can with infection so that they get immunity that way. The procedure that Ed Bohl has described precipitates this method by pouring in the cultures. I think you can achieve the same end fairly well without having to do that, by keeping the sows fairly close together.

One major objection to Ed Bohl's method is that it does involve putting lots of entero-pathogens into the environment which may spread to other environments. An additional objection is that most of the pathogenic characteristics of entero pathogenic strains are plasmid determined. In most pig strains, entero pathogens have the K88 antigen which makes the *coli* stick to the bowel wall; they produce enterotoxin; most are haemolytic. Those are all pathogenic characteristics which are plasmid controlled so there is a possibility not only of retaining that one strain in the environment but also of building up other strains with these characteristics.

There is one factor which is of interest that occurs in this country but I don't know about the United States. That is we have some pigs with genetic resistance to K88 adhesion. In other words, some pigs have a specific genetic mechanism which stops the *E. coli* adhering to the small intestines.

When problems arise in developing herd immunity, it would appear from work done at Compton that this occurs in herds where some of the sows are genetically resistant and some are not. The genetic resistance is determined by two alleles on one locus acting in a simple Mendelian manner. For example, we can say that 'S' is the dominant gene which is able to stick to the epithelial cell. In these herds there will be some sows which

are homozygous for sticking, some which are heterozygous, but
they will stick, and others which are 'S'. These are the ones
that are the problems in producing immunity because when you
give the *coli* to these pigs they will not stick to the epithelial
cells and so you will not get a very good immunity produced in
those cells. If sow ('S') is bred with a boar ('S'), all of the
piglets will be susceptible to adhesion and therefore to diarrhoea. I think that is really an interesting concept.

With regard to Ed Bohl's method, it can also be argued
that there are now competent vaccines available which should be
used instead. One other thing I would say is that when the
farmers are experiencing these outbreaks, normally they control
the diarrhoea as well as they can with antibiotics, over the
period until there is herd immunity.

It is interesting that in spite of the fact that many of
us have been working on diarrhoea in piglets for the last 15
or 20 years, and we now have much new information, the method
of controlling the disease in piglets is now the same as when
we started.

DISCUSSION

B.A. Bokhout   *(Netherlands)*

    I would like to make two comments. If I understood you correctly, Dr. Bienenstock, you said that the intraperitoneal route was not practical.

J. Bienenstock   *(Canada)*

    Well, it certainly is not practical in man.

B.A. Bokhout

    I agree with you but in piglets it certainly is. You can inject 100 to 120 piglets, intraperitoneally, in 20 minutes.

    The second comment I would like to make is that I think it would be worthwhile to study the factor which we often know in animal husbandry, which is the time at which the animal will be confronted with a certain antigen. If the antigen is there, you don't need to use it in your vaccine. So if you take an adjuvant for two or three days and bring the immune response to a higher level, it may be possible to use the antigen which is introduced naturally. I think we will publish results in the near future on weaning diarrhoea in the pig which indicate a very high level of protection not only against *coli* but against a whole range of pathogenic organisms.

J. Bienenstock

    Can you give us more information about the method you are talking about?

B.A. Bokhout

    Well, as I said, it will be published shortly. It is an adjuvant which, in rabbits, gives a response 5 to 10 times higher than incomplete Freund's adjuvant. It is a question of introducing the adjuvant into the animal at the appropriate time. But there is still a lot we don't know about, a lot more work to be done.

F.J. Bourne   *(UK)*

Dr. Williams Smith suggested that the isolation of sows, particularly in the UK, or any pig industry, leads to problems in relation to disease control in that it does not lead to a rapid biological spread of a pathogen through a population. He also indicated that bringing in a large number of young animals does increase the incidence of *E. coli* disease - which is certainly true. However, we do have a problem in the British pig industry which is not going to be easily overcome, in that the majority of sows are housed in stalls, either tethered or confined in such a way that there is minimum contact during the gestation period when you would hope that these animals would be exposed to pathogenic *coli*. In addition to that, because of genetic improvements within the industry, farmers regularly turn over 33% of stock per year. It would be possible, but extremely difficult, to reduce this to 25% per year. So you have a potentially dangerous situation where a minimum of 25% and more likely 30%+ of the animals are young animals, in addition to the fact that they are isolated from each other. Whatever we say we are not going to alter that situation. In the light of this, obviously we must resort to vaccinal policies. Some farms do this, not by using the approach indicated by Ed Bohl, namely feeding live *coli* which are cultured in the laboratory, but by developing a feedback system whereby they feed faeces from sows and particularly, scouring piglets, back to their dry sows. It could be argued that that is equally dangerous as the feeding of pathogenic *coli* but it is a common practice which does seem to work and which does seem to have some effect not only with *coli* but with some of the entero viruses. The alternative, of course, is to develop suitable vaccines coupled with sound husbandry practices. Dr. Morein suggested that they have suitable vaccines in Sweden. I would question whether we have suitable vaccines in the UK.

B. Morein   *(Sweden)*

I can only quote what they say at the slaughter organisation. When they follow this vaccination procedure, using the right strains and so on, they say they can control the disease in the newborn to a level of 80%. However, in many cases they get the same disease, with exactly the same strains, at three weeks. It may be that if you use this live immunisation you get more antibodies in the milk and protect for a longer period. There might be the same problem at weaning but when they are older they are more resistant.

E. Bohl (USA)

There are several comments I could make but I will try to keep them brief. Firstly I would say to Dr. Morein that they must have much better vaccines in Sweden than we have in the United States and you could make a tremendous amount of money exporting them to us! We don't have anything to give us that type of immunity in pregnant swine, although there is a lot of work being done and I am sure progress will be made.

Now, I am not advocating, and I never have advocated, the approach which I described, as a routine extensive programme. This method is used in those herds where there is a distinct problem. It is very well controlled. There is nothing hap-hazard about it. As I said, we are only using those organisms that are already on the farm but we are making sure that the animals are being exposed and I don't really see too much wrong with this approach if it is done in this way. These are enzootic infections - you have to keep this in mind. I don't know that there is any hope of ever eradicating pathogenic E. coli from an animal population. The only approach I know to control it is to have, routinely, a good level of immunity in all animals. By exposing them at the right time you have a good chance of getting a decent immunity in 100% of the animals, in contrast to 50% of the animals which would have it naturally.

B.A. Bokhout

I don't think that the vaccines Dr. Morein is talking about should be introduced in America. The problem is that we wean too early so the maternal immunity is at a relatively high level.

Therefore the antigen does not contact the immune system of the young animal. This is why the same problems arise with the same *coli* bacteria later on. I think the answer is to choose a method whereby you give your maternal immunity at a low level. There will be some problems with diarrhoea in the early weeks of life and the farmer will have to live with that but the results prove that this eliminates the problems after weaning.

F.J. Bourne

Dr. Bokhout suggests that maternal immunity would have an adverse effect on developing immunity of the piglet; I would suggest that there is no evidence for this at all in relation to *E. coli* infections. This is one area where research is demanded.

J. Bienenstock

There is a little evidence in man to support the fact that if the mother is immune then the child cannot be immunised.

J. Soothill   *(UK)*

The tiny bit of evidence is in polio, and that is only in Africa. It really does not seem to work in individuals who have not got an enormous amount of IgA antibody in their milk.

J. Hall   *(UK)*

There is some evidence from cows that the maternal colostrum will actually suppress the development of the immune response.

F.J. Bourne

Equally, one can provide evidence where the maternal anti-body enhances the immune development in the young offspring, I believe that we must be far more specific since different effects may be apparent with different infectious agents.

J. Bienenstock

In pigs there is certainly some evidence that this is the

case. This raises this whole very big area that we really have
not gone into of what it is in colostrum, for example, and
potentially not just colostrum, that does promote the development of a B cell or other immune mechanisms, promote the retention of those cells in the appropriate places, and so on. Jarrett
has information about suppressive effects in colostrum; other
workers have evidence for enhancement. This is an enormous area
that requires further study.

502

SUMMARY

J. Soothill   *(UK)*

Clearly it is very difficult to summarise what we have
discussed in the past few days. We have had a mass of information most of which is of considerable practical importance.

In developing immunisation programmes for the individual
animal and on a herd basis we are trying to achieve a number of
factors:

Individual freedom from disease
Individual recovery from infection
Freedom of the herd from infection
Possible elimination of the infectious agent
Maximal levels of colostral antibody for passive transfer

We have heard a good deal about the above but really what
they are aimed at doing in Agricultural Systems is to increase
animal performance at reduced cost. Thus we must in addition
to infectious disease consider all aspects that influence growth
rate and food conversion ratios and we have heard something of
the influence that allergic reactions, particularly to food
antigens, may have on gut integrity and one would assume animal
performance.

Besides considering the beneficial effects of vaccination
we must beware that we do not make infections worse either by
generating allergic effects as has been done with RSV or by
generating tolerance about which we have heard a lot following
oral immunisation although it can be achieved by other routes too.

We are faced with an interesting comparison between human
infants and those of farm animals in their breast feeding methods.

The majority of farm species are weaned extremely early, so
until recently were human infants but now the vast majority of
human infants are breast fed with little supplement. This has

arisen because of the recognised immunological importance of breast feeding and the emotions of the mothers.

The early weaning of farm animals might be expected to lead to immunological problems and this is an area that needs actively researching with well thought out experimental design.

Further factors that are likely to influence the immune status are hygiene, nutrition and prophylactic chemotherapy - these factors lie outside the real subject matter of this meeting, which is immunisation.

We heard from Professor Bohl of the importance of the interaction of passive and active immunisation. Further work is necessary to explore this interaction, and how appropriate means of active immunisation should be modified to take into account the passive immunisation that may be present. Clearly the effect of giving antigen parenterally will depend on the passive IgG that is present in serum and oral presentation will depend on the IgA antibody in milk.

The presentation of antigen to stimulate active immunity may be subcutaneous, intra-peritoneal or oral. We had very interesting discussions on this interaction - intra-peritoneal immunisation seems to stand mid-way between oral and subcutaneous immunisation. Most interesting of all in this area is the information from Dr. Carlsson that with cholera vaccination it depends on whether you are talking about the primary or the secondary dose in terms of the pattern of response that occurs. The fact that you can boost a local immunity by a parenteral dose when you cannot initiate it must be important in our forward planning, but so must that worrying information of Dr. Stokes that under certain circumstances dietary changes can interfere with antibody production - this could be important. So, route is important.

We must also consider the nature of the vaccine. Dr. Morein's rather sophisticated approach was to get the right

immunogen on a truly appropriate molecule for presentation.
Much more is needed in that field. We had the worrying information from Dr. Newby that oral tolerance can arise to bacterial
antigens. That is new to me and I think it is a very important
observation.

An important consideration that arose from this meeting was
the relationship between antigen presentation and the use of
adjuvants, particularly adjuvants in the gastro intestinal tract.
Dr. Bienenstock told us of this but has told us also what I think
we all know, that our actual knowledge of adjuvants for oral
antigens is extremely limited. We have the startling half story
from Dr. Bokhout that you can give the adjuvant without the
antigen if the individual already has the antigen. Work on
adjuvants has usually assumed that, in general, you have to give
the adjuvant and the antigen together but there is already
experimental evidence for questioning this. Then for oral
immunisation, Anne Ferguson directed our attention towards the
possibility of suppressing suppressors. We have the special
tendency for mucosal immunisation to generate tolerance. Dr.
Ferguson told us that if we give the antigen plus cytophosphamide
then the response is far more positive. I do think that that
would be a very real field for research. It is a mode of
immunisation which we are unlikely to apply to humans where
killing an animal is regarded as really a rather bad thing to do!
But the occasional risk is, I imagine, more acceptable in an
agricultural situation if you can make a widespread benefit in
conversion ratio to the majority. I don't know whether I have
judged your priorities correctly, but I am trying to.

Another important factor was discussed that relates to
'antigen presentation' by Dr. Newby, Dr. Bienenstock and others
and raised the question of how to get the antigen past the acid
in the stomach, this has not been worked out in detail.

These are all important fields of work.

Understanding mechanisms of protection has been the subject of most of the presentations - Bienenstock, Hall, Vaerman,
Brandtzaeg, Stokes, have all been talking about rather fundamental immunology, and then we had the attractive superimposition
of rather more bizarre immunology from Clamp and Miller, of the
way in which IgA and mucus interact. This is a very intriguing
field that warrants further study. Immunologists have spent far
too long describing the effects of an experience of an antigen.
A mass of passive transfer experiments are going to be needed
if we want to understand the mechanism, which I think we do
because we now know that different immunisation regimes vary in
the type of response that is generated. The clearest example
of this is the secretory response. We really must explore in
greater detail how each individual immune mechanism achieves
protection in each individual infection. This will be a
staggering mass of work which, I suspect, has not gone very far
yet.

Allergy was considered by Jarrett, Levinsky, André and
Kilshaw. Kilshaw's remarks were very pleasing to me because I
spend a lot of time on food allergy in humans - a very big problem in human medicine but occurring in only a minority of the
population. I fear Kilshaw is right, that the right way of
handling food allergy in animals is to say, "Well, if this
particular food is sufficiently allergenic to cause trouble, just
cook it a bit more and then maybe it won't be". That is the sort
of philosophy he has outlined and I will stick my neck out and
say that I do not think that you are going to have food allergy
as the kind of big problem it is in human medicine.

I want to close by reminding you that we are only 30 miles
from where immunology started in Gloucestershire where Jenner did
his first immunological experiments. Immunisation is much older
than immunology and was done initially with virulent organisms.
I had intended to put the case for considering virulent organisms
as an immunising agent in agriculture but Professor Bohl has
already done it for *E. coli*. However, I think he has chosen
rather an odd example because of the extreme complexity of

bacterial variations, virulence and so on. It was a virus that
was first handled in this way, the smallpox virus. I think all
of us predicted that getting an attenuated rubella virus was
going to take a very long time and I suggested that we ought to
use virulent rubella virus to prevent congenital abnormality,
with the concept, of course, that the disease is trivial unless
you happen to be pregnant and pregnancy is something that can
be manipulated nowadays. In veterinary medicine you have a
number of similar examples, of which rotavirus and gastro
enteritis virus seem to be the most obvious. Smith and Bohl
have taken diametrically opposite views, very pleasantly, in our
discussions but presumably if you have to be at one pole or another
for each individual organism, and of course, hygiene is the best
way of dealing with many infections - Dr. Smith is a hygienist,
Professor Bohl is an immuniser - these are two rather opposed
positions and it would be perfectly possible, as I see it, to
give all known strains of rotavirus to all female pigs, as adults,
before they are mated, and then present the virus to the offspring while they are still being fed. You could eliminate the
whole problem by that sort of approach before you get the
attenuated vaccine that people are asking for. I don't know
which you should do, but do remember that that is where immunisation started.

I have tried to summarise the major points and to give a
forward look. I know that many people would disagree with what
I have said, are there any suggestions for future work?

FINAL DISCUSSION

E. Bohl (USA)

I think it would be very interesting to know more about the role of cell mediated immunity in overcoming an infection, and specifically, the effect that cold stress has on interfering with the manifestation of cell mediated immunity.

J. Soothill (UK)

I think the relevance of the environment to the particular response is very important but to answer that question precisely we need a passive transfer experiment. Simply to observe that CMI is present is not enough. Passive transfer experiments of cell mediated immunity require inbred strains - it can't be done in the domestic animal, it is something that would have to be done in mouse.

F.J. Bourne

Inbred strains of miniature pigs could well be available in the next few years for scientific experiment.

J. Soothill

That is a very important statement of advance; I didn't realise that. So, we know how to do it Professor Bohl.

Dr. Bokhout, I know you have thoughts on the problems of experimental design, can you tell us more?

B.A. Bokhout (Netherlands)

I think a lot of you are familiar with the fact that if you wish to test a vaccine, you use a laboratory model or use a suitable group of farm animals and divide them as nearly as possible into two halves, half of the animals being vaccinated and the other half unvaccinated. If the vaccine is successful you don't see disease. The problem is that no two farms are the same. Our approach is different - we had a farm on which about 25% of the piglets died after weaning and 100% had diarrhoea and none of them died. We vaccinated half of one litter in the infected litter - none of them got diarrhoea and none of them died. We next vaccinated 20%, two out of ten piglets - none of them got diarrhoea and none of them died. We were simply using an immunostimulant, an adjuvant. But the thing is we only vaccinated two animals out of ten.

F.J. Bourne

What was your problem disease in this case?

B.A. Bokhout

Post weaning diarrhoea with K88 - *E. coli*. K88 was still present in the faeces of vaccinated animals but not at such a high level as in the other animals in the litter. It is a general observation that you can have pathogenic organism in your herd but problems only arise when it gets above a certain level. I think it is the same with TGE, it is there but you won't get problems unless it gets above a certain level. I believe we are reducing environmental load by this practice.

J. Soothill

The word 'elimination' of an infectious agent is wrong but I do think that 'control' of an infectious agent is an important goal for immunisation that we forget about.

J. Bienenstock

I think it is a very interesting observation that Dr. Bokhout has made and I would like to make a philosophical comment. You might say that immunity as a protective mechanism has evolved not to eliminate an organism but, in fact, to regulate and to control its level. If that is the case, then only in the rare instance, such as smallpox, should we be interested at all in trying to eliminate the infectious agent. This is a very important issue.

J. Soothill

Yes, I would like to develop that thought which I think is important. I used the word 'eliminate' meaning elimination from the herd, not elimination from the world. Control would be a better word in that context. But, we do believe that the small-pox organism has been eliminated from the world. The important factor there, of course, is that there is no alternative host. Now, you might consider individual attempts at true elimination of pathogens of that type and it ought to be easier with farm animals than with humans, where you have infections confined to your farm animals. But are there any viruses which are confined to farm animals?

E. Bohl   (USA)

Sure, hog cholera has been eradicated in the United States, that is a good example.

J. Soothill

But it still exists somewhere else?

E. Bohl

Well yes, it exists in Europe. Our concern was whether other species are infected with hog cholera; if that was the case we probably would not have been successful. As far as we know, swine was the only species in the United States that was susceptible.

J. Soothill

Do you have wild swine in the United States?

E. Bohl

No, not really, escaped domestic swine, yes.

J. Soothill

Was it by immunisation or by slaughter that you eliminated this disease, or by both?

510

E. Bohl

Both.

F.J. Bourne

In the UK it was purely by slaughter, vaccination did not eradicate the disease - you would not expect it to do so.

J. Soothill

I regret that I must bring this session to a close but before doing so I would like to take this opportunity to thank John Bourne and his colleagues for an absolutely fascinating and enjoyable time here. I think there is an exciting programme getting going here with John, Tim Newby and Chris Stokes. We congratulate them on the achievement of the meeting.

F.J. Bourne

Thank you for your kind comments. On behalf of the University of Bristol, and Tim Newby and Chris Stokes my colleagues who have put so much effort into ensuring its success, we are extremely happy to have been able to invite you here to this meeting. I feel, as you do, that it has been a success and I thank you all very much for the extremely hard work you have put into it. Finally, I believe that I speak for all of you in thanking Dr. Connell of the EEC Agricultural Division for the keen interest that he has taken in helping to organise the meeting and to ensure that we received adequate support that was necessary for its success.

POSTER PRESENTATIONS

HOMING OF LYMPHOCYTES AFTER ORAL VACCINATION OF THE SOW

Netty Kortbeek-Jacobs and Hans van der Donk
Department of Immunology, Faculty of Veterinary Medicine,
Utrecht, The Netherlands.

ABSTRACT

Migration of sensitised lymphocytes in swine was studied by measuring the lymphocyte proliferative response to K88 antigen and to class specific antisera.

Oral administration of antigen (E. coli 08 : 087 : K88ab) resulted in the appearance of K88 positive cells in peripheral and mammary lymph nodes In lactating sows these cells appear preferentially in mammary lymph nodes. The most effective vaccination schedule was found to be frequent vaccination over a long period.

A route of migration of lymphocytes is postulated and we conclude that oral vaccination of pregnant sows results in K88 positive cells, which – during lactation – home to the mammary lymph nodes.

INTRODUCTION

Protection of the newborn piglet can only be acquired via antibodies from colostrum and milk of the sow. Oral vaccination results in high titre of specific antibody, since immunisation by this route causes local antibody production (Bourne, 1976; Kortbeek-Jacobs and van der Donk, 1978; Kortbeek-Jacobs and van der Donk, in press). Oral administration of antigen leads to stimulation of lymphocytes in the gut, after which these cells selectively migrate to the mammary glands (Goldblum et al., 1975).

The aim of this study was to demonstrate the route of migration of lymphocytes after sensitisation in the gut.

MATERIALS AND METHODS

Animals

Pregnant sows were inoculated orally with 200 ml *E. coli* O8 : K87 : K88ab 10^9 viable organisms/ml). *E. coli* cultures were fed on each of 3 consecutive days at intervals indicated in Table 3. One pregnant sow was used as a non-vaccinated control. Five days after parturition the animals were killed and lymphoid organs asceptically removed. Heparinised blood samples were taken before slaughter.

To study the influence of lactation, a non lactating sow was also vaccinated once and killed five days later.

Lymphocyte stimulation test

The development of sensitised lymphocytes after vaccination was studied by lymphocyte stimulation tests (Shimizu and Shimizu, 1979). Cell suspensions were prepared from Peyers' Patches (PP), mesenteric lymph nodes (MLN), mammary lymph nodes (MaLN), peripheral lymph nodes (PLN) and the spleen. Lymphocytes from these tissues and from peripheral blood (PBL) were separated by Ficoll-Isopaque centrifugation (Dam et al., 1978). Cells (2×10^5/200 μl) were cultured in RPMI-1640 medium containing 10% newborn piglet serum, 1% 0.2 M L-glutamine, 0.2% penicillin (100 U./ml) and 0.2% streptomycine (0.1 mg/ml) for 3 days, and labelled with ^{3}H-thymidine (0.4 μ Ci/culture, spec. act. 1.0 Ci/mmole) for the last 18 h.

Lymphocyte proliferative response to K88 antigen was measured in cultures containing 5 μg purified antigen. The response to class specific antisera was measured at concentrations of 8, 15 and 33 μg/200 μl respectively of anti-α, -μ and -γ (IgG-fractions of the class specific goat antisera). The results of the assays were expressed as the ratio

$$\frac{\text{mean cpm of triplicate stimulated cultures}}{\text{mean cpm of triplicate control cultures}} \text{(stimulation index, SI)}$$

RESULTS AND DISCUSSION

The lymphocyte proliferative response to K88 antigen is shown in Table 1. Vaccination results in the appearance of K88 positive cells: in peripheral lymph nodes and mammary lymph nodes of non lactating sows, but preferentially in mammary lymph nodes of lactating sows. Table 2 shows the lymphocyte proliferative response to class specific antisera. The effect of vaccination is an increase of IgM positive cells and in lactating sows, to a lesser extent, of IgA positive cells. IgM positive cells are found in PLN of non lactating sows and in MaLN of lactating sows, while the sites of IgA positive cells are PP and MLN.

The influence of the vaccination schedule is demonstrated in Table 3. Oral vaccination is most effective if it is done frequently and over a long period. Not only does the number of K88 positive cells increase but also the proportion of these cells in the mammary lymph nodes.

LYMPHOCYTE PROLIFERATIVE RESPONSE

TABLE 1

TO K88 ANTIGEN

	Lactating not vaccinated K88	Lactating vaccinated K88	Not lactating* vaccinated K88
PBL	2.7**	2.8	4.6
PLN	1.3	4.1	7.0
PP	nd	1.8	2.4
MLN	2.2	4.1	4.0
Spleen	2.9	< 1	< 1
MaLN	1.5	12.0	7.9

TABLE 2

TO CLASS SPECIFIC ANTISERA

	Lactating not vaccinated			Lactating vaccinated			Not lactating* vaccinated		
	α	μ	γ	α	μ	γ	α	μ	γ
PBL	1.5**	12.0	1.6	1.4	3.2	8.2	< 1	2.0	5.5
PLN	< 1	3.1	< 1	2.1	25	5.4	4.2	65	18
PP	nd	nd	nd	nd	1.5	1.8	1.2	2.2	1.0
MLN	< 1	10.0	3.8	5.8	34	5.2	1.9	26	3.5
Spleen	< 1	1.1	< 1	< 1	< 1	< 1	< 1	1.2	1.0
MaLN	< 1	4.5	< 1	2.5	133	15.0	1.0	25	3.4

PBL : peripheral blood lymphocytes

PLN : peripheral lymph nodes

PP : Peyers' Patches

MLN : mesenteric lymph nodes

MaLN : mammary lymph nodes

* two weeks after delivery

** stimulation index

TABLE 3

EFFECT OF VACCINATION SCHEDULE ON LYMPHOCYTE STIMULATION

		Vaccination		parturition⌐		LST	K88 + cells (SI)		
days	-28	-21	-14	-7	0	+5	MaLN	PLN	MLN
schedule I	+	+	+	+	+		19	9.9	6.5
II	+				+		12	4.1	4.1
III			+		+		7.5	4.3	12
IV							1.5	1.3	2.2

The evaluation of these results suggests a route of migration, which is shown in Figure 1. Oral administration of antigen causes traffic of sensitised lymphocytes from PP via MLN to MaLN and/or PLN depending on lactation. We did not find stimulation of lymphocytes by K88 antigen in the spleen of vaccinated sows. Therefore we suggest that homing lymphocytes bypass this organ.

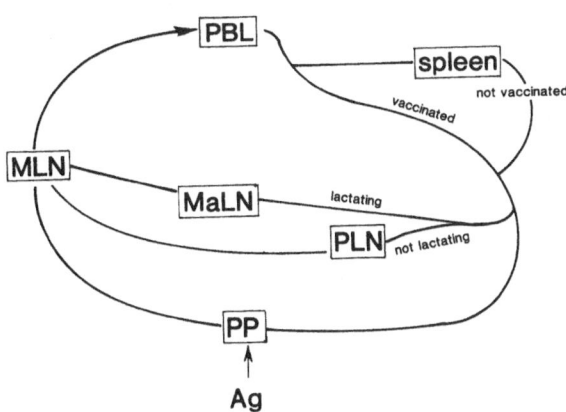

Fig. 1. Suggested route of migration.

518

Finally, we conclude that oral vaccination of pregnant sows results in K88 positive cells, which - during lactation - home to the mammary glands. There is a positive correlation between the amounts of K88 positive cells and of IgM positive cells.

ACKNOWLEDGMENT

We thank Dr. J.E. van Dijk for performing the surgery involved in this study.

REFERENCES

Bourne, F.J., 1976. Vet. Rec., 98, 499.

Dam, R.H.v., van Kooten, P.J.S. and van der Donk, J.A., 1978. J. Immunol. Meth. 21, 217.

Goldblum, R.H. et al., 1975. Nature, 257, 797.

Kortbeek-Jacobs, N. and van der Donk, H., 1978. J. Immunol. Meth. 24, 195.

Kortbeek-Jacobs, N. and van der Donk, H., manuscript in preparation.

Shimizu, M. and Shimizu, Y., 1979. Infect. Immun., 23, 239.

IMMUNE MECHANISMS IN THE RESPIRATORY TRACT

P.J. Quinn

Department of Veterinary Preventive Medicine and Food Hygiene,
Veterinary College, Ballsbridge,
Dublin, 4, Ireland.

INTRODUCTION

Mucous membranes are constantly challenged by micro-
organisms resident on body surfaces or present in the environment.
Under favourable health and environmental conditions relatively
few organisms are found deep in the respiratory tract. While
viable organisms may occasionally evade the respiratory defence
mechanisms, normal clearance mechanisms usually prevent their
establishment and tracheal secretions normally contain few
bacteria. The size of inhaled particles often determines the
sites they may reach in the respiratory tract. The 'filtration'
system inherent in the anatomical features of the nose and
turbinate bones ensures that larger particles are trapped in
the mucus covering the epithelium or settle out in the upper
respiratory tract. Smaller particles may reach the alveolar
spaces. Because the nasal passages are continually exposed
to a variety of micro-organisms, bacteria can be frequently
recovered from this area. Microbial contamination of the
environment strongly influences the numbers and types of
organisms found in this location. The nasal flora is usually
composed of a resident bacterial population and a transient
population. In calves, organisms frequently include *Pasteurella*,
Micrococcus and *Corynebacterium* spp. Resident microflora of the
host tend to prevent colonisation by bacterial interaction.
Infectious processes involving the lower respiratory tract or the
lung may occur when environmental conditions or host factors
allow infectious agents to penetrate the physical barriers of
the upper respiratory tract. Below the larynx, the mucociliary
blanket operates as an efficient trapping and clearing defence
mechanism. Naturally occurring factors present in mucus which
contribute to non-specific immunity, together with immunoglobulins

and pulmonary-alveolar macrophages offer substantial protection in the lower respiratory tract and alveoli against infectious agents. The immunoglobulin classes present in respiratory secretions are significantly different from those in serum. Of the immunoglobulins present in respiratory secretion, IgA in its secretory form is the predominant immunoglobulin. There is evidence for independent regulation of serum and secretory antibody either through selective transport or local synthesis. Since the respiratory tract is continually challenged by infectious agents from the environment, local immune mechanisms play an important role in combating respiratory disease.

DEPOSITION OF PARTICLES IN THE LUNGS

Particles 10 - 20 µm in diameter tend to settle in the nasopharyngeal region, but deposition in this region approaches zero as particle sizes decrease to 1 µm. Particles less than 3 µm may settle in the tracheobronchial region or pulmonary region (Stuart, 1973). In man, whole pollen grains measuring 25 µm were not deposited below the oropharynx, whereas fragments 1 - 5 µm in size could easily penetrate deeply into the lungs. (Busse et al., 1972).

DEFENCE MECHANISMS OF THE NOSE

Particle trapping in the nose by impaction is enhanced by the conformation of the turbinate bones covered with nasal mucosa rendered sticky by mucus-secreting cells.

Following nasal installation of Coxsackie virus in humans, interferon could be demonstrated in nasal wash solutions in 24 hours (Cate et al., 1969). Protection against virus shedding and illness was achieved by administration of interferon one day before and three days after challenge with rhinoviruses (Soloviev, 1968). During acute infections with viruses, transudation from the vascular tree occurs and IgA concentrations increase progressively in relation to other proteins. In two separate studies, volunteers with high levels of IgA in nasal secretions were better able to resist infection but the mechanism

of protection was not established (Rossen et al., 1970). Virus
neutralising antibody, usually in the form of secretory IgA,
appears in nasal secretions two weeks after infection becomes
established. Although the role of secretory IgA in limiting
natural infection is uncertain, protection mediated by
secretory IgA is demonstrable in previously immunised hosts
(Smith et al., 1966). The role of cell-mediated immunity in
nasal infections is still unclear.

Microbial antagonism suppresses the growth of many
potentially pathogenic bacteria and fungi at superficial
sites where they might otherwise initiate disease. A wide
range of 'normal' nasal bacteria flora are encountered in
different species. In humans, 40 to 70% of the adult population
carry one or more serological types of pneumococci in their
throats, yet epidemics of pneumococcal pneumonia are rare
(Davis et al., 1973). Bacterial antagonism involving
α haemolytic streptococci, tends to limit the growth of
pneumococci in the pharynx. Other mechanisms that influence
nasal flora seem to have an immunological basis both in their
mediation and specificity (Ehrenkranz, 1966).

The antibacterial activity of serum through the
co-operation of antibody and complement is long established.
In respiratory secretions it is doubtful if a similar anti-
bacterial mechanism could operate due to the limited
concentration of complement components present in these secretions
in the absence of inflammation (Rossen et al., 1966). That IgA
per se in the presence of adequate complement levels can effect
bacterial killing is disputed (Hauptman and Tomasi, 1978).

DEFENCE MECHANISMS OF THE AIRWAYS

Defence barriers in the airways and lower respiratory
tract include the epiglottal reflex which prevents gross
aspiration of foreign material and a mucociliary blanket which
covers most of the surface of the lower respiratory tract.
Mucociliary clearance moves infected material upwards into the
pharynx and the cough reflex clears accumulated mucus from the

lower respiratory tract. The terminal portions of the lower
respiratory tract, the alveoli, are protected by pulmonary-
alveolar macrophages, the resident mononuclear phagocytes of the
lung, which function as primary defence against inhaled
particulate matter. Collections of lymphoid cells in the
submucosal area of the bronchii are described (Nagaishi, 1972),
and these probably serve for both antigen processing and local
antibody production. Apart from secretory immunoglobulins,
non-specific antibacterial substances such as lysozyme which
contributes to the lysis of some gram negative organisms, and
lactoferrin which inhibits growth of bacteria dependent on iron
by chelating soluble iron salts, are present in airway
secretions. The immune response in the upper respiratory
tract relating to protection, appears to involve secretory IgA
and limited cellular activity. In the lower respiratory tract
cellular mechanisms are more actively involved in immune
responses.

Although cellular immune mechanisms may operate in either
the upper or lower repiratory tract, thymus derived cells
(T cells) are not ordinarily present on the air side of the
respiratory epithelium (Cohen and Gold, 1975). Certain
infectious agents with an affinity for the respiratory tract
are able to evade airway defences. Myxoviruses have a
haemagglutinin on their surface which specifically reacts with
a receptor substance on the epithelial cells (Mimms, 1976),
and both rhinoviruses and *Mycoplasma pneumoniae* have their own
receptors on epithelial cell surfaces. Certain micro-organisms
that infect the respiratory tract directly depress ciliary
activity thereby facilitating infection. *Bordetella pertussis* and
Haemophilus influenzae inhibit ciliary activity and damage respiratory
epithelium (Mimms, 1976).

DEFENCE MECHANISMS OF THE ALVEOLI

Immune responses can be demonstrated with lymphocytes
recovered from the lung after immunisation via the respiratory
tract but not by the systemic route. Although lymphocytes
lavaged from the lungs of animals sensitised via the respiratory

tract can function as antibody producing cells (B cells) or T cells, lymphocytes normally residing in the lung appear to have only B cell characteristics (Cohen and Gold, 1975). Accordingly, the T cells must be recruited from the blood. The rapid clearance of bacteria from the lungs of animals after exposure to bacterial aerosols is well documented (Robertson, 1941; Green and Kass, 1964; Laurenzi et al., 1964; Lillie and Thomson, 1972), and the contribution of the pulmonary-alveolar macrophage to this process area is clearly established (Hocking and Golde, 1979). The cellular and humoral immune mechanisms that operate in the lung, combined with an effective phagocytic system usually render the alveolar regions microbiologically sterile in normal animals. Small numbers of potentially pathogenic bacteria can, however, be frequently isolated from the lungs of normal calves (Allan, 1978).

THE SECRETORY IMMUNE SYSTEM

The role of local immunity in body defences has been known since the beginning of this century. The mechanism of resistance to infection at mucous membranes can how be shown frequently to operate independently of systemic immunity. The demonstration of IgA as the predominant immunoglobulin in many secretions, in contrast to its relatively lower concentration in serum led to the concept of a distinct immune system operating through external secretions, sometimes referred to as the mucosal immune system. Species and age differences are well recognised, however, and while IgA is the predominant immunoglobulin in bovine nasal secretions (Duncan et al., 1972). IgG1 is the immunoglobulin present in the highest concentration in the bovine respiratory tract during the first six weeks of life (Morgan and Bourne, 1978). Evidence for local production of IgA has been well documented for the salivary glands, the gastrointestinal tract, the mammary gland and the respiratory tract. The site of synthesis of IgA is primarily in submucosal plasma cells. In human serum, IgA exists mainly as a monomer, whereas in external secretions it exists mainly as a dimer. Secretory IgA is composed of an IgA dimer, a molecule of secretory component and a molecule of J chain. Secretory component is produced locally. IgA and J chain are produced in submucosal plasma cells (Hauptman and Tomasi, 1978). IgA in bovine serum appears to be in the dimeric form only (Duncan et al., 1972).

Biological Activity of the Secretory Immune System

Immunity to many respiratory viruses which produce disease locally in the respiratory tract of man seems to be mediated to a large extent by locally produced, mostly secretory IgA activiral antibodies (Ogra and Karzon, 1969). In adult volunteers challenged intranasally with Type 1 parainfluenza virus, the presence of antibodies in nasal secretions proved to be a better index of host resistance to infection than the level of serum antibody (Smith et al., 1966). Studies with an inactivated rhinovirus vaccine in human volunteers indicated that the intranasal route of immunisation stimulated a protective immunity in over 60% of recipients to challenge with the live virus. Less than 20% of those given vaccine intramuscularly were protected (Perkins et al., 1969). Only the group which developed nasal antibody showed significant protection against challenge with the live virus. The majority of calves inoculated with infectious bovine rhinotracheitis by the nasal route showed a local antibody response in two weeks (Le Jan and Asso, 1978). Following administration of a local booster inoculation an increase in the level of neutralising activity was demonstrable between the fifth and fifteenth day. No correlation between local and systemic response was evident. Results of vaccination trials with agents incriminated in bovine respiratory diseases have yielded conflicting results. A field trial with an inactivated vaccine containing adenoviruses, reoviruses and parainfluenza viruses given subcutaneously conferred substantial protection against bovine enzootic pneumonia (Wizigmann, 1978). In another trial with an inactivated virus vaccine containing strains of five viruses associated with respiratory diseases of cattle and given intramuscularly, there was no evidence that the vaccine provided any protection for the calves (Morzaria et al., 1978).

The large numbers of viral strains potentially pathogenic in the respiratory tract, the possibility of 'antigenic drift' occurring in individual strains and the uncertain contribution of bacteria and mycoplasma to the pathogenesis of respiratory disease have proved to be serious obstacles to the development of reliable viral vaccines for use in cattle.

The function of the mucosal immune system in anti-bacterial defences is still unresolved. The inability of IgA to fix complement via the classical pathway in a manner similar to IgM or IgG makes it less likely that the anti-bacterial effect of IgA is complement-mediated. The low levels of complement components on most mucosal surfaces support this view. Activation of complement by IgA through the alternative pathway may be possible but it is not clear if there are sufficient concentrations of complement and alternative pathway components in respiratory secretions to allow this system to operate at a significant level. The role of secretory IgA as an opsonin is also in doubt. Although this antibody can combine and coat bacteria *in vivo* evidence that this enhances phagocytosis is not totally accepted (Hauptman and Tomasi, 1978). Nevertheless, there is experimental evidence which demonstrates greater opsonic activity for IgA against *E. coli* than either IgM or IgG (Wernet et al., 1971).

The abiltiy of secretory IgA to inhibit bacterial adherence to epithelial cells is one of the few antibacterial functions conclusively demonstrated for this immunoglobulin. Since mucous membranes are often the site of many bacterial infections and portals of entry for more generalised disease, establishment of such infections usually requires initial colonisation by bacteria. Adherence to an epithelial surface is a prerequisite for colonisation. Adherence, therefore, constitutes a virulence mechanism and the ability of secretory IgA to inhibit the attachment of certain strains of streptococci to human buccal epithelial cells may be a significant method of mucosal protection (Williams and Gibbons, 1972). Motility of bacteria may also be a potential invasive advantage on mucosal surfaces, and the ability of secretory IgA in the vaginal mucus of heifers to immobilise *C. foetus* may be yet another protective mechanism (Corbeil et al., 1974).

THE PULMONARY-ALVEOLAR MACROPHAGE

Tissue macrophages of various organs derive from stem cells in the bone marrow (van Furth, 1970). Macrophages found in different tissues exhibit regional differences in their biochemistry, morphology and function (Walker, 1976). Pulmonary-alveolar macrophages are unique among mononuclear phagocytes in several ways. These cells differ metabolically from peritoneal macrophages in that they rely largely on aerobic glycolysis for energy requirements, whereas peritoneal macrophages depend primarily on anaerobic glycolysis (Wing and Remington, 1978). Although the lysosomal content of alveolar macrophages is generally higher than that of peritoneal macrophages, the former do not destroy bacteria as readily as the latter (Pavillard, 1963). Alveolar and peritoneal macrophages respond differently to chemotactic agents. Rabbit alveolar macrophages do not respond to chemotactic agents with activity for peritoneal macrophages (Ward, 1968). Guinea pig pulmonary-alveolar macrophages do not respond to migration inhibition factor and fail to absorb activity from culture supernatants (Leu et al., 1972). The ability of pulmonary-alveolar macrophages to replicate *in vitro* is clearly established (Fox 1973; Soderland and Naum, 1973), and cell division of alveolar macrophages *in vivo* is also recorded (Wing and Remington, 1978). The life-span of alveolar macrophages in the mouse is 50 days compared with 40 days for peritoneal macrophages and 60 days for Küpffer cells (Fauve, 1978).

Antimicrobial Activity of Pulmonary-Alveolar Macrophages

Surface membrane receptors for various serum components have been identified on alveolar macrophages and these receptors have functional importance in the initiation of phagocytosis by mononuclear cells (Mantovani et al., 1972). Receptors for the Fc portion of IgG and the third component of complement C3 have

been demonstrated on both human and rabbit alveolar macrophages
(Daughaday and Douglas, 1976). The number of IgG receptor sites
on rabbit pulmonary-alveolar macrophages increases after repeated
administration of Freund's adjuvant (Arend and Mannik, 1973)
Macrophages in an 'activated' state show an enhanced capacity
to ingest opsonised micro-organisms. BCG vaccination of rabbits
resulted in an increase in both the number of pulmonary-alveolar
macrophages possessing complement and IgG receptors and the
number or affinity of the receptors on each cell (Montarroso
and Myrvik, 1978).

The precise mechanisms involved in microbial destruction
by alveolar macrophages are not fully elucidated. Evidence for
the involvement of hydrogen peroxide, catalase, lysosomal cationic
proteins and other components is documented (Hocking and Golde,
1979). Whatever the steps involved in bacterial destruction by
alveolar macrophages, these are facilitated by specific antibody
which enhances postphagocytic killing (Reynolds et al., 1975).
The cell free portion of bronchopulmonary lavage fluid is known
to enhance bacterial destruction by alveolar macrophages (La Force
et al., 1973), and the factor(s) responsible cannot be supplied
by serum.

Viral infections of the lung frequently predispose to
subsequent bacterial pneumonias. This sequence of events has
generally been considered to result from impaired mucociliary
clearance mechanisms (Mimms, 1976). Studies in mice have shown
that postviral susceptibility to bacterial infection may relate
to impaired bactericidal activity as a result of either
defective phagocytosis or killing (Jakab and Green, 1972).

Immunological Functions of the Pulmonary-Alveolar Macrophage

Resistance to certain infectious agents such as intracellular micro-organisms depends on cell-mediated immune
mechanisms. 'Activated' macrophages are the principal effector
cells in this line of defence. The resident alveolar
macrophage population may participate in cell-mediated immunity

in the lung but recruitment of circulating monocytes into the
alveolar spaces may also occur (Truitt and Mackaness, 1971).
Activation of macrophages may occur directly or through
soluble mediators released from sensitised T lymphocytes
following contact with antigen. Macrophage migration inhibitory
factor is believed to be largely responsible for macrophage
activation after antigenic stimulation. Pulmonary lymphoid
cells are capable of releasing macrophage migration inhibitory
factor after antigenic stimulation (Gadol et al., 1974) and
alveolar macrophages of some species do respond to this factor
(Moore and Myrvik, 1974) but not in the guinea pig (Leu et al.,
1972). Pulmonary-alveolar macrophages exhibit cytotoxic activity
for virus-infected cells (Stott et al., 1975) and may thereby
limit viral infections in the lung. Interferon production by
rabbit alveolar macrophages has been demonstrated also (Acton
and Myrvik, 1966). Other soluble factors released by
pulmonary-alveolar macrophages stimulate granulocyte and
monocyte production by the bone marrow and induce migration of
these cells to the lung (Golde and Cline, 1974).

REFERENCES

Acton, J.D. and Myrvik, Q.N., 1966. Production of interferon by alveolar
    macrophages. J. Bacteriol. 91, 2300.

Allan, E.M., 1978. Pulmonary bacterial flora of pneumonic and non-
    pneumonic calves. In: Respiratory Diseases in Cattle (Ed. by
    W.B. Martin), p. 345. Martinus Nijhoff, The Hague.

Arend, W.P. and Mannik, M., 1973. The macrophage receptor for IgG:
    number and affinity of binding sites. J. Immunol. 110, 1455.

Busse, W.W., Reed, C.E. and Hoehne, J.H., 1972. Where is the allergic
    reaction in ragweed asthma? II. Demonstration of ragweed antigen in
    airborne particles smaller than pollen. J. Allergy Clin. Immunol.
    50, 289.

Cate, T.R., Douglas, R.G. Jr. and Couch, R.B., 1969. Interferon and
    resistance to upper respiratory virus illness. Proc. Soc. exp. Biol.
    Med. 133, 631.

Cohen, A.B. and Gold, W.M., 1975. Defense mechanisms of the lungs. Annu.
    Rev. Physiol. 37, 325.

Corbeil, L.B., Schurig, G.D., Duncan, J.R., Corbeil, R.R. and Winter, A.J.,
    1974. Immunoglobulin classes and biological functions of *Campylobacter*
    (Vibro) fetus antibodies in serum and cervicovaginal mucus. Infect.
    Immun. 10, 422.

Daughaday, C.C. and Douglas, S.D., 1976. Membrane receptors on rabbit and
    human pulmonary-alveolar macrophages. J. Reticuloendothel. Soc.
    19, 37.

Davis, B.D., Dulbecco, R., Eisen, H.N., Ginsberg, H.S. and Wood, W.B. Jr.,
    1973. Microbiology, p. 701. Harper and Row, New York.

Duncan, J.R., Wilkie, B.N., Hiestand, F. and Winter, A.J., 1972. The serum
    and secretory immunoglobulins of cattle: characterization and
    quantitation. J. Immunol. 108, 965.

Ehrenkranz, N.J., 1966. Nasal rejection of experimentally inoculated
    Staphylococcus aureus: evidence for an immune reaction in man.
    J. Immunol. 96, 509.

Fauve, R.M., 1978. Phagocytes. In: Immunology (Ed, by J.-F. Bach),
    p. 93. John Wiley and Sons, New York.

Fox, M.L., 1973. The bovine alveolar macrophage. I. Isolation, *in vitro*
    cultivation, ultrastructure and phagocytosis. Can. J. Microbiol. 19,
    1207.

Gadol, N., Johnson, J.E. III and Waldman, R.H., 1974. Respiratory tract
cell-mediated immunity: comparison of primary and secondary response.
Infect. Immun. 9, 858.

Golde, D.W. and Cline, M.J., 1974. Regulation of granulopiesis. N. Engl.
J. Med. 291, 1388.

Green, G.M. and Kass, E.H., 1964. The role of the alveolar macrophage in
the clearance of bacteria from the lung. J. exp. Med. 119, 167.

Hauptman, S.P. and Tomasi, T.B. Jr., 1978. The secretory immune system.
In: Basic and Clinical Immunology (Ed. by H.H. Fudenberg, D.P. Stites,
J.L. Caldwell and J.V. Wells), p. 215. Lange Medical Publications,
Los Altos, California.

Hocking, W.G. and Golde, D.W., 1979. The pulmonary-alveolar macrophage.
N. Engl. J. Med. 301, 580.

Jakab, G.J. and Green, G.M., 1972. The effect of Sendai virus infection on
bactericidal and transport mechanisms of the murine lung. J. clin.
Invest. 51, 1989.

La Force, F.M., Kelly, W.J. and Huber, G.L., 1973. Inactivation of staphylo-
cocci by alveolar macrophages with preliminary observations on the
importance of alveolar lining material. Am. Rev. resp. Dis. 108, 784.

Laurenzi, G.A., Berman, L., First, M. and Kass, E.H., 1964. A quantitative
study of the deposition and clearance of bacteria in the murine lung.
J. clin. Invest. 43, 759.

Le Jan, C. and Asso, J.M., 1978. Immunology in calf respiratory disease.
In: Respiratory Diseases in Cattle (Ed. by W.B. Martin), p. 457.
Martinus Nijhoff, The Hague.

Leu, R.W., Eddleston, A.L.W.F., Hadden, J.W. and Good, R.A., 1972.
Mechanisms of action of migration inhibitory factor (MIF). J. exp.
Med. 136, 589.

Lillie, L.E. and Thomson, R.G., 1972. The pulmonary clearance of bacteria
by calves and mice. Can. J. comp. Med. 36, 129.

Mantovani, B., Rabinovitch, M. and Nussenzweig, V., 1972. Phagocytosis of
immune complexes by macrophages. Different roles of the macrophage
receptor sites for complement (C3) and for immunoglobulin (IgG).
J. exp. Med. 135, 780.

Mimms, C.A., 1976. The Pathogenesis of Infectious Disease, p. 12.
Academic Press, London.

Montarroso, A.M. and Myrvik, Q.N., 1978. Effect of BCG vaccination on the
    IgG and complement receptors on rabbit alveolar macrophages. J.
    Reticuloendothel. Soc. 24, 93.

Moore, V.L. and Myrvik, Q.N., 1974. Inhibition of normal rabbit alveolar
    macrophages by factor(s) resembling migration inhibition factor.
    J. Reticuloendothel. Soc. 16, 21.

Morgan, K.L. and Bourne, F.J., 1978. The respiratory tract immune system.
    In: Respiratory Diseases in Cattle (Ed. by W.B. Martin), p. 440.
    Martinus Nijhoff, The Hague.

Morzaria, S.P.; Maund, E.A., Richards, M.S. and Harkness, J.W., 1978.
    Results of a small field trial with a multicomponent inactivated
    respiratory viral vaccine. In: Respiratory Diseases in Cattle
    (Ed. by W.B. Martin) p. 497. Martinus Nijhoff, The Hague.

Nagaishi, C., 1972. Functional Anatomy and Histology of the Lung. p.5.
    University Park Press, Baltimore, Md.

Ogra, P.L. and Karzon, D.T., 1969. Distribution of poliovirus antibody in
    serum, nasopharynx and alimentary tract following segmental
    immunization with poliovaccine. J. Immunol. 102, 1423.

Pavillard, E.R.J., 1963. *In vitro* phagocytic and bactericidal ability of
    alveolar and peritoneal macrophages of normal rats. Aust. J. exp.
    Biol. med. Sci. 41, 265.

Perkins, J.C., Tucker, D.N., Knopf, H.L.S., Wenzel, R.P., Hornick, R.B.,
    Kapikian, A.Z. and Chanock, R.M., 1969. Evidence of protective
    effect of an inactivated rhinovirus vaccine administered by the nasal
    route. Am. J. Epidemiol. 90, 319.

Reynolds, H.Y., Kazmierowski, J.A. and Newball, H.H., 1975. Specificity of
    opsonic antibodies to enhance phagocytosis of *Pseudomonas aeruginosa*
    by human alveolar macrophages. J. clin. Invest. 56, 376.

Robertson, O.H., 1941. Phagocytosis of foreign material in the lung.
    Physiol. Rev. 21, 112.

Rossen, R.D., Butler, W.T., Vannier, W.E., Douglas, R.G. Jr. and Steinberg,
    A.G., 1966. The sedimentation and antigenic properties of proteins
    in nasal and other external secretions. J. Immunol. 97, 925.

Rossen, R.D., Butler, W.T., Waldman, R.H., Alford, R.H., Hornick, R.B.,
    Togo, Y. and Kasel, J.A., 1970. The proteins in nasal secretions.
    J. Ad. med. Ass. 211, 1157.

Smith, C.B., Purcell, R.H., Bellanti, J.A. and Chanock, R.M., 1966. Protective
    effect of antibody to Parainfluenza, Type I virus. N. Engl. Med. 275, 1145.

Soderland, S.C. and Naum, Y., 1973. Growth of pulmonary-alveolar
     macrophages *in vitro*. Nature (Lond.). 245, 150.

Soloviev, V.D., 1968. Some results and prospects in the study of
     endogenous and exogenous interferon. In: The Interferons, An
     International Symposium (Ed. by G. Rita), p. 233. Academic Press,
     New York.

Stott, E.J., Probert, M. and Thomas, L.H., 1975. Cytotoxicity of alveolar
     macrophages for virus-infected cells. Nature (Lond.). 255, 710.

Stuart. B.O., 1973. Deposition of inhaled aerosols. Archs. intern. Med.
     131, 60.

Truitt, G.L. and Mackaness, G.B., 1971. Cell-mediated resistance to
     aerogenic infection of the lung. Am. Rev. resp. Dis. 104, 829.

van Furth, R., 1970. Origin and kinetics of monocytes and macrophages.
     Semin, Haematol. 7, 125.

Walker, W.S., 1976. Funtional heterogeneity of macrophages. In:
     Immunobiology of the Macrophage (Ed. by D.S. Nelson), p. 91.
     Academic Press, New York.

Ward, P.A., 1968. Chemotaxis of Mononuclear cells. J. exp. Med. 128, 1201.

Wernet, P., Breu, H., Knop, J. and Rowley, D., 1971. Antibacterial action
     of specific IgA and transport of IgM, IgA and IgG from serum into the
     small intestine. J. infect. Dis. 124, 223.

Williams, R.C. and Gibbons, R.J., 1972. Inhibition of bacterial adherence
     by secretory immunoglobulin A : mechanism of antigen disposal.
     Science 177, 697.

Wing, E.J. and Remington, J.S., 1978. Delayed hypersensitivity and
     macrophage functions. In: Basic and Clinical Immunology (Ed. by
     H.H. Fudenberg, D.P. Stites, J.L. Caldwell and J.V. Wells), p. 96.
     Lange Medical Publications, Los Altos, California.

Wizigmann, G., 1978. Vaccination against bovine enzootic pneumonia. In:
     Respiratory Diseases of Cattle (Ed. by W.B. Martin), p. 509.
     Martinus Nijhoff, The Hague.

CHANGES OF SYSTEMIC HYPERSENSITIVITY DUE TO ENTERALLY APPLIED ANTIGEN *

J. Seifert, T. Eberle, K. Hallfeld, G. Enders and
W. Brendel

Institute for Surgical Research at the University of Munich,
Klinikum Grosshadern, Marchioninistr. 15, 8000 Munich 70,
Federal Republic of Germany.

ABSTRACT

With enteral antigen application it is possible to manipulate the local immune response in animals. The aim of the experimental investigations was to test the influence of enterally applied antigen on a systemic immune response. Immunised rabbits were fed with the antigen and afterwards i.v. challenged with the antigen. Circulatory disorders like blood pressure decrease or blood flow reduction after challenge was markedly improved by antigen feeding. An explanation for this observed phenomenon is a significant reduction of circulating antibodies during the absorption of the antigen. The reduction of antibodies is due to a fixation within the layers of the gut and an elimination into the lumen. These mechanisms are probably also involved in a successful desensitisation in allergic patients.

* Supported by a grant from Deutsche Forschungsgemeinschaft.

INTRODUCTION

Investigations published by Thomas and Parrot (1974), André et al. (1978), Bazin (1978) and Walker et al. (1975) have shown that it is possible to influence the immune response via the gut. On one hand, immunological tolerance was observed, and on the other, a local immunisation was induced by enteral antigen application. For clinical and practical purposes it seems of more interest to change a stage of sensitisation into a stage of unresponsiveness by enteral antigen administration, because this way of application is without any risk with regard to side reactions. In the literature there are a few reports (De Weck and Girard, 1972; Hedin et al., 1976; Messmer et al., 1980) which indicate that it is possible to eliminate antibodies by degraded antigen - so called haptens - without the initiation of the immune response. Since food antigens are naturally degraded in the gut, it was speculated that it might be possible to reduce circulating antibodies by enterally applied antigen.

MATERIALS AND METHODS

For this purpose adult rabbits were actively immunised with human gamma globulin (HGG) + Freund's Adjuvant, until precipitating antibodies could be detected in the serum of the animals (Figure 1). Afterwards the animals were divided into 3 groups. Group 1 remained untreated, group 2 was orally pretreated with 1 g human gamma globulin, and group 3 was orally pretreated with 1 g pepsin digested human gamma globulin, that is with Fab_2 and Fc-fragments. All animals were intravenously challenged with 50 mg HGG. Blood pressure was measured with a Statham strain gauge transducer and blood flow with the microsphere technique (Seifert et al., 1979). To observe quantitatively the antibody content in the serum of the rabbits, a radioimmunoassay was developed to record changes during the feeding period and after i.v. challenge.

536

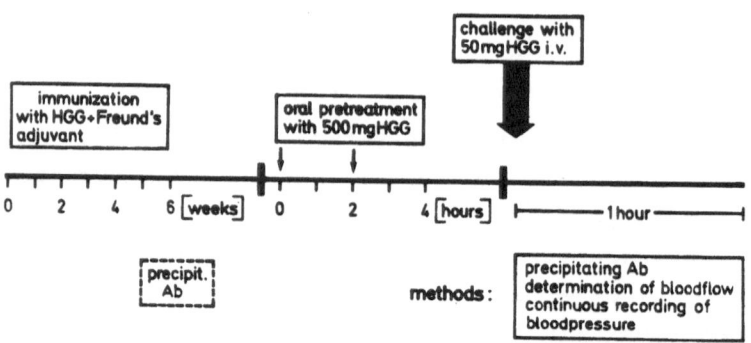

Fig. 1. Immunisation and test procedures in rabbits to test the influence of antigen feeding on circulatory disorders after i.v. antigen challenge.

To follow the fate of circulating antibodies, 50 mg rabbit anti-HGG antibodies were radioactively labelled (Franks et al., 1962) and intravenously injected into untreated rabbits. Control animals received the same amount of radioactively labelled rabbit IgG, but without the anti-HGG component. Both groups were fed HGG at dose rates of 25 mg, 250 mg or 1 000 mg HGG enterally applied. After an absorption time of 4 to 6 h the radioactivity was determined in the layers of the duodenum, jejunum, ileum and colon and also in the Peyer's Patches.

In both the control and the treated groups the radioactivity in the lumen of the gut was determined, in order to gain an impression of the direction of transport of the radioactivity. Sephadex chromatography (G-25) was used to determine the percentage of intact labelled protein and the proportion of degraded protein. The radioactivity was expressed as a percentage of the applied dose. For statistical analysis mean values and SEM were calculated and if necessary Students' t-test performed.

RESULTS

If animals are immunised and intravenously challenged
with the same antigen severe circulatory disorders can be observed. In control animals (Figure 2) with precipitating
antibodies against HGG the i.v. challenge induced a marked
blood pressure decrease from 100 mmHg to 40 mmHg. Within the
short observation time of 30 min these animals did not recover
from this severe anaphylactic reaction. After feeding and
absorption of HGG the blood pressure decrease is reduced. Mean
values were found at 60 mmHg and all animals recovered from
this decrease within 30 min to nearly normal values. Virtually
no change in blood pressure was observed in animals orally pretreated with pepsin digested human gamma globulin. This group
had a blood pressure decrease to values of only 80 mmHg, which
was followed by an instant recovery.

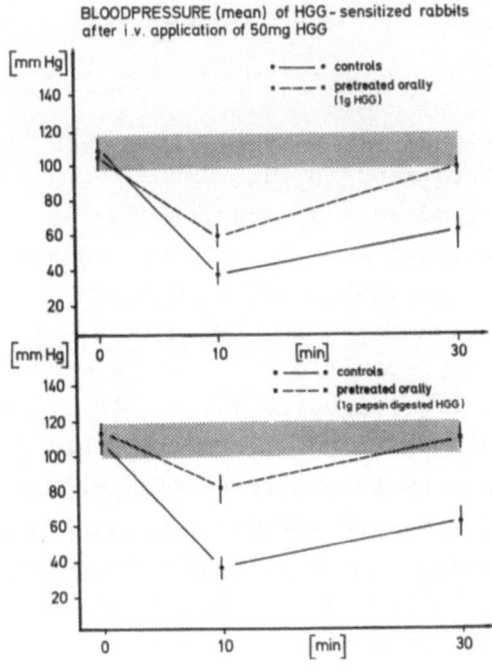

Fig. 2. Behaviour of blood pressure of immunised rabbits after i.v. challenge.

The mortality after intravenous challenge in animals with
precipitating antibodies corresponds to the behaviour of the
blood pressure and also blood flow changes (Table 1). Sixty
per cent of control animals die within 60 - 90 min as a consequence of circulatory disorders. Following oral pretreatment
with HGG this mortality is reduced to 30%. However, a short
term mortality rate of sera was observed in animals treated
with pepsin digested HGG (Figure 3).

TABLE 1

BLOOD FLOW VALUES (ml/min/g ORGAN) AFTER i.v. ANTIGEN CHALLENGE IN IMMUNISED
RABBITS

	Orally pretreated		Control	
	$\bar{x}$	$s\bar{x}$	$\bar{x}$	$s\bar{x}$
Duodenum	0.4 ±	0.1	0.2 ±	0.1
Gastric wall	0.2 ±	0.05	0.1 ±	0.04
Lung	3.5 ±	0.5	1.8 ±	0.8
Kidney	2.5 ±	0.5	1.0 ±	0.5

The prevention of the circulatory disorders must be a
consequence of alterations in the immune response. Therefore
the content of antibodies was determined using Ouchterlony's
agar diffusion technique and by radioimmunoassay. Whereas no
changes in antibody content could be detected by the Ouchterlony's
technique, a marked decrease in circulating antibody could be
found with the highly specific and sensitive radioimmunoassay.
As shown in Figure 4 circulating antibodies are reduced by antigen feeding from 350 µg/ml to 275 µg/ml. This decrease is even
more pronounced in animals orally treated with pepsin digested
antigens (Figure 5). There the decrease is from 550 µg/ml to
150 µg/ml. This reduction can be explained by antigen antibody
processes, which probably take place in the layers of the gut,
since the antigen was enterally applied.

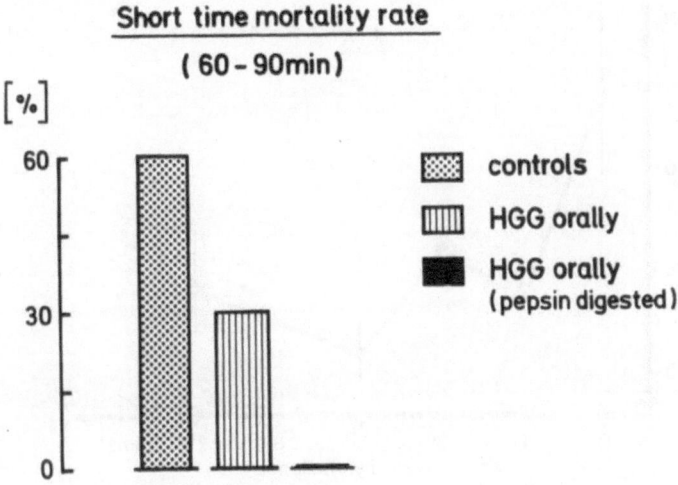

Fig. 3. Short time mortality rate after i.v. challenge in immunised rabbits with and without oral pretreatment.

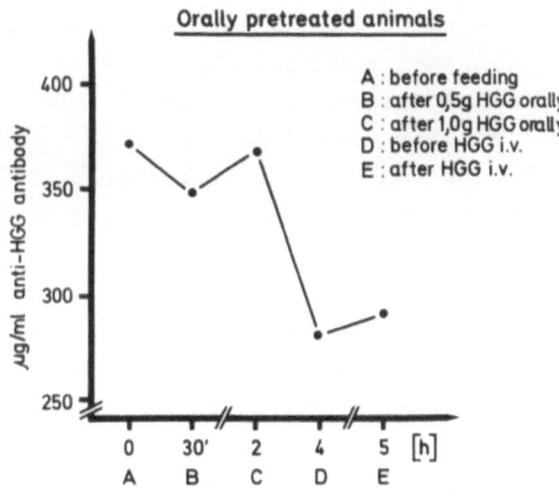

Fig. 4. Circulating antibodies in immunised and antigen fed animals.

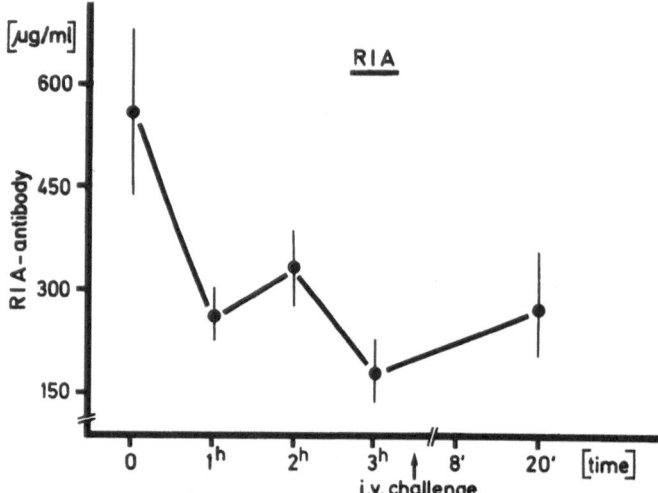

Fig. 5. Circulating antibodies in immunised animals fed with pepsin digested antigen.

To test this possibility untreated rabbits were injected with radioactively labelled anti-HGG-IgG and control animals with labelled IgG without the antibody component. If antigen antibody reactions take place in the layers of the gut the radioactivity must be higher and dose dependent in the test animals compared to control animals. Figure 6 shows the results of this experiment. A clear dose dependent fixation of the radioactively labelled antibody after oral dosage of 25, 250 and 1 000 mg HGG could be observed in duodenum, jejunum and ileum of the test animals.

To get more information on the fate of the radioactively labelled antibody, radioactivity was also measured in the fluid of the lumen of the gastrointestinal tract. Figure 7 shows a representative example of the radioactivity in the lumen of a test animal and a control animal. The very high amount of radioactivity in the lumen of the gut of animals, in which antigen antibody processes could take place, indicates that the circulating antibody is mainly transported in the direction of the lumen probably after the fixation of the antigen. It seems likely that the antigen antibody complex is enzymatically degraded, because the measured radioactivity in the lumen of the gut is not bound to high molecular size protein as indicated by Sephadex chromatography (G-25).

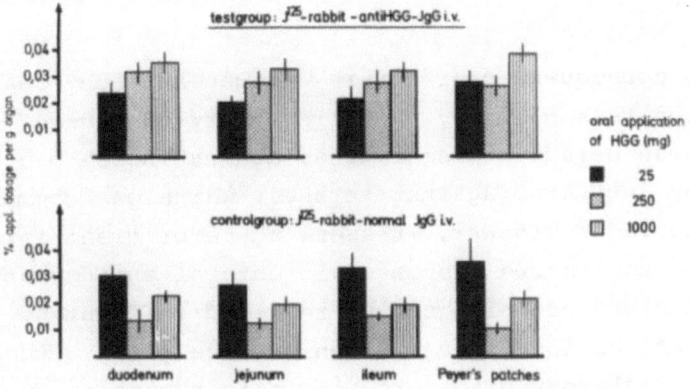

Fig. 6. Radioactively labelled antibodies in the layers of the gut after varying doses of enterally applied antigen. Control experiments were performed with normal IgG without the anti HGG component.

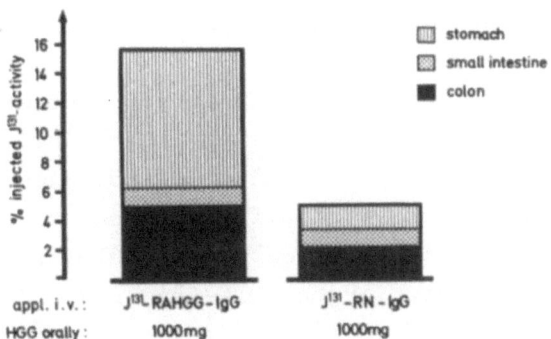

Fig. 7. Radioactivity in the lumen of the gut in test and control animals.

DISCUSSION

The consequences of severe antigen antibody reactions in living organisms normally are circulatory disorders. Since a lot of human beings are sensitised against horse protein, for example by antiserum against tetanus, which was commonly used during the 2nd World War, it seems to be of great interest to manipulate the immune response via enteral antigen application. If an immunised organism can be rendered tolerant by enteral antigen application, then antigens can be given without the risk of circulatory disorders, if it is necessary for therapeutic reasons to do so. For some antigens such as dextran (Hedin et al., 1976; Messmer et al., 1980) or penicillin (De Weck and Girard, 1972) it has been demonstrated that the immune response could be altered by intravenous application of degraded split products of the original antigen. Since antigens are naturally degraded during absorption from the gut, it was speculated that those absorbed split products can also alter the immune response after or during absorption. The effect of antigen feeding on blood pressure during intravenous challenge shows that this speculation is confirmed by a reduced blood pressure decrease in antigen fed animals. This effect is even more pronounced after the enteral application of pepsin digested antigen, i.e. Fab_2 and Fc-fragments indicating that the degradation of the antigen is of great importance.

The pathomechanism of this observed phenomenon seems to be partly influenced by humoral immune reactions. The increase of radioactivity in the intestinal wall indicates that enteral applied antigen can bind circulating antibodies within the layers of the gut. By this fixation the circulating antibodies are reduced markedly as shown by the RIA-findings. If circulating antibodies are decreased to a certain limit, antigen antibody reactions and circulatory disorders cannot be observed. The exact limit of circulating antibodies in the serum, which is responsible for circulatory disorders was not evaluated by this investigation. However, the observed decrease of the values determined by the radioimmunoassay leads to the conclusion

that this limit of circulating antibodies must be expected
between 100 and 200 μg antibody/ml in this experiment.

If antigen antibody reactions take place in the layers
of the gut one possibility is that these complexes are delivered
again back into the circulating blood. As complexes are able to
induce certain diseases this would be without any advantage.
This was, however, not observed. On the contrary the maximum
amount of radioactivity is delivered into the lumen of the gut
indicating that the antigen antibody complex is degraded and
eliminated in this natural way. The degradation of antibody
could be shown by Sephadex radiochromatography. From these
results it can be concluded that it is possible to desensitise
an organism by enteral antigen application for at least a short
time. How long this desensitisation lasts, must be a matter for
further investigations.

REFERENCES

Andre, C., Vaerman, J.P. and Heremans, J.F., 1978. Oral immunization of
    rats with human serum albumin. Interference with intestinal
    absorption and tolerogenic effect. In: Antigen Absorption by the
    Gut. Ed. W.A. Hemmings, MTP Press, Lancaster.

Bazin, H., 1979. Specific tolerance obtained by local antigenic stimulation
    of mucosal surfaces. In: Protein Transmission through Living Mem-
    branes. Ed. W.A. Hemmings, Elsevier/North-Holland Biomedical Press.

De Weck, A.L. and Girard, J.P., 1972. Specific inhibition of allergic
    reactions to penicillin in man by monovalent hapten. II. Clinical
    studies. Int. Archs. Allergy appl. Immunol. 42, 798-803.

Franks, J.J., Takeda, V. and Reeve, E.B., 1962. Preparation of autologous
    J-131-albumin for metabolic studies in man. J. Lab. Clin. Med.
    60, 619-628.

Hedin, H., Richter, W. and Ring, J., 1976. Dextran-induced Anaphylactoid
    Reactions in Man. Role of Dextran Antibodies. Int. Archs. Allergy
    appl. Immunol. 52, 145-159.

Messmer, K., Seemann, C., Hedin, H., Richter, W. and Peter, K., 1980.
    Anaphylaktoide Reaktionen nach Dextran. II. Tierexperimentelle und
    klinische Ergebnisse der Prophylaxe durch Hapten-Hemmung.
    Allergologie 3, 59-66.

Seifert, J., Welter, H., Lenz, J. and Brendel, W., 1979. Absorption of
    Horse-Gamma-Globulin: Correlation between Immune-Response and Micro-
    circulation in the Gastrointestinal-Tract of Dogs. In: Protein
    Transmission through Living Membranes. Ed. W.A. Hemmings, Elsevier/
    North Holland Biomedical Press.

Thomas, H.C. and Parrot, D.M.W., 1974. The induction of tolerance to a
    soluble protein antigen by oral administration. Immunology 27,
    631-638.

Walker, W.A., Wu, M., Issebacher, K.J. and Bloch, K.J., 1975. Intestinal
    uptake of macromolecules. III. Studies on the mechanism by which
    immunization interferes with antigen uptake. J. Immunol. 115,
    854-861.

AEROGENIC VACCINATION WITH LIVE BACTERIA - IMMUNE REACTIONS OF GNOTOBIOTIC PIGLETS AGAINST *ERYSIPELAS**

K. Petzoldt[1], W. Leibold[1], S. Jeckstadt[1], K.L. Morgan[2] and Ch. von Benten[1]

[1] Institut für Mikrobiologie und Tierseuchen and Institut für Pathologie der tierärztlichen Hochschule Hannover, D-3000-Hannover, Federal Republic of Germany.

[2] Department of Animal Husbandry, School of Veterinary Science, Langford House, Bristol, UK.

ABSTRACT

In gnotobiotic piglets a single aerosol exposure to live Erysipelas vaccine induced a strong protection against an infectious challenge with highly pathogenic Erysipelas bacteria. As the local and humoral antibody response was low if not undetectable the response of lymphoid cells was evaluated. In vaccinated animals suppressor effects of autologous thymocytes and remarkable differences in the reactivity of lymphoid cells depending on the presence or absence of the homologous antigen were observed. Therefore locally induced cellular immune mechanisms seem to be acting in vivo.

* Presented - in part - at the 4th International Pig Veterinary Society Congress, Copenhagen, 1. - 4.7.1980.

[1] Supported by the Fraunhofer Gesellschaft, München (In San I-1173-V-043) and by the Deutsche Forschungsgemeinschaft (SFB 54, C5).

INTRODUCTION

About two weeks after a single aerogenic vaccination
with live bacteria (*Erysipelothrix rhusiopathiae* = ER) gnotobiotic
piglets are protected against a strong infectious challenge
with highly pathogenic ER bacteria. The antibody response in
those piglets is only weak. Therefore, preliminary studies
were performed to detect local and/or cellular immune mechanisms
which may explain this strong protection. The model used for
these studies was developed as described previously (Petzoldt
et al., 1976; Petzoldt, 1979).

MATERIAL AND METHODS

Animals

Outbred, gnotobiotic, German Landrace piglets aged 3 - 4
weeks, were used in these experiments. The investigation of
cellular immune response was carried out in six animals. The
investigation of antibody in respiratory tract secretions and
the proliferative response to bacterial antigen components was
carried out in two animals.

Immunisation

Aerosol immunisation with 0.13 ml of a suspension of
avirulent ER in broth (5 x 10^8 organisms/ml of N-strain B 10)
was performed as previously described (Petzoldt et al., 1976).
For intranasal immunisation the same number of bacteria in a
total of 1 ml was sprayed in both nostrils. Sterile broth was
administered to control animals in a similar manner.

Challenge

The piglets were challenged with 100 LD_{50} of highly pathogenic ER bacteria (1.6 x 10^7 organisms/ml of A-strain FFA),
12 - 14 days after immunisation.

Collection of samples

Heparinised blood was collected from the anterior *vena*

cava, allowed to sediment (Waithe and Hirschorn, 1973) and centrifuged on Ficoll-Hypaque at 400 g for 40 minutes (Boyum, 1968). The plasma and lymphocyte rich interface were then collected. Lymphoid cells from thoracic lymph nodes, spleen, thymus and bone marrow were collected in a similar manner after homogenising these organs. Respiratory tract secretions were collected by lavage, centrifuged sonicated and concentrated by ultrafiltration (Morgan and Bourne, 1980). For sampling the piglets were anaesthetised with Saffan (Glaxo Limited) administered intramuscularly (20 - 25 mg/kg).

Serum was taken from clotted blood sampled at the same time and in the same manner as the heparinised blood samples described above.

Antibody assay

The agglutination test (Widal test) for monitoring the antibody response in blood was performed with dead ER bacteria in a conventional manner. The antiglobulin haemagglutination assay (Coombs and Fiset, 1954) modified for use in microtitre plates was used for antibody determinations in blood serum and respiratory tract secretions. Tanned sheep erythrocytes were sensitised with a sonicated preparation of heat killed ER bacteria.

Preparation of bacterial antigen

A protein antigen was prepared from ER bacteria by sonication, ammonium sulphate precipitation and gel filtration chromatography on Sephadex G 100 (Pharmacia). For studies on the proliferative response of lymphoid cells from different organs to mitogens in presence of bacterial antigen mitomycin treated whole bacteria (ER strain T 28 preparation) were used.

Lymphocyte proliferation assay

With lymphocytes of four animals immunised and in two control animals the H^3-thymidine incorporation after stimulation was measured. Besides these examinations of the mitogenic response to LAG, ConA and PWM in presence or absence of bacterial antigen the percentages of E-rosetting cells of lymphocytes were estimated. In addition, the effect of autologous thymocytes on proliferative capacity of lymphoid cells from peripheral blood, spleen and lymph nodes were assayed.

Another proliferation assay was carried out also in microtitre plates as described by Penhale et al. (1973). In this assay 100 μl of a lymphocyte suspension containing 1 x 10^6 cells/ml and 50 μl of the protein antigen solution (16 g/ml) were cultured for 7 days in RPMI medium containing 10% heat inactivated pig serum at 37°C in an atmosphere containing 8% Co$_2$. For further methodological details see Petzoldt et al. (1980).

RESULTS

No marked serum agglutinin titres occurred following the priming immunisation neither after 15 minutes nor after 30 minutes of aerosol vaccination time. The titres increased slightly after challenge (Table 1). No antibody was detected in respiratory tract secretions and serum of control or unimmunised animals. IgM antibody was detected in serum seven days after immunisation. No antibody was detectable in secretions at this time.

Following challenge the level of serum IgM antibody increased slightly and IgA antibody was detected in respiratory tract secretions. IgA antibody was also detected in serum six days after challenge. No differences in the proportion of E-rosetting and Ig bearing cells were observed in control and immunised animals. After challenge bone marrow cells of two immunised animals exhibited reduced proliferative response in contrast to a non-immune control animal (Figure 1). Furthermore in contrast to a non-immune control autologous thymocytes from immunised animals showed suppressor effects on the mitogenic response of lymphocytes *in vitro* (Figure 2).

TABLE 1

ONE TIME VACCINATION AGAINST ERYSIPELAS - SEROLOGICAL RESPONSE OF
GNOTOBIOTIC PIGLETS

Aerosol vaccination	Group n	Lowest and highest agglutination titre			
		After vaccination		After challenge	
30'	4	negative 1: 5 (1:10)	1:10 1:40	(1: 40) 1:160	(1: 80) 1:160
15'	6	negative negative 1:20	1:20 1:80	1: 40 1:320	1: 80 1:320
control	4	negative negative negative			

2w   2w   1w   1w

vaccination   challenge

The proliferative response of peripheral blood lymphoid
cells (PBL) to the mitogens Leucoagglutinine (LAG), Concanavaline
A (Con A) and Pokeweed mitogen (PWM) was very differently modul-
ated by killed ER bacteria, depending on the lapse of time after
immunisation and challenge respectively. At day 0 only the LAG
showed an inhibition of mitogen response in comparison with the
response in the absence of ER bacteria. At day 6 there was an
increasing inhibition of the proliferative response of PBL in
cultures if antigen was present. The inhibition was even
stronger when more antigen was added to the culture. On the
other hand at day 20 with all three mitogens the proliferative
response was even stronger when more antigen was given (Figure 3).

Employing a fractionated protein antigen from ER bacteria
only borderline proliferative responses of peripheral blood
lymphoid cells were induced. Up till now a relative optimum
was observed *in vitro* three days after challenge. A significant
proliferative response (SI 3) only appeared to occur following
challenge (Figure 4).

550

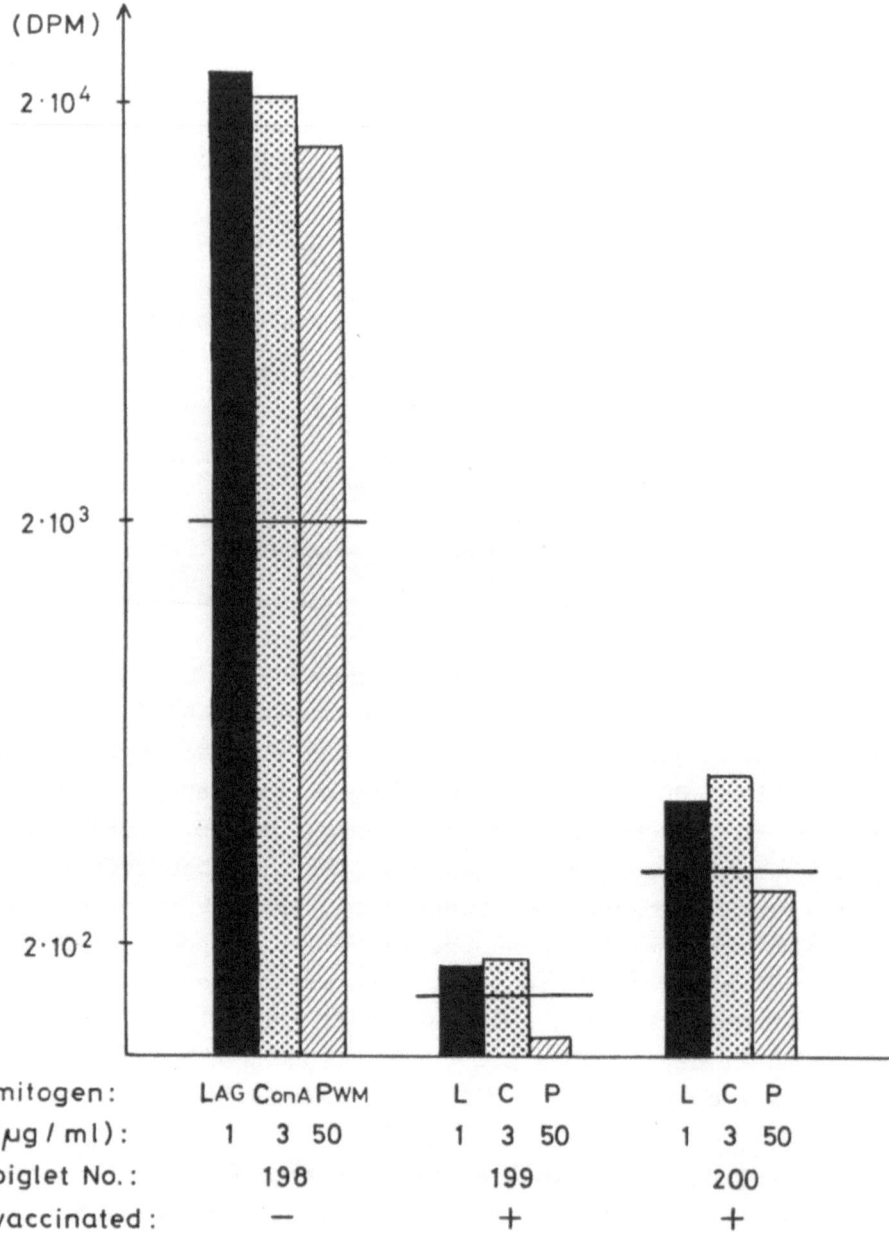

Fig. 1. Mitogenic stimulation of bone marrow cells from gnotobiotic piglets after infection with a virulent strain of *E. rhusiopathiae*.

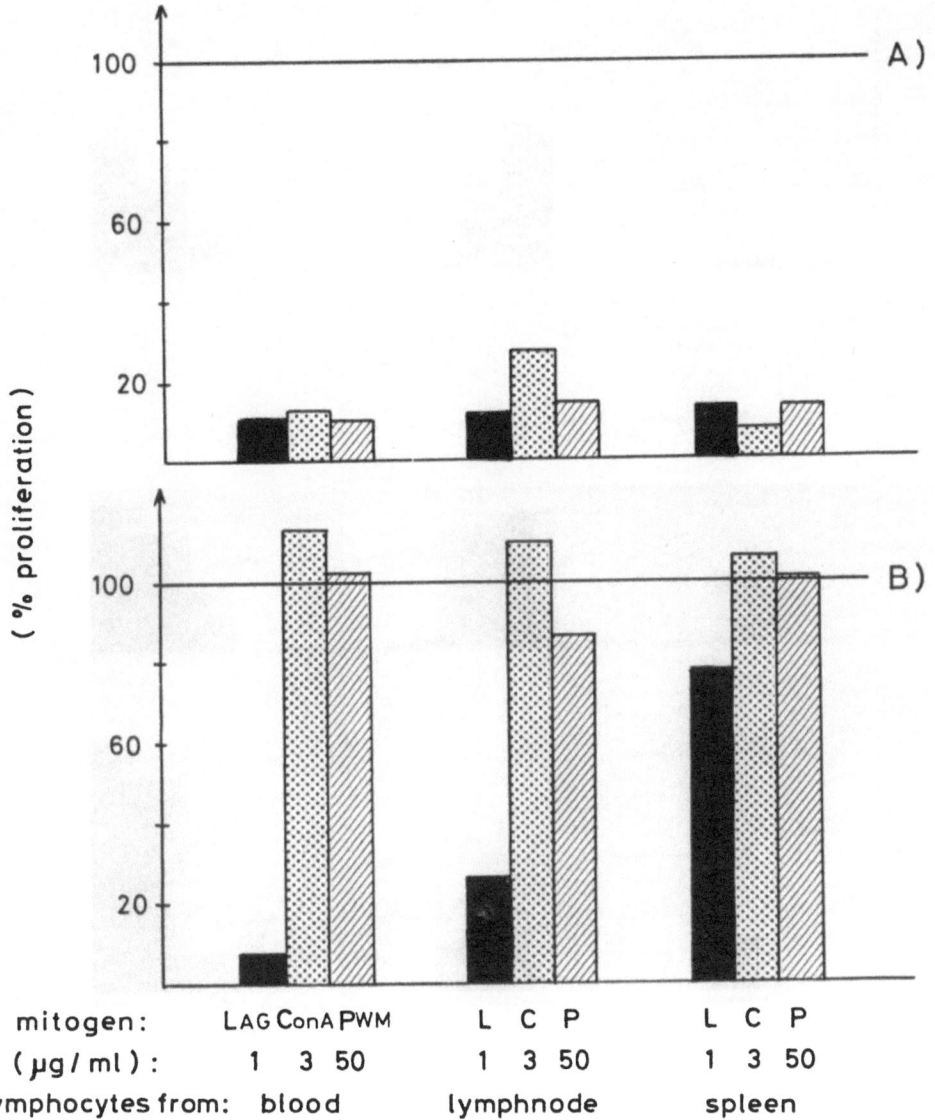

Fig. 2. Effect of 20% autologous thymocytes on the mitogen response of lymphocytes from a non-vaccinated (A) and an aerosol vaccinated (B) gnotobiotic piglet after infection with a virulent strain of *E. rhusiopathiae* (day 20).

552

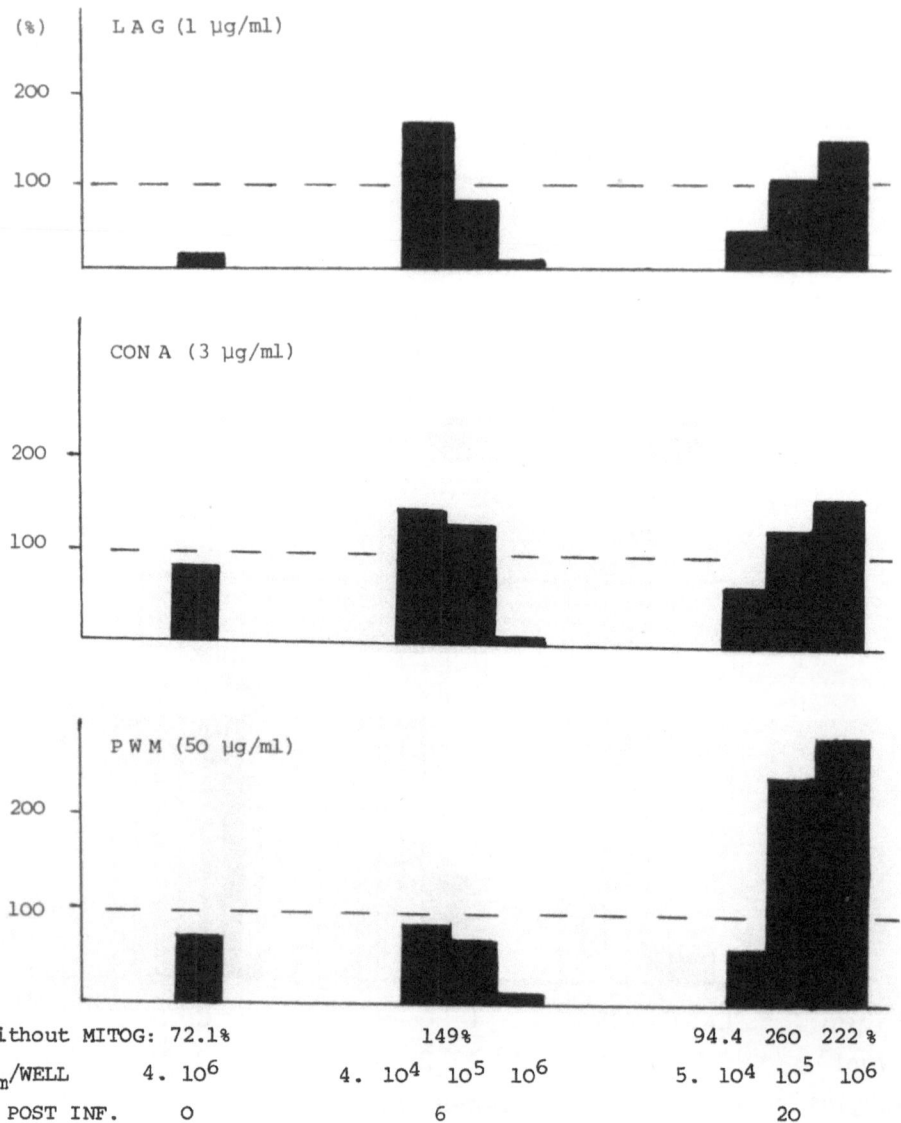

Fig. 3. Influence of dead *Erysipelas* bacteria (T 28) on the proliferative response of PBL from aerosol-vaccinated gnotobiotic piglets.

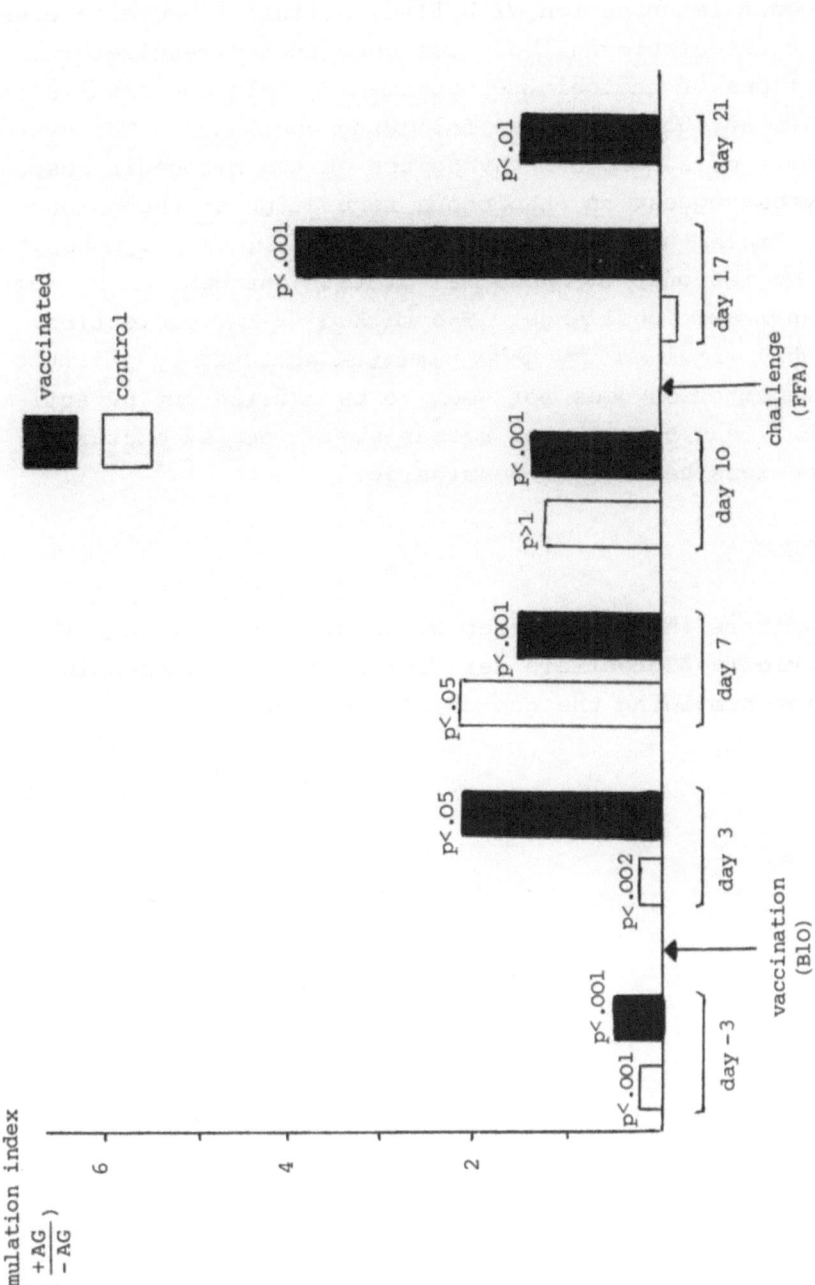

Fig. 4. The proliferative response of peripheral blood lymphocytes cultured *in vitro* with a protein antigen prepared from *E. rhusiopathiae* (B 10).

CONCLUSIONS

Aerogenic immunisation with live, avirulont bacteria does not induce a detectable antibody response in the respiratory tract secretions of gnotobiotic unprimed animals but results in a mucosal IgA antibody response following challenge. The suppressor effects of autologous thymocytes on the mitogenic response of lymphocytes suggest an autologous regulation of the defence mechanism. Preliminary results suggest that *in vitro* lymphocyte proliferative response to bacterial protein antigens might occur following antigenic challenge. The marked *in vivo* protection against highly virulent *Erysipelas* strains achieved by a single aerogenic vaccination does not seem to be carried out by antibodies rather than by cellular mechanisms. Complex bacteria-cell interactions have to be considered.

ACKNOWLEDGMENT

The authors thank Professor W. Schulze and his co-workers, Klinik für kleine Klauentiere der Tierärztlichen Hochschule Hannover, for providing the gnotobiotic piglets.

REFERENCES

Boyum, A., 1968. A one-step procedure for isolation of granulocytes and
    lymphocytes from human blood. Scand. J. Clin. Lab. Invest. 21,
    Suppl. 97.

Coombs, R.R.A. and Fiset, M.L., 1954. Detection of complete and incomplete
    antibodies to egg albumin by means of sheep red cell-egg albumin
    antigen unit. Brit. J. Exper. Path. 35, 472.

Morgan, K.L. and Bourne, F.J., 1980. Immunoglobulin levels in porcine nasal
    and tracheal secretions - the influence of the method of collection.
    J. Immunol. Meth. (in press).

Penhale, W.J., Farmer, A., McKenna, R.P. et al., 1973. Spontaneous thyroid-
    itis in thymectomized and irradiated Wistar rats. Clin. Exp. Immunol.
    15, 225.

Petzoldt, K., 1979. Development of an experimental animal model of aerogenic
    immunization with bacterial antigens. Z. Erkrank. Atm.-Org. 153, 232.

Petzoldt, K., Floer, W., von Benten, Ch. and Stühmer, A., 1976. Experiments
    with a model of aerosol immunization of mice and swine against
    Erysipelothrix insidiosa (E.i.). Develop. biol. Standard. 33, 57.

Petzoldt, K., Jeckstadt, S., Leibold, W., Plonait, H. and Sailer, J., 1980.
    Studies on aerogenic immunization against bacterial infections. Zbl.
    Vet. Med. (in preparation).

Waithe, W.I. and Hirschhorn, K., 1973. Lymphocyte response to activators.
    In Handbook of Experimental Immunology 3rd Ed. Chapter 26 p. 26.1
    Edit. Weir, D.M., Blackwell Scientific Publications.

LIST OF PARTICIPANTS

Dr. C. André
Unité de Recherches de Physio-Pathologie Digestive
INSERM U-45
Hôpital Edouard-Herriot Pavilion H B13
69374 Lyon Cedex
FRANCE

Dr. J. Asso
Institut National de la Recherche Agronomique
Station de Recherches de Virologie et d'Immunologie
Route de Thiverval
78850 Thiverval-Grignon
FRANCE

Dr. H. Batten
University of Bristol
Veterinary School
Park Row
Bristol
UK

Dr. H. Bazin
University of Louvain
Faculty of Medicine
Experimental Immunology Unit
Clos Chapelle-aux-Champs 30
B-1200 Brussels
BELGIUM

Dr. J. Bienenstock
McMaster University Health Sciences Centre
1200 Main Street West
Hamilton
Ontario L8N 3Z5
CANADA

Prof. E.H. Bohl
Department of Veterinary Science
Ohio Agricultural Research and Development Center
Wooster
Ohio 44691
USA

Dr. B.A. Bokhout
Central Veterinary Institute
Prof. Poelslaan 35
3028 EP Rotterdam
THE NETHERLANDS

Prof. F.J. Bourne
Department of Animal Husbandry
Langford House
Langford
Bristol BS18 7DU
UK

Dr. P. Brandtzaeg
Institute of Pathology
Immunohistochemical Laboratory
The National Hospital
Rikhospitalet
Oslo 1
NORWAY

Dr. F. Cancellotti
Istituto Profilattico
Via G. Orus 2
35100 Padua
ITALY

Dr. Barbro Carlsson
Department of Clinical Immunology and
    Department of Pediatrics
University of Göteborg
Göteborg
SWEDEN

Prof. J. Clamp
Department of Medicine
University of Bristol
UK

Dr. J. Connell
Commission of the European Communities
DG VI
200 rue de la Loi
B-1049 Brussels
BELGIUM

Dr. de la Croce
University of Pisa
Via di Gello 29
Pisa
ITALY

Dr. K. Dalsgaard
State Veterinary Institute for Virus Research
Lindholm
DK-4771 Kalvehave
DENMARK

Dr. Anne Ferguson
Western General Hospital
Gastro-intestinal Unit
Crewe Road
Edinburgh EH4 2XU
UK

Dr. J. Hall
Block X
Chester Beatty Research Institute
Institute of Cancer Research
Downs Road
Sutton
Surrey SM2 5PX
UK

Prof. J. Hannon
University College Dublin
Faculty of Veterinary Medicine
Ballsbridge
Dublin 4
IRELAND

Dr. Heppell
Agricultural Research Council
National Institute for Research in Dairying
Shinfield
Reading RG2 9AT
UK

Dr. G. Hess   Institut für Med. Mikrobiologie, Infektions
                          und Seuchermedizin
                      Ludwiq-Maximillians Universität
                      Veterinärstrasse 13
                      D-8000 München 22
                      FEDERAL REPUBLIC OF GERMANY

Dr. Ellen E.E. Jarrett   Wellcome Laboratory for Experimental Parasitology
                      University of Glasgow
                      Veterinary Hospital
                      Bearsden Road
                      Bearsden
                      Glasgow G61 1QH
                      UK

Dr. P.T. Jensen   State Veterinary Serum Laboratory
                      Bulowsvej 27
                      DK-1870 Copenhagen V
                      DENMARK

Dr. P.J. Kilshaw   Nutrition Department
                      National Institute for Research in Dairying
                      Shinfield
                      Reading RG2 9AT
                      UK

Dr. J.M. Kortbeek-Jacobs Department of Immunology
                      Faculty of Veterinary Medicine
                      Yaleaan 1
                      3584 CL Utrecht
                      THE NETHERLANDS

Dr. W. Leibold   Institut für Mikrobiologie
                      und Tierärztliche Hochschule
                      Hanover
                      FEDERAL REPUBLIC OF GERMANY

Dr. R. Levinsky   Institute of Child Health
                      University of London
                      Department of Immunology
                      30 Guildford Street
                      London WC1N 1EH
                      UK

Dr. G. Mayrhofer   MRC Cellular Immunology Unit
                      Sir William Dunn School of Pathology
                      University of Oxford
                      Oxford OX1 3RE
                      UK

Dr. H. Miller   Moredun Institute
                      408 Gilmerton Road
                      Edinburgh EH17 7JH
                      UK

Dr. B. Morein   Statens Veterinarmedicinska Anstalt
                                Fack
                                104 05 Stockholm 50
                                SWEDEN

Dr. K.L. Morgan   Department of Animal Husbandry
                                Langford House,
                                Langford
                                Bristol BS18 7DU
                                UK

Dr. T.J. Newby   Department of Animal Husbandry
                                Langford House
                                Langford
                                Bristol BS18 7DU
                                UK

Dr. J. Nielsen   State Veterinary Institute for Virus Research
                                Lindholm
                                DK-4771 Kalvehave
                                DENMARK

Prof. Dr. K. Petzoldt   Institut für Mikrobiologie
                                   und Tierärztliche Hochschule
                                Hanover
                                FEDERAL REPUBLIC OF GERMANY

Prof. N.F. Pierce   Department of Medicine
                                Baltimore City Hospital
                                Johns Hopkins University
                                4940 Eastern Avenue
                                Baltimore
                                Maryland 21224
                                USA

Dr. Podoerigora   WHO Headquarters
                                Immunology Unit
                                Geneva
                                SWITZERLAND

Dr. J. Quinn   University College Dublin
                                Faculty of Veterinary Medicine
                                Ballsbridge
                                Dublin 4
                                IRELAND

Mrs. M.J. Robins   Janssen Services
                                33a High Street
                                Chislehurst
                                Kent BR7 5AE
                                UK

Prof. Dr. J. Seifert   Institut für chirurgische Forschung
                                Ludwig-Maximillians Universität
                                Klinikum Grosshadern
                                D-8000 München 70
                                FEDERAL REPUBLIC OF GERMANY

Prof. J. Soothill   Institute of Child Health
                           University of London
                           Department of Immunology
                           30 Guildford Street
                           London WClN 1EH
                           UK

Dr. C.J. Stokes   Department of Animal Husbandry
                           Langford House
                           Langford
                           Bristol BS18 7DU
                           UK

Miss. C.M. Swale   Janssen Services
                           33a High Street
                           Chislehurst
                           Kent BR7 5AE
                           UK

Dr. Geraldine Taylor   Agricultural Research Council
                           Institute for Research in Animal Diseases
                           Compton
                           Nr. Newbury
                           Berks
                           UK

Dr. J.P. Vaerman   Université Catholique de Louvain
                           74 avenue Hippocrate
                           B-1200 Brussels
                           BELGIUM

Dr. C. Valente   Istituto di Malatto Infettive
                           Facoltà di Medicina Veterinaria
                           Via S. Costanzo
                           I-06100 Perugia
                           ITALY

Dr. J.F. Vautherot   Institut National de la Recherche Agronomique
                           Grignon
                           FRANCE

Dr. H. Williams Smith   Houghton Poultry Research Station
                           Houghton
                           Huntingdon
                           Cambs PE17 2DA
                           UK

Dr. D. van Zeane   Central Veterinary Institute
                           Virology Department
                           Houtribweg 39
                           8221 RA Lelystad
                           THE NETHERLANDS

Manuscript prepared by:

JANSSEN SERVICES, 33a High Street, Chislehurst, Kent BR7 5AE, UK.